SUDDEN CARDIAC DEATH

Sidney Goldstein, MD
Head, Division of Cardiovascular Medicine
Henry Ford Hospital
Detroit, Michigan
Professor of Medicine
Case Western Reserve University
Cleveland, Ohio

Antonio Bayés-de-Luna, MD
Professor of Cardiology
University Autonomous Barcelona
Head, Department of Cardiology
Hospital Sant Pau
Barcelona, Spain

J. Guindo-Soldevila, MD
Department of Cardiology
Hospital Sant Pau
Barcelona, Spain

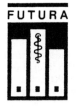

**Futura Publishing
Company, Inc.**
Armonk, N.Y.

Library of Congress Cataloging-in-Publication Data

Goldstein, Sidney, 1930-
    Sudden cardiac death / Sidney Goldstein, Antonio Bayés de Luna,
J. Guindo Soldevila.
        p.   cm.
    "Revision of the original monograph, published in 1972"—Introd.
    Includes bibliographical references and index.
    ISBN 0-87993-589-8
    1. Cardiac arrest.   I. Bayés, de Luna, Antonio.   II. Guindo
Soldevila, J.   III. Title.
    [DNLM: 1. Death, Sudden, Cardiac.   WG 205 G624s 1994]
    RC685.C173G65   1994
    616.1'23025—dc20
    DNLM/DLC
    for Library of Congress   94-9562
                                                                  CIP

Published by
Futura Publishing Company, Inc.
P.O. Box 418
135 Bedford Road
Armonk, New York 10504

L.C. No.: 94-9562
ISBN No.: 0-87993-589-8

Every effort has been made to ensure that the information in this book is as up to date and accurate as possible at the time of publication. However, due to the constant developments in medicine, neither the author, nor the editor, nor the publisher can accept any legal or any other responsibility for any errors or omissions that may occur.

Printed in the United States of America on acid-free paper.

Introduction

Death, like birth, is a secret of nature.
The Meditations of Marcus Aurelius Antonius[1]

The growing awareness among physicians and surgeons concerning sudden death has prompted a revision of the original monograph published in 1972. In this revision, we have added to our previous work and expanded our discussion to include the broader issue of sudden death as it relates to heart disease. Coronary heart disease remains the preeminent issue, however. Of the 600,000 deaths due to coronary heart disease each year in the United States, approximately half are sudden. These deaths represent a staggering public health statistic. The magnitude of this problem has led the medical profession to embark on a number of programs directed at the treatment and prevention of sudden death. These efforts run the entire spectrum from diet modification to the surgical excision of portions of the myocardium and the implantation of a variety of electronic devices. All of these approaches are directed at the important issue of prevention. These efforts have been based on a varying degree of scientific evidence, some of which has been twisted and turned in the mind of the therapist to provide a rationale for proceeding on a therapeutic course. The turning away from the age-old exhortation to the physician of *do no harm* has found a rationale and legitimacy in the fear of the unknown and of the unexpected death. The fearful clinical dilemma surrounding the choice of treatment for the patient with accelerating angina, frequent premature contractions, or one who has experienced a previous cardiac arrest is increasingly important as we realize how large a factor sudden death is in the total picture of coronary heart disease. Because of this unknown, therapeutic programs of dubious scientific basis have been justified to prevent sudden death.

We have little information about the identity of those who are at risk of dying suddenly and yet the medical community has embarked upon therapeutic programs, often based on superficial and inferential evidence. Coronary heart disease is clearly epidemic in the western world and sudden death is its usual expression. The control of this and other causes of sudden death therefore could significantly modify the overall mortality rates from this disease. Unfortunately, with coronary heart disease in particular, "prospective and retrospective studies indicate that sudden death victims share most of the major risk factors for coronary artery disease, but none of these factors thus far identified can be used to distinguish sudden death victims from those whose deaths are less precipitous."[2] Since the same factors that predispose to sudden death also define the presentation of coronary artery disease, the key to prevention appears to be the reduction of all risk factors.

The clinical dilemma as to why an individual's first expression of coronary heart disease is angina pectoris, others myocardial infarction, and others sudden death remains. Is it merely the magnitude of the experience, the size of the infarct, or is it the biological milieu in which the ischemic process takes place?

We will review our success and failures in altering the biological milieu in which the ischemic process occurs. We will also review pharmacological and surgical interventions in cardiac disease, other than coronary heart disease, which lead to sudden death. At the present time we have no clear answers. Many risk factors including age, diastolic pressure, hypertensive status, obesity, and smoking are all significant predictors of both total and sudden cardiac death in coronary heart disease. In other disease states, predictors are less evident. Our inability to identify sudden death victims from those who will survive the acute infarction or who have advanced heart failure, regardless of its etiology, continues to pose a major challenge to the scientist.

In this era of medical therapeutics, it will probably be impossible to halt or restrain the enthusiasm for many of the medical and surgical approaches. In this book, however, we hope to describe the current state of knowledge about sudden death due to cardiovascular disease. From this framework, perhaps, we can then develop the foundations for rational therapeutic programs.

There are three major problems related to sudden death that exist at the present time. The first is the primary prevention of sudden cardiovascular collapse in the general population. This depends upon the identification of risk factors and the prevention of the major cause, coronary heart disease. The solution of the latter is not within the scope of this monograph, although its solution clearly will make these writings obsolete. For the foreseeable future, however, atherosclerosis and its primary mortal event, sudden death, will be major medical problems to our society. The second issue is secondary prevention of coronary heart disease in those people who have already "joined the coronary club."[2] In this group we already have a high-risk population who may be approachable through therapeutic endeavors. The third problem of sudden death is handling the event itself. It is imperative that we act expeditiously and effectively with the occurrence of acute cardiovascular collapse in the community. The emergency medical squads have provided major advances in medical care in many communities. We will review some of the factors that determine the effectiveness of these units.

My interest in this area developed from the First Pre-Hospital Phase Symposium on Acute Myocardial Infarction held in Rochester, New York in 1969[3] and was nurtured by the intellectual stimulation of my coinvestigators at that time, Dr. Arthur Moss and Dr. William Greene, in our exploration of the pre-hospital phase of acute myocardial infarction and sudden death. The studies by Lewis Kuller[4] describing the epidemiologic significance of out-of-hospital deaths helped us focus on the magnitude of this important public health program. A subsequent symposium, held again in Rochester in 1971,[5] further emphasized the importance of the pre-hospital phase of acute myocardial infarction and refocused attention on sudden death. The symposium on sudden cardiac death organized in Barcelona in 1989 by Dr. Antonio Bayes-de-Luna[6] provided the stimulus for the creation of this revision. My enthusiasm for the revision of the original text was stimulated by Professor Bayes-de-Luna and Dr. J. Guindo Soldevila, and all three of us have revised the original text and created this new edition.

Sidney Goldstein, MD

References

1. Marcus Aurelius Antonius. Meditations IV, 5; trans. by Morris Hickey Morgan (1859–1910). In: Bartlett J, ed. *Bartlett's Familiar Quotations, 14th ed.* Little, Brown and Company, Boston, Toronto: Little Brown and Company; 1968;141b.

2. Warren JV. A revolution in coronary artery disease. *J Chronic Dis* 1973;26:547.

3. Goldstein S, Moss AJ. Symposium on the pre-hospital phase of acute myocardial infarction. *Am J Cardiol* 1969;24:609:830.

4. Kuller L, Lilienfield A, Fisher R. Epidemiological study of sudden and unexpected deaths due to arteriosclerotic heart disease. *Circulation* 1966;34:1056.

5. Moss AJ, Goldstein S. Symposium on the pre-hospital phase of acute myocardial infarction. *Arch Intern Med* 1972;129:713–830.

6. Bayes de Luna A, Guindo J. *Sudden Cardiac Death.* Barcelona: MCR Editors; 1989. Spanish version; Barcelona: Doyma SA; 1990.

Contents

Chapter I

Historical Survey of Sudden Death

From the vantage point of the last half of the 20th century, it is difficult to appreciate the major change in clinical emphasis that occurred in coronary heart disease at the turn of this century: from that of sudden death to the clinical description of acute myocardial infarction. Prior to the 20th century, with the exception of the description of angina by Heberden, clinical descriptions of coronary heart disease emphasized sudden death as its major sequelae. In 1901, Ludwig Krehl,[1] a leading figure in German medicine, set the stage for this change when he wrote: "Occlusion is compatible with survival; the patient survives, unaware of the abyss which he has crossed." This observation was a forerunner to the important work by Obrastzow and Straschesko,[2] two Russian clinicians from Kiev, in 1910 and by James B Herrick[3] of Chicago in 1912. All three described the syndrome of acute myocardial infarction and emphasized that survival was possible after the acute episode. Subsequent investigations in the early 20th century described the clinical pathology including the leucocytosis and febrile response, electrocardiographic findings and more recently, the hemodynamic and angiographic sequelae of acute myocardial infarction. Herrick attempted to dispel the dogmatic adherence to the principle that sudden death was the inevitable sequel to coronary heart disease. He described four groups of acute coronary heart disease: (1) a sudden death group, (2) a group representing anginal attacks with severe pain in which death might follow in some minutes, (3) a nonfatal group with mild symptoms but without the usual causes precipitating attack, and (4) a group show-

From: S. Goldstein, A. Bayés-de-Luna, J. Guindo-Soldevila: *Sudden Cardiac Death.* Armonk, NY: Futura Publishing Co., Inc., © 1994.

ing severe symptoms, usually fatal but not immediately. Although Herrick published his findings in 1912 he states that, "The publication aroused no interest; it fell like a dud." In order to prove his theory, he called upon his resident, Fred Smith, to ligate the coronary artery in a dog, reproducing the same electrocardiographic pattern as that seen in his patients with a "heart attack." He spent much of the next two decades attempting to inform physicians about this new clinical entity that "was later to become a household word translated by the layman into 'heart attack.'[4]"

Yet, for the previous 2000 years, sudden death was associated with pain in the chest and heart disease. The Egyptians over 4000 years ago were aware of sudden death and coronary ischemia. They provided the first classic description of coronary ischemia: "If thou examinest a man for illness in his cardia and he has pain in his arm and breast and in one side of his cardia . . . . it is death threatening him."[5] In China in 500 BC, Pien Chio wrote that intermittency of pulse was a predictor of death and when every other pulse was felt, death could occur within days.[6] Hippocrates wrote of the importance of chest pain and sudden death: "Sharp pains irradiating soon towards the clavical and towards the back, are fatal."[7] Expounding for the first time on risk factors in coronary heart disease, he stated that, "Those who are constitutionally very fat are more apt to die quickly than those who are thin;"[8] and "Frequent recurrence of cardialgia, in an elderly person, announces sudden death."[9] Those concepts of sudden death were held from the time of Hippocrates through the Middle Ages and were reemphasized during the Renaissance and in the 17th century.

An early layman's description of sudden death is reported in Froissart's *Chronicles*[10] in which he recounts the sudden death of the Count de Foix (1331–1391). The death of Count Gaston de Foix (Fig. 1), who was a patron of the arts, is colorfully described by Froissart as follows:

> The day he died, he had all the forenoon been hunting bear. The weather was marvelously hot, even for the month of August. In the evening (at the Inn) he called for water to wash and stretch out his hands; but no sooner had his fingers . . . touched the cold water, then he changed colour, from an oppression at his heart and his legs failing him, fell back on a seat, exclaiming, 'I am a dead man: Lord God, have mercy on me!' He never spoke after this, though he did not immediately die, but suffered great pain . . . in less than a half an hour he was dead, having surrendered his soul very quietly."

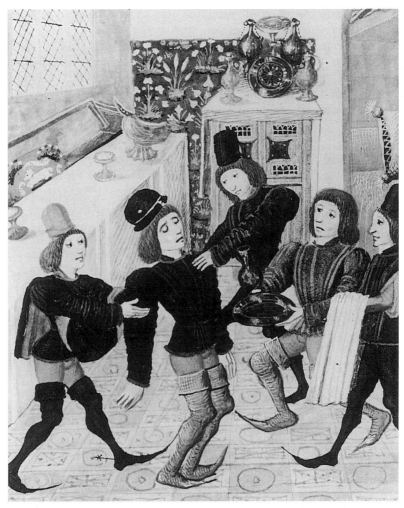

Figure 1. The death of Count Gaston de Foix.[10]

The intriguing aspect of this description is the possibility of the reflex relationship between the cold water and coronary arterial spasm. Immersion of the hand in ice water is now often used to produce coronary spasm in the laboratory.

To Leonardo da Vinci (1452–1519)[11] has been attributed the first autopsy examination of a sudden death victim due to what appears to have been coronary heart disease. He witnessed the death of a hundred-year-old man and sought "the cause of so peaceful a death."

A contemporary of Vesalius, Amatus Lusitanus (1511–1568),[12] provided us with one of the earliest clinical descriptions of sudden death due to myocardial infarction. Although a postmortem examination is not described, the death, attributed by Amatus to obstruction in the heart, represents an unusual diagnosis for the time.

"A reverend Abbot from the Isle of Croma, one or two miles distant from Ragusa, when he was in good health and talking to several persons, said that he suddenly felt pain in his heart and with his hand moved rapidly toward the region of the heart, he fell, though slowly, to the earth and rapidly lost all his animal faculties. When called in I said he was dead. Not only was the pulse at the metacarpium and the temples missing, but even no motion upon the heart could be perceived. In order to satisfy the assistants, I brought to the nostrils a burning candle whose flame did not move at all. Also a bright mirror was advanced near the mouth and nothing of respiratory contraction was seen on it. We then applied a glass vessel filled with water upon the thorax but the water was unmoved. Thereupon I ordered to keep him unburied until the next day; and if nothing happened, I advised them to dismiss him till the third day, since, as you know, the humours complete their motion within seventy-two hours which denotes three days. (Scholia) Some people contended that this Abbot met his death from apoplexy, but verily not without error, since this (man) ended his day due to syncope, his heart lancinated, and his spirits dissolved, either through some venomous humour or, to be more precise, through some obstruction engendered in the heart which is attested by the following signs. First, because he had pain in the heart and as you know from Hippocrates: where the pain is, say there is the disease. Secondly, since no froth was brought to the mouth, nor was there any distortion of the mouth or retraction of the limbs. The mouth even remained almost open, so that he had his teeth not tightly closed. Therefore it may be rightly and with greater probability asserted that, his nerves being without lesion, he died not from apoplexy, but suddenly and unexpectedly from a primarily affected heart. If somebody contends this comes from the nerves and he supposes that in a vehement apoplexy some kind of dissolution of the limbs may occur without retractions (an assertion which we contest) then he may be aware that an apoplexy cannot supervene without lesion of the brain and the nerves, which in his violent and sudden death did not appear. Therefore, since this (man) suffered from pain in the heart, and no damage of the nerves became visible, it seems to me more plausible that he died from a badly damaged heart than from apoplexy."

This case history is not only lucid in its description of a clinical entity but unusually prophetic in view of our current concepts of mechanisms of sudden death.

A student of Galen, Petrus Salius Diversus,[13] also in the 16th century, emphasized the importance of pulse irregularity as a prodrome of sudden circulatory collapse in the fourth chapter of his book *Desyncope Cardiaca*:

> "Two signs indicate impending cardiac syncope and sudden death, first, a sensation of sudden constriction of the heart associated with collapse, pallor and perspiration, and the second, that in those (patients) an intermittent pulse sometimes occurs; if the intermission extends beyond one pulse great danger threatens and it signifies that such syncope is imminent; which intermission, as well as the feeling of suffocation, originates nowhere else but from the amount of thickened blood which obstructs and impairs those vessels and internal part."

The latter reference to thickened blood which obstructs and impairs vessels may be a Renaissance description of the modern day concept of coronary arterial thrombosis as the cause of myocardial infarction. The suggestions regarding pulse irregularity may well be one of the first suggestions of the relationship between ventricular premature contractions and ventricular fibrillation, or perhaps the first clinical description of Stokes-Adams syndrome.

In the 17th century the physiologist Harvey described the pathophysiology of coronary heart disease in his *Second Disquisition to John Riolan* (1649):[14]

> "I add another observation. A noble knight Sir Robert Darcy, when he reached to about middle period of life, made frequent complaint of a certain distressing pain in the chest especially in the night season; so that dreading at one time syncope, and at another suffocation in his attacks he led an unquiet and anxious life. He tried many remedies in vain, having had the advice of almost every medical man. His disease going from bad to worse, he by-and-by became cachectic, dropsical, and finally grievously distressed, he died in one of his paroxysms. In the body of this gentleman, we found the wall of the left ventricle of the heart ruptured, having a rent in it of size sufficient to admit any of my fingers, although the wall itself appeared sufficiently thick and strong. This laceration had apparently been caused by an impediment to the passage of blood from the left ventricle into the arteries."

This is an interesting description of the progressive cardiac decompensation due to coronary heart disease beginning with angina, congestive heart failure, and ultimately sudden death associated with myocardial rupture.

In 1612, Paolo Grassi, a physician of Corregio, Italy, wrote *Mortis Repentinae Examen* ("Examination of Sudden Death"),[15] in which he not only described the clinical syndrome of sudden death, but also discussed the risk factors including obesity and sedentary life style that could lead to sudden death. Grassi made his deductions without the aid of autopsy. He was the first to express concern about smoking as a risk factor. In order to prevent sudden death, he wrote that the "soul should be treated with words and the body with drugs."

The first epidemiologic study of sudden death and noncommunicable diseases was commissioned by Pope Clement XI in the early 18th century. He assigned his physician Lancisi (1655–1720) to investigate the large number of sudden deaths that were occurring in Rome using postmortem examination. Lancisi, in his book *De Subtaneis Mortibus*,[16] developed the first link between coronary heart disease and sudden death and reemphasized the observation of Hippocrates in regard to the relationship between pain, dyspnea, and sudden death. In addition, his population study indicated that the elderly, the obese, and those with recurrent pain were more prone to die suddenly. According to Roelandt,[17] Lancisi's book became a classic because of its integration of anatomical pathology with clinical observations. Lancisi also dealt with the issue of the definition of sudden death. He wrote:

> "Indeed this absolutely complete cessation of animal movements and the departure of the soul from the body even though it happens at all times more swiftly than itself, is nevertheless divided for the sake of common parlance and for greater clarity of teaching into natural, untimely and violent death, and these again into slowly and sudden deaths, into those as are foreseen and 'forcefelt' and finally into such as are unforeseen, unperceptible and unexpected."

In addition to calling attention to the risks of smoking and urban pollution, he suggested that eating chocolate, which was at that time used as an aphrodisiac, could also lead to sudden death.

Later in the 18th century the importance of angina and its relationship to sudden death was emphasized by the Quaker physician John Fothergill (1712–1780). In his report "Case of an angina pectoris, with remarks,"[18] he describes spasm of the chest related to sudden death:

> "I soon suspected angina pectoris, a disease which I had too often met with. I saw the patient in the evening, he described a stricture around his chest, sharp pain, (breast, elbow left), difficulty in breathing. Death very suddenly in the morning. Postmortem: mediastinum loaded with fat under the lungs a quart of water in each side. Heart; near the apex, a small white spot as big as a sixpence resembling a cicatrix."

In a later report he describes a patient 63 years old whose complaints began three to four years before his death and who ultimately "in a sudden and violent transport of anger he fell down and expired immediately."[19] When William Heberden of London in 1772, rendered his description of angina pectoris,[20] he more than likely was aware of its relationship to early death, if not sudden death. He noted that "most of those, with whose cases I have been acquainted were buried, before I had heard that they were dead." According to Kligfield,[21] shortly after the publication of Heberden's book, he received a letter from an anonymous English physician, later identified by Dr. KD Keele[22] as Dr. Haygarth of Chester. Haygarth described his own characteristic symptoms of angina pectoris, but with a unique feature which "have frequently led me to think that I should meet with a sudden death . . . I have often felt what I can best express by calling it a universal pause within me of the operations of nature for perhaps three or four seconds; and when she has resumed her functions, I felt a shock at the heart, like that which one would feel from a small weight being fastened by a string to some part of the body, and falling from the table to within a few inches of the floor." Kligfield suggests that this is the first description of the relationship of angina pectoris, ventricular premature beats and sudden death. It is possible that his interpretation is correct although I would offer an alternative interpretation that the description is more compatible with short periods of asystole than with ventricular premature beats. Haygarth offered his body for postmortem examination in order "to show the course of it; and perhaps, tend at the same time to a discovery of the origin of that disorder, which is the subject of this letter and be productive of means to counteract and remove it." He died a half-hour after the onset of symptoms during an after-dinner walk.[21] Heberden arranged to have Mr. John Hunter, recently appointed as Surgeon to St. George's Hospital, perform the autopsy. He was assisted by Edward Jenner, the developer of the small pox vaccine. Jenner stated he was almost positive that the coronary arteries of this patient were not examined. Jenner, however, performed the autopsy on his next angina pectoris patient himself and observed that, while making a transverse section through the heart near its base, his knife struck against something so hard and gritty that it notched the scalpel: "I will remember looking up to the ceiling, which was old and crumbling, conceiving that some plaster had fallen down. But on further scrutiny the real cause appeared: The coronaries had become bony canals." Because Jenner's good friend John Hunter began to suffer from angina himself and wishing not to cause Hunter any unnecessary anxiety, he chose not to publish his own observations until Hunter ultimately succumbed to the disease. The association between emotions and sudden death was noted in the description of the death of John Hunter by his brother-in-law, Sir Everard Home,[23] which occurred in a fit of anger after many years of angina pectoris. Hunter often remarked "that his life was in the hands of the rascal who chose to annoy or tease him."

A further description of angina and sudden death by Johnstone[24] tells of a man in 1785 who suffered from "shortness in breathing, pain in his chest, and across his arms, on ascent; symptoms returned until the fatal attack. On the second August 1785, after being sometime in bed, he complained he was ill; early in the morning third August his wife was roused by noise of expiring groan, death in an instant." At autopsy by Mr. Gunter, a surgeon, it was observed "the heart very putrid, admitting my fingers passing through it with very little pressure."

In 1799, Caleb Perry proposed a new syndrome entitled "Syncope Anginosa." He states: "All circumstances in Angina Pectoris preceding the actual syncope are approaches toward it: and in every uncombined and recent case, like those I described, the patient probably dies of no other symptoms than those which show an irrecoverable diminution of the motion of the heart"[25] and further, "the Angina Pectoris is a mere case of Syncope or Fainting, differing from the Common Syncope only in being preceded by an unusual degree of anxiety or pain in the region of the heart, and in being readily excited, during a state of apparent health, by any general exertion of the muscles, more especially that of walking."[25]

The studies in the latter part of the 19th century by von Bezold[26] and by Cohnheim[27] indicated that the experimental occlusion of the coronary arteries resulted in decrease in left ventricular function and cardiac arrest. Von Bezold[26] demonstrated in 1867 that the left ventricular contractions slowed following occlusion and observed that when a ligature was loosened the heart action could be restored. In 1881 Cohnheim[27] published his experimental data on coronary occlusion and observed that ligation of one of the branches of the coronary artery resulted in progressive arrhythmia and after 105 seconds, blood pressure fell suddenly while the auricles continued to function. Cohnheim theorized that the coronary arteries were "end arteries" and that the interruption of heart action was due to metabolites elaborated during the ischemic episode. His theory had to wait almost one hundred years for general acceptance.

In 1884, von Leyden published a paper entitled "On the sclerosis of the coronary arteries, and the morbid states arising from them"[28] in which he describes (according to Leibowitz[29]) three groups of patients suffering from coronary arterial disease: acute cases with sudden death who "do not always feature angina pectoris but are often marked by collapse;" subacute cases who have recurrent thrombosis but not complete necrosis, and chronic cases complicated by cardiac asthma and dropsy. He emphasized the different stages of coronary heart disease starting with angina and progressing to left ventricular failure.

In the later part of the 20th century, the emphasis turned from sudden death to the clinical description of acute myocardial infarction as a result of the observations by Herrick.[3] The importance of sudden death had almost totally been lost sight of, until the observation of Lewis Kuller[30] reemphasized its relationship to coronary heart disease. In the last three decades, there has been an animated controversy in regard to the mechanism and prevention of sudden death. This has largely revolved around the importance of ventricular ectopy or ischemia as the genesis of cardiac arrest, particularly in coronary heart disease. Much of this controversy will be discussed in this text.

It is important for us to realize that others have walked these paths before us. Although our techniques of investigation are more sophisticated, many of the early physicians, using little more than deductive reasoning, made important observations regarding sudden death and its relationship to heart disease.

References

1. Krehl L: *Die Erkrankungen des Herzmuskels.* Vienna: Holder,A; 1901.
2. Obrastzow WP, Straschesko ND: Zur Kenntnis der Thrombose der Koronararterien des Herzens. *Z Klin Med* 1910;71:116. Russian original in Russk, Vrach, 1910, reproduced in *Z Klin Med* (Mosk) 1949;27:15.
3. Herrick JB: Clinical features of sudden obstruction of the coronary arteries. *JAMA* 1912;59:2015.
4. Herrick JB: *Memories of Eighty Years.* Chicago: University of Chicago Press, 1949.
5. Ebbel B. *The Papyrus Ebers.* Copenhagen: Levin and Munksgaard; 1937:191.
6. Hubotter F. *Die chinesische Medizin zu Beginn des Jahrhunderts und ihr Historischer Entwicklungsgang, Asia Major.* Leipzig: Schindler; 1929.
7. Littre E: *Ouevres Complètes d'Hippocrates.* (Traduction nouvelle avec le texte grec. Baillière 1839–1861). Paris: Con Prenotions, Vol V:601, para 70.
8. Littre E: *Ouevres Complètes d'Hippocrates.* (Traduction nouvelle avec le texte grec. Baillière 1839–1861). Paris: Aphorism II, 41, Vol IV:483.
9. Littre E: *Ouevres Complètes d'Hippocrates.* (Traduction nouvelle avec le texte grec. Baillière 1839–1861). Paris: Con Prenotions, Vol V:647, para 280.
10. Froissart J, Johnes T, trans. *Chronicles of England, France, Spain, etc.* (Two vols). London: Bohn, 1849.
11. MacCurdy E, ed: *The notebooks of Leonardo da Vinci*, New York:Reynal and Hitchcock; 1938:I:125.
12. Amatus Lusitanus. *Curationum Medicalium Centuria Sexta.* Venice: Valgrisius; 1560.
13. Diversus PS. *DeFebre Pestilenti Tractatus, et Curationes Quorundam Particularium Morborum, etc.* Frankfurt: Heirs of A Wechel; 1586.
14. Harvey W, Willis R, trans. *The Works of William Harvey.* London: The Sydenham Society; 1847.
15. Grassi P. *Mortis Repentinae Examen.* Molena: Presso Guiliano Cassiano; 1612.
16. Lancisi GM. *De Subitaneis Mortibus.* Rome: Buagni F, 1706.
17. Roelandt H. Two paragon books on sudden death. *Thorax-Centre Journal* 1990;2:17.
18. Fothergill J. Case of angina pectoris with remarks. *Med Obsns Inquir* 1776;5:233.
19. Ibid. Farther account of the angina pectoris. *Med Obsns Inquir* 1776;5:252.
20. Heberden W. Some account of disorder of the breast. *Med Trans Coll Phys* (London) 1772;2:59.

21. Kligfield P. The frustrated benevolence of "Dr. Anonymous." *Am J Cardiol* 1981;47:185.
22. Keele KD. John Hunter's contribution to cardiovascular pathology. *Ann Royal Coll Surg Engl* 1966;39:248.
23. Hunter J. *A Treatise on the Blood, Inflammation and Gun–shot. To which is prefixed a short account of the author's life by his brother-in-law, Everard Home.* London: Richardson; 1794.
24. Johnstone J: Case of angina pectoris from an unexpected disease in the heart. *Mem Med Soc Lond* 1792;1:376.
25. Parry CH. *An Inquiry into the Symptoms and Causes of the Syncope Anginosa, Commonly called Angina Pectoris, Illustrated by Dissections.* Bath and London: R Crutwell; 1799;60.
26. von Bezold A. Von den Veranderungen des Herzchlages nach Verschliessung der Coronar–arterien. *Unters Physiol Lab Wurzburg* 1867;2:256.
27. Cohnheim J, Schulthess-Rechberg A. Uber die Folgen der Kranzarterienverschliessung fur das Herz. *Virchow Arch Path Anat* 1881;85:503.
28. von Leyden E: Uber die sclerose der Coronar–Arterien und die von abhangigen Krankheitszustande. *Z Klin Med* 1884;7:459–539.
29. Leibowitz JO. *The History of Coronary Heart Disease.* Berkeley and Los Angeles: University of California Press; 1970:151.
30. Kuller L, Lilienfield A, Fisher R. An epidemiological study of sudden and unexpected deaths in adults. *Medicine* 1967;46:341.

Chapter II

Sudden Cardiac Death:
A Multifactorial Problem

Sudden cardiac death is one of the most serious problems facing modern cardiology, not only because of its dramatic presentation, but because of its frequency in the general population and its socio-economic implications.[1,2] Although more than 80% of sudden death events occur in individuals with coronary artery disease, there is usually no specific anatomical distribution that singles them out. Markers and triggers of sudden cardiac death do exist, however. They differ on whether the final event is a malignant ventricular arrhythmia or a bradyarrhythmia. In this section we will emphasize a multifactorial approach to both the identification of the markers present in individuals at risk of sudden death and the occurrence of the triggers which lead to it.

Markers of Sudden Cardiac Death Due to Malignant Ventricular Arrhythmias

Sudden cardiac death is usually a result of a cumulative effect of several factors[3–5](Fig. 1). From a clinical point of view, it is clear that the final cause of sudden death is usually a ventricular tachyarrhythmia, and less frequently, a bradyarrhythmia. These malignant arrhythmias are induced by a series of triggering events acting upon a myocardium that is prone or vulnerable to a malignant ar-

From: S. Goldstein, A. Bayés-de-Luna, & J. Guindo-Soldevila: *Sudden Cardiac Death*. Armonk, NY: Futura Publishing Co., Inc., © 1994.

rhythmia. Ventricular tachyarrhythmias are responsible for 80% of ambulatory sudden death.[6,7]

Clearly we know many markers of a vulnerable myocardium and some triggering events that lead to malignant ventricular arrhythmias. We do not, however, completely understand all their interactions. At one moment, perhaps with a slight increase in heart rate, the appearance of a pause, or a slight increase in myocardial ischemia, a malignant ventricular arrhythmia can appear and cause sudden death. At other times, a change in heart rate has no importance. The interaction between vulnerable myocardium and triggered events is not the same in all diseases, and even in a seemingly homogeneous disease state it is continuously in flux.

Markers in Ischemic Heart Disease

A patient who experiences an acute myocardial infarction may present a series of markers of a vulnerable myocardium such as premature ventricular contractions, residual ischemia, or a decreased ejection fraction without suffering any malignant ventricular arrhythmia for days, weeks, and even years. At one moment in time, however, the occurrence of an old or new triggering factor can produce a malignant ventricular arrhythmia and precipitate a sudden death event.

A number of hypotheses[3] have been generated to explain the multifactorial problem of sudden cardiac death due to malignant ventricular arrhythmias in postmyocardial infarction patients. These include not only the sequence of events leading to sudden death secondary to malignant ventricular arrhythmias in patients with coronary heart disease as shown in Figure 1, but also the interaction among the three angles of the so-called "triangle of risk" (Fig. 2): residual ischemia, left ventricular dysfunction, and electrical instability. Each of these three factors includes others (Fig. 3) that can be considered as markers. Markers of electrical instability that can explain the appearance of malignant arrhythmias and sudden death are anatomical alterations (substrate), the presence of premature ventricular complexes (PVC), and other electrical alterations of the autonomic nervous system. These markers can be detected by different methods (Table 1).

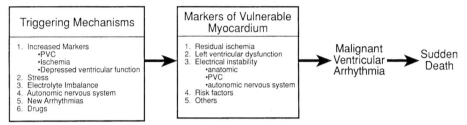

Figure 1. Principal triggering factors and markers of vulnerable myocardium in postmyocardial infarction patients. One or several triggering factors acting upon a vulnerable myocardium induce malignant ventricular arrhythmias and sudden cardiac death PVC = premature ventricular contractions.(from Bayés-de-Luna et al.[3]).

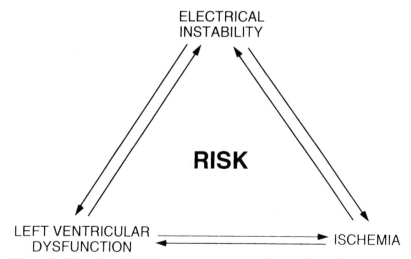

Figure 2. Triangle of risk. The three angles are the most important factors related to major complications in the postmyocardial infarction patient. There is strong interaction among these three factors.

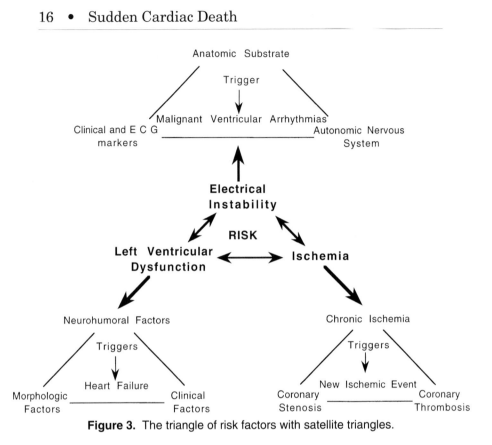

Figure 3. The triangle of risk factors with satellite triangles.

Ischemia

The importance of myocardial ischemia as a marker of sudden death cannot be over-emphasized. Many studies[8–13] support the relationship of both symptomatic and asymptomatic ischemia as markers of a vulnerable myocardium. Theroux[8] demonstrated that the presence of ST segment depression in postmyocardial infarction patients during exercise stress tests predicts a poor prognosis, including sudden death. The evidence of ST segment depression in ambulatory electrocardiographic recording is also a marker of poor prognosis both in unstable[9,10] and in chronic angina patients.[11] In patients with positive exercise stress tests, Rocco[12] observed that the presence of ST segment depression with or without symptoms during ambulatory electrocardiographic recording identifies patients

Table 1

Parameters and Techniques Used to Stratify Risk in Postmyocardial Infarction Patients

	Parameters	*Techniques*
Electrical instability	• Ventricular arrhythmias	• Holter ECG
	• Autonomic nervous system —Heart rate variability	• Programmed electrical stimulation
	—QT interval	• Holter ECG
	• Anatomic substrate	• Late potentials (conventional or Holter techniques)
Ischemia	• Coronary flow	• Exercise testing • Holter ECG • Imaging techniques
	• Coronary stenosis	• Coronary angiography
	• Prethrombotic state	• Blood test
Left ventricular dysfunction	• Diastolic function	• Echo-Doppler
	• Systolic function	• Echocardiography and angiography and isotropic techniques
	• State of Renin-angiotensin system	• Blood test

with poor prognoses. In addition, patients resuscitated from out-of-hospital cardiac arrest, a group of patients known to have an increased recurrence of cardiac arrest, have been shown to express an increased incidence of silent ST segment depression.[13]

Left Ventricular Dysfunction

Depressed left ventricular function and heart failure[14–17] are considered the strongest markers for a poor prognosis and sudden death in postmyocardial infarction patients. Their presence can activate the neuroendocrine system which may also have an adverse affect on arrhythmias.

Anatomical Alterations

The anatomical markers of sudden death in postmyocardial infarction patients include postinfarction scarring, ventricular aneurysms, and left ventricular hypertrophy, in addition to extent of coronary artery stenosis.[18-22]

Premature Ventricular Contractions

Premature ventricular contractions are one of the preeminent predictors of sudden death, particularly in the presence of left ventricular dysfunction.[15,16,23-25] Although it is clear that premature ventricular contractions are markers of vulnerable myocardium, their importance as a direct cause of sudden death has been strongly questioned after the Cardiac Arrhythmia Suppression Trial (CAST).[26] That study suggests that despite the eradication of ventricular premature beats, the occurrence of sudden death continues and in fact is increased.

Autonomic Nervous System Alterations

The integrity of the autonomic nervous system and its control of the heart rate[27-31] is also an important marker of a vulnerable myocardium. The loss of autonomic control of cardiac function, expressed as a loss of R-R interval variability,[27] prolongation of the QT interval,[28,29] and baroreflex insensitivity[30,31] have been shown to identify the sudden death patient.

These markers of the vulnerable myocardium do not exist in isolation. The combinations of markers can improve the sensitivity, specificity, and predictive accuracy of defining a patient at risk.[32-34] Future studies must assess the problem of sudden death from a multifactorial approach in order to determine the total risk of each patient. Using information obtained from the clinical laboratory, including exercise testing, ambulatory electrocardiographic recording, signal-averaged ECG, and a variety of cardiac imaging techniques, we can further stratify the risk of sudden death in postmyocardial infarction patients[32-34] (see also Chapters VII and VIII).

Markers in Patients Without Ischemic Heart Disease

These patients comprise approximately 20% of all sudden death events and represent a varied mixture of electrical and myocardial dysfunction.

Chronic Hypertension

Chronic hypertension resulting in left ventricular hypertrophy can create a vulnerable myocardium in which ventricular arrhythmias and sudden cardiac death[35] are recognized sequelae. The relationship of these events to relative or actual ischemia has not been fully evaluated (see also Chapter XVI).

Hypertrophic Cardiomyopathy

Hypertrophic cardiomyopathy, with its associated myocardial vulnerability due to hypertrophy, appears to have unique characteristics associated with its increased ventricular mass. It is further complicated by the special derangement of the myocardial fibers[36,37] which can result in abnormalities in ventricular depolarization and repolarization (see Chapter X).

Idiopathic Dilated Cardiomyopathy

The myocardium is particularly vulnerable to arrhythmias in the setting of depressed left ventricular function. Ventricular arrhythmias[17,38] can result from abnormal stretch or diffuse fibrosis leading to interference with homogeneous ventricular depolarization and reentry arrhythmias (see Chapter X).

Wolff-Parkinson-White Syndrome[39,40]

Wolff-Parkinson-White syndrome, due to the presence of anomalous conduction pathways with very fast conduction, can convert a normally functioning heart to an inefficient and life-threatened organ. The important markers in this group, characterized by Klein et al.[39] and Torner et al.[40] will be discussed in subsequent sections (see Chapter XIII).

Prolonged QT Syndrome

Prolonged QT syndrome, leading to irregular repolarization, facilitates the appearance of malignant ventricular arrhythmias.[41,42] This phenomenon often occurs in the setting of physical or psychic stress (see Chapter XII).

Other forms of heart disease such as mitral valve prolapse, aortic stenosis, and right ventricular dysplasia also have a part in the total description of the sudden death victim (see Chapters X to XVI).

Despite improved diagnostic procedures, it is not always possible to find a specific cause of the sudden death event.[43] Explanations of this enigma suggest that myocarditis undetected by usual diagnostic methods may play a role as a cause of sudden death.

Triggering Mechanisms of Malignant Ventricular Arrhythmias

It is apparent that patients may have one or several markers of ventricular vulnerability for many years without the appearance of a malignant arrhythmia. A triggering mechanism acting on a vulnerable myocardium at a given moment is required in order to precipitate a malignant ventricular arrhythmia. What are the known mechanisms?

Alterations of the Autonomic Nervous System

Modulation of the autonomic nervous system can facilitate the appearance of malignant ventricular arrhythmias.[27-31] We have observed an increase in heart rate in patients during ambulatory electrocardiographic recording[6,7] prior to the occurrence of malignant ventricular arrhythmia, which may be an expression of sympathetic overdrive. Nevertheless, prolongation of the QT interval has not been observed in patients prior to the onset of ventricular arrhythmias in the setting of acute myocardial infarction.[44]

Physical and Mental Stress

On occasion, sudden cardiac death can be triggered by both physical and mental stress.[45,46] Mental stress is an especially important trigger in long QT syndrome. It has also been shown that exercise can trigger malignant ventricular arrhythmias,[47] although the incidence of malignant ventricular arrhythmias during exercise testing is very low.

Symptomatic, Silent Ischemia, and Arrhythmias

Symptomatic and silent ischemia are responsible for the majority of sudden deaths in acute myocardial infarction and other acute ischemic syndromes.[48,49] Although acute ischemia has been demonstrated during recordings of ambulatory sudden death,[50,51] its specific role remains uncertain.[6,7] Using ambulatory electrocardiographic recording technology, new exacerbations of silent or symptomatic ischemia explain only 30%–40% of all cases of recorded ambulatory sudden death.[6,7] Pathological studies by Davies et al.,[52] however, suggest that thrombosis or acute ischemia occur in most episodes of sudden death. Coronary arterial spasm associated with coronary stenosis may also play a role as a trigger mechanism of sudden death. The difference between the pathological evidence of ischemia and the ambulatory electrocardiographic recording evidence of ischemia as a triggering mechanism of sudden death may be due to the different patients studied. Patients who are studied with ambulatory recordings usually have frequent ventricular premature contractions and have significant left ventricular dysfunction and complex electrocardiographic abnormalities of the QRS, ST segment, and T wave. In this setting, subtle changes in the ST segment indicating ischemia may not be apparent. In addition, the techniques used to detect ischemia are also different. The recording of one or two specific precordial leads, as is the usual routine with ambulatory recording, may not record the specific area of ischemia, and the degree of ischemia required to produce ventricular fibrillation in a scarred ventricle may be quite small. The increased number of PVCs and/or the appearance of supraventricular arrhythmias, a pause induced by a premature ventricular or, less often, a supraventricular contraction, may also trigger malignant ventricular arrhythmias.[6,7,53-55] This has been observed in patients with ischemia, and particularly in patients with Wolff-Parkinson-White syndrome (see Chapter XIII).

Electrolyte or metabolic imbalance can also act as a trigger of malignant ventricular arrhythmias, particularly in the presence of premature ventricular contractions and a vulnerable myocardium.[56] Recent investigations suggest that magnesium and potassium depletion may also be important precipitating causes for ventricular tachy-arrhythmias in patients with severe left ventricular dysfunction. In this setting, arrhythmia vulnerability is markedly heightened by preexisting structural, hemodynamic, or neurohormonal factors.

Drugs

The administration of drugs, particularly antiarrhythmic agents, may also trigger ambulatory sudden death. Proarrhythmia may be enhanced in the setting of electrolyte imbalance or ischemia. In our experience,[6,7] proarrhythmia is suspected in approximately 66% of cases of ambulatory sudden death due to "torsade de pointes." It is less likely to be implicated in the setting of primary ventricular fibrillation or classic ventricular tachycardia. The results of the study of encainide and flecainide in CAST[26] suggest that this phenomenon may be more frequent than previously recognized. The observations by Moosvi and Goldstein[57] in high-risk resuscitated patients suggest that both quinidine and procainamide also have potential for proarrhythmic responses.

Markers and Triggers of Sudden Death Due to Bradyarrhythmias

Patients whose cardiac arrest is associated with bradyarrhythmia usually have very advanced heart disease and successful resuscitation is unlikely even if the bradyarrhythmia is corrected by implantation of a pacemaker. These patients often have evidence of advanced sinoatrial or atrioventricular dysfunction. Patients with bradyarrhythmic cardiac arrest, however, account for approximately 20% of arrhythmic deaths in our series.[6,7] In these patients, ischemia or an increase of left ventricular dysfunction can precipitate electrical instability and malignant ventricular arrhythmias.

Malignant bradyarrhythmia can be reversible in some instances. Increased vagal tone or the administration of antiarrhythmic drugs are particularly important as triggers of reversible malignant bradyarrhythmias. All antiarrhythmic agents, as well as cardioactive drugs including digitalis and calcium blocking agents, can induce severe bradyarrhythmia. Malignant bradyarrhythmias induced by drugs may explain at least some cases of late proarrhythmia and sudden death detected in the CAST study.[58]

In this chapter, a variety of potential markers and triggers of cardiac arrest have been reviewed.Our main objective is to emphasize the complexity and the multifactorial issues that lead to sudden death. Simplistic solutions for prevention should be avoided. The complexity of the biological environment in which sudden death occurs must be appreciated.

References

1. Goldstein S. *Sudden Death and Coronary Heart Disease.* New York: Futura Publishing Company; 1974.
2. Lown B. Sudden cardiac death: The major challenge confronting contemporary cardiology. *Am J Cardiol* 1979;43:313.
3. Bayés de Luna A, Guindo J, Fiol M, et al. Sudden cardiac death. In: Fisch C, Surawicz B, eds. *Advances in Cardiac Electrophysiology and Arrhythmias.* New York: Elsevier; 1991.
4. Coumel P. Factors responsible for sudden death: Triangle or polygon? In: Piccolo E, Raviele A, Alboni P, eds. *Aritmie Cardiache.* Venice: Centro Scientifico Editore; 1989:279.
5. Wellens HJJ, Brugada P. Sudden cardiac death: A multifactorial problem. In: Brugada P, Wellens HJJ, eds. *Cardiac Arrhythmias: Where To Go From Here?* New York: Futura Publishing Company; 1987:391.
6. Bayés de Luna A, Coumel PH, Leclercq JF. Ambulatory sudden death: mechanisms of production of fatal arrhythmia on the basis of data from 157 cases. *Am Heart J* 1989;117:151.
7. Bayés de Luna A, Guindo J, Rivera I. Ambulatory sudden death in patients wearing Holter devices. *J Ambulat Monitoring* 1989;2:3.
8. Theroux P, Waters D, Halphen C, et al. Prognostic value of exercise testing soon after myocardial infarction. *N Engl J Med* 1979;301:341.
9. Gottlieb LS, Weisfeldt M, Ouyang P, et al. Silent ischemia as a marker for early unfavorable outcomes in patients with unstable angina. *N Engl J Med* 1986;314:1214.
10. Nademanee K, Intarachot V, Josephson M, et al. Prognostic significance of silent myocardial ischemia in patients with unstable angina. *J Am Coll Cardiol* 1987;10:1.
11. Tzivoni D, Gavish A, Gottlieb S, et al. Prognostic significance of ischemic episodes in patients with previous myocardial infarction. *Am J Cardiol* 1988;62:661.
12. Rocco MB, Nabel EG, Campbell S, et al. Prognostic significance of myocardial ischemia detected by ambulatory monitoring in patients with stable coronary artery disease. *Circulation* 1988;78:877.

13. Sharma B, Asinger R, Francis G, et al. Demonstration of exercise-induced painless myocardial ischemia in survivors of out-of-hospital ventricular fibrillation. *Am J Cardiol* 1987;59:740.
14. Ahnve S, Gilpin E, Henning H, et al. Limitations and advantages of the ejection fraction for defining high risk after acute myocardial infarction. *Am J Cardiol* 1986;58:872.
15. Bigger JT, Fleiss JL, Kleiger R, et al. The relationships among ventricular arrhythmias, left ventricular dysfunction, and mortality in the 2 years after myocardial infarction. *Circulation* 1984;69:250.
16. Mukharji J, Rude RE, Poole WK, et al. The MILIS study Group. Risk factors of sudden death after acute myocardial infarction: Two-year follow-up. *Am J Cardiol* 1984;54:31.
17. Packer M. Sudden unexpected death in patients with congestive heart failure: A second frontier. *Circulation* 1985;72:681.
18. Miller JM, Vassallo JA, Kussmaul WG, et al. Anterior left ventricular aneurism: Factors associated with the development of sustained ventricular tachycardia. *J Am Coll Cardiol* 1988;12:375.
19. Breithardt G, Schartzmaier J, Borggrefe M, et al. Prognostic significance of late ventricular potentials after acute myocardial infarction. *Eur Heart J* 1983;4:487.
20. Roubin GS, Harris PJ, Bernstein R, et al. Coronary anatomy and prognosis after myocardial infarction in patients 60 years of age and younger. *Circulation* 1983:67:743.
21. Cooper RS, Simmons BE, Castaner A, et al. Left ventricular hypertrophy is associated with worse survival independent of ventricular function and number of coronary arteries severely narrowed. *Am J Cardiol* 1990;65:441.
22. Sanz G, Castaner A, Betriu A, et al. Determinants of prognosis in survivors of myocardial infarction: A prospective clinical angiographic study. *N Engl J Med* 1982;306:1065.
23. Ruberman W, Wienblatt E, Golberg J. Ventricular premature complexes and sudden death after myocardial infarction. *Circulation* 1981;64:297.
24. The Multicenter Postinfarction Research Group. Risk stratification and survival after myocardial infarction. *N Engl J Med* 1983;309:331.
25. Kostis JB, Byington R, Friedman LM, et al. for the BHAT Study Group. Prognostic significance of ventricular ectopic activity in survivors of acute myocardial infarction. *J Am Coll Cardiol* 1987;10:231.
26. CAST Investigators. Preliminary report: Effect of encainide and flecainide on mortality in a randomized trial of arrhthymia suppression after myocardial infarction. *N Engl J Med* 1989;321:406.
27. Kleiger RE, Miller JP, Bigger JT, et al. Decreased heart rate variability and its association with increased mortality after acute myocardial infarction. *Am J Cardiol* 1987;59:256.
28. Schwartz PJ, Wolf SW. QT interval prolongation as predictor of sudden death with myocardial infarction. *Circulation* 1978;57:1074.
29. Martí V, Bayés de Luna A, Arriola J, et al. Value of dynamic QTc in arrhythmology. *New Trends Arrhyth* 1988;4:683.
30. Billman GE, Schwartz PJ, Stone HL. Baroreceptor reflex control of heart rate: A predictor of sudden death. *Circulation* 1982;66:874.

31. Bigger JT, La Rovere MT, Steinman RC, et al. Comparison of baroreflex sensitivity and heart period variability after myocardial infarction. *J Am Coll Cardiol* 1989;14:1511.
32. Gomes JA, Winters SL, Stewart D, et al. A new noninvasive index to predict sustained ventricular tachycardia and sudden death in the first year after myocardial infarction: Based on signal-averaged electrocardiogram, radionuclide ejection fraction and Holter monitoring. *J Am Coll Cardiol* 1987;10:349.
33. Kuchar DL, Thorburn CW, Sammel NL. Prediction of serious arrhythmic events after myocardial infarction: Signal-averaged electrocardiogram, Holter monitoring and radionuclide ventriculography. *J Am Coll Cardiol* 1987;9:531.
34. Cripps T, Bennet D, Camm J, et al. Prospective evaluation of clinical assessment, exercise testing and signal-averaged electrocardiogram in predicting outcome after acute myocardial infarction. *Am J Cardiol* 1988;62:995.
35. Messerli FH, Ventura HO, Elizari DJ, et al. Hypertension and sudden death, increased ventricular ectopic activity in left ventricular hypertrophy. *Am J Med* 1984;77:18.
36. Nicod P, Polikar R, Peterson KL. Hypertrophic cardiomyopathy and sudden death. *N Engl J Med* 1987;316:780.
37. Maron BJ, Roberts WC, Epstein SE. Sudden death in hypertrophic cardiomyopathy: A profile of 78 patients. *Circulation* 1982;65:1388.
38. Unverferth DV, Magorien RD, Moechsberger ML, et al. Factors influencing one year mortality of dilated cardiomyopathy. *Am J Cardiol* 1984;54:147.
39. Klein GJ, Bashore TM, Sellers TD, et al. Ventricular fibrillation in the Wolff-Parkinson-White syndrome. *N Engl J Med* 1979;301:1080.
40. Torner-Montoya P, Brugada P, Smeets J, et al. Ventricular fibrillation in the Wolff-Parkinson-White syndrome. *Eur Heart J* 1991;12:144.
41. Surawicz B, Knoebel SB. Long QT: good, bad or indifferent? *J Am Coll Cardiol* 1984;4:398.
42. Schwartz PJ, Locati E. The idiopathic long QT syndrome: Pathogenetic mechanisms and therapy. *Eur Heart J* 1985;6:103.
43. Sugrue DD, Holmes DR, Gersh BJ, et al. Cardiac histologic findings in patients with life-threatening ventricular arrhythmias of unknown origin. *J Am Coll Cardiol* 1984;4:952.
44. Fiol M, Marrugat J, Bergadá J, et al. Ventricular fibrillation markers on admission to hospital for acute myocardial infarction. *Am J Cardiol* 1993;71:117.
45. Lown B. Mental stress, arrhythmias and sudden death. *Am J Med* 1982;72:177.
46. Greene WA, Goldstein S, Moss AJ. Psychosocial aspects of sudden death. *Arch Intern Med* 1972;129:725.
47. Maron BJ, Epstein SE, Roberts WC. Causes of sudden death in competitive athletes. *J Am Coll Cardiol* 1986;7:204.
48. Lie KJ, Wellens HJJ, Dorsnar E, et al. Observations on patients with primary ventricular fibrillation complicating acute myocardial infarction. *Circulation* 1975;52:755.

49. Adgey AA, Devlin JE, Webb SW, et al. Initiation of ventricular fibrillation outside hospital in patients with acute ischemic heart disease. *Br Heart J* 1982;47:55.

50. Hong R, Bhandari A, McKay C, et al. Life-threatening ventricular tachycardia and fibrillation induced by painless myocardial ischemia during exercise test. *JAMA* 1987;257:1937.

51. Pepine CJ, Morganroth J, McDonald JT, et al. Sudden death during ambulatory ECG monitoring. *Am J Cardiol* 1991;68:785.

52. Davies MJ, Thomas A. Thrombosis and acute coronary artery lesions in sudden cardiac ischemic death. *N Engl J Med* 1984;310:1137.

53. Leclerq JF, Maisonblanche P, Cuchemezand B, et al. Respective role of sympathetic tone and of cardiac pauses in the genesis of 62 cases of ventricular fibrillation recorded during Holter monitoring. *Eur Heart J* 1988;9:1276.

54. Wang Y, Scheinman MM, Chien W, et al. Patients with supraventricular tachycardia presenting with aborted sudden death: Incidence, mechanism and long-term follow-up. *J Am Coll Cardiol* 1991;18:1711.

55. Anderson JL. Supraventricular tachyarrhythmias: Not always so benign. *J Am Coll Cardiol* 1991;18:1720.

56. Hollenberg NK, Hollifield JW. Potassium/magnesium depletion: Is your patient at risk of sudden death? *Am J Med* 1987;82:1.

57. Moosvi AR, Goldstein S, Medendorp SV, et al. Effect of empiric antiarrhythmic therapy in resuscitated out-of-hospital cardiac arrest victims with coronary artery disease. *Am J Cardiol* 1990;65:1192.

58. Bayés de Luna A, Guindo J, Borja J, et al. Recasting the approach of treatment of potentially malignant ventricular arrhythmias after CAST study. *Cardiovasc Drugs Ther* 1990;4:651.

Chapter III

Sudden Cardiac Death:
Final Events

The final or explicit sudden death phenomenon has had, until recent years, a mystical quality about it. The mechanism of death in the coronary care unit during an acute myocardial infarction is well known.[1-3] We also have information concerning the final lethal arrhythmia responsible for death in the prehospital phase of acute coronary attack.[4] In addition, the events that occur in the terminal stage of noncardiac disease[5] have also been recorded. Until recently, however, we lacked information about final events in ambulatory patients dying of heart disease. In this chapter, we will review the final arrhythmic events leading to sudden cardiac death and provide a global view of events recorded in patients who die while wearing ambulatory electrocardiographic recorders.

Ambulatory Sudden Death Recorded By Ambulatory Electrocardiographic Recording

In a recent publication,[6,7] we surveyed the ambulatory electrocardiographic recordings of 233 patients who died suddenly. The results of these and other studies have contributed to a better understanding of the arrhythmic events of sudden death.[8-15] Most deaths were recorded out-of-hospital, although a few patients were hospitalized at the time of the final event. The in-hospital recordings

From: S. Goldstein, A. Bayés-de-Luna, J. Guindo-Soldevila: *Sudden Cardiac Death*. Armonk, NY: Futura Publishing Co., Inc., © 1994.

were obtained in patients admitted to the hospital in order to determine the best therapeutic approach to their arrhythmias.

In describing these recordings, there is a need to clarify several points. Confusion exists as to the difference between ambulatory sudden death and sudden death recorded by ambulatory electrocardiogram. Ambulatory cardiac arrest is the unforeseen sudden death of a patient in a stable state of health. Many of these patients have heart disease, usually coronary heart disease. We excluded patients admitted to the coronary care unit in the acute phase of myocardial infarction or unstable angina. Patients in the terminal stage of any disease were also excluded. Although these patients may die while wearing a recording device, they are deaths recorded on a magnetic tape rather than cases of ambulatory sudden death. Recordings such as these have been reported in previous studies[5,16] and it is doubtful that such cases are appropriate to the study of the mechanism of ambulatory sudden death. We did not exclude patients hospitalized for adjustment of their antiarrhythmic regimen since these patients die unexpectedly and provide information regarding the proarrhythmic phenomena associated with antiarrhythmic agents.

Cardiac arrests were divided into three groups[6,7] (Fig. 1, Table 1): group I had ventricular tachyarrhythmias which included primary ventricular fibrillation, classic sustained ventricular tachycardia degenerating into ventricular fibrillation, or directly into asystole (143/233, 61.4%); group II had torsade de pointes terminating in ventricular fibrillation (41/233, 18%); group III had bradyarrhythmias (48/233, 20.6%). Although we have drawn heavily on the results of our survey, we have added appropriate observations from other researchers.[8–15]

Group I: Primary Ventricular Fibrillation and Ventricular Tachyarrhythmia Leading to Ventricular Fibrillation

This group includes 60% to 70% of instances of cardiac arrest and approximately 80% of all ambulatory cardiac arrest.[6,7] The mean age was 70 years; 76% were male (Figs. 2 to 4). Eighty-four percent had evidence of coronary heart disease; 12% had other forms of heart disease. The remaining 4% had no apparent heart disease, but were

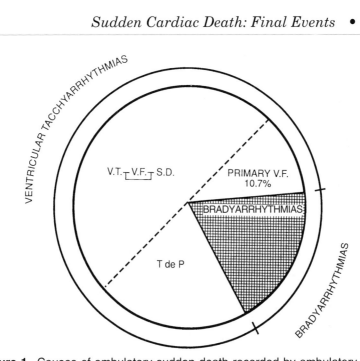

Figure 1. Causes of ambulatory sudden death recorded by ambulatory electrocardiography. T de P = torsade de pointes; VF = ventricular fibrillation; VT = ventricular tachycardia; SD = sudden death (from Bayés de Luna A, et al[7]).

Table 1

Clinical Characteristics of Recorded Cardiac Arrest by Ambulatory Electrocardiography

	Ventricular Tachyarrhythmias		
	Group I Primary VT and VT→VF	Group II Torsade de Pointes	Group III Brady-arrhythmias
	n = 143	n = 42	n = 48
Mean age (yrs)	70	60	70
Sex (males)	76%	40%	39%
Coronary patients	84%	50%	70%
No known heart disease	4%	22%	10%
Resuscitated	20%	28.5%	4%
Prior antiarrhythmic treatment	64%	76%	—

VT = systained monomorphic ventricular tachycardia; VF = ventricular fibrillation (Adapted from Bayes de Luna et al.[7])

E.M. 57 y.o. ♂
Recurrent sudden death

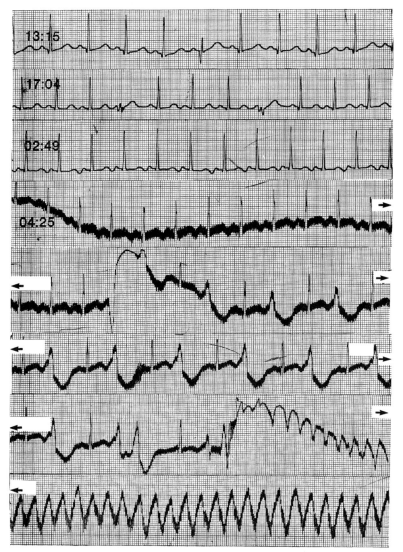

Figure 2. Sudden deaths as result of primary ventricular fibrillation initiated by a ventricular extrasystole with short coupling interval.

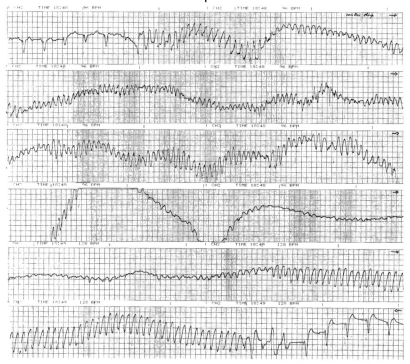

Figure 3. Ventricular fibrillation with spontaneous reversion occurring in a patient with a permanent pacemaker precipitated by an R-on-T beat.

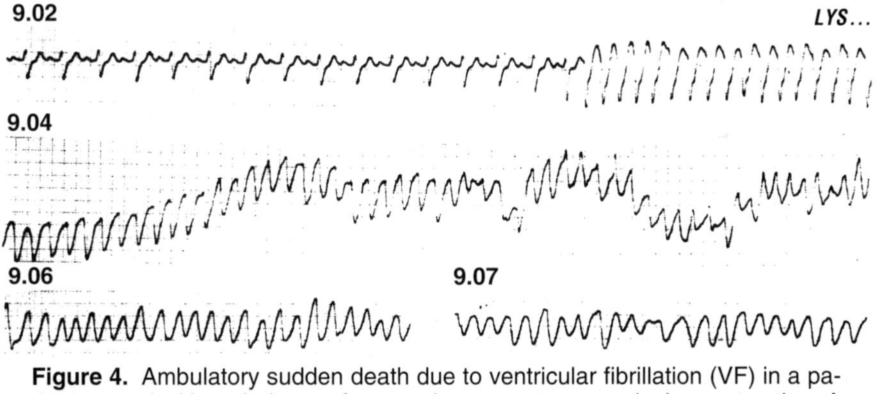

Figure 4. Ambulatory sudden death due to ventricular fibrillation (VF) in a patient treated with amiodarone for complex premature ventricular contraction. A monomorphic sustained ventricular tachycardia (VT) occurred at 9:02 AM and ventricular fibrillation ensued at 9:04 AM after an increase of ventricular tachycardia rate and QRS width (from Bayés de Luna et al.[6]).

recorded because of the presence of frequent ventricular premature beats. Compared to the torsade de pointes group II (Table 1), patients in group I were slightly older, more often male, and frequently had coronary or other cardiac disease.

The presence of heart failure varied considerably. The mean ejection fraction calculated by isotopic ventriculography was approximately 35%. Ejection fraction was less than 40% in 80% of the patients.[13] Lewis[14] reported that the mean ejection fraction was less than 30% in only 20% of the patients in a similar study.

We observed that 63% of the patients were taking class I antiarrhythmic drugs, 17% were not taking antiarrhythmic drugs, and information was lacking in the remaining 20%. It is difficult to ascertain the degree to which antiarrhythmic drugs may have induced sudden death. Proarrhythmic effects have been suspected by several researchers. The incidence of proarrhythmia varies considerably in different series.[8,15] The incidence of proarrhythmia as a triggering mechanism of sudden death in patients with ventricular fibrillation appears to be lower than in patients with torsade de pointes. The results of the Cardiac Arrhythmia Suppression Trial (CAST) suggest, however, that proarrhythmic phenomena may be more important than previously realized.[17,18]

The increased occurrence of ischemic events and sudden death in the morning upon awakening has been recently emphasized. Various explanations have been proposed for this phenomenon. However, ambulatory sudden cardiac death was not related to a circadian pattern in our study.[6,7] Although patient activity at the time of death varied, it was not related to exercise and occurred with equal frequency during rest or sleep. Only 2 of the 19 patients reviewed by Roelandt[12] died suddenly during exercise. Since most of these patients had advanced heart disease, they were capable of mild effort only. Although the time of sudden death in patients with ventricular fibrillation was distributed homogeneously throughout the 24 hours, Pratt[13] noted that 10 of the 15 patients died between 13:16 hours and 19:28 hours.

Ventricular fibrillation was the primary mechanism of sudden death in patients with Wolff-Parkinson-White syndrome, valvular heart disease, and cardiomyopathies. In patients with Wolff-Parkinson-White syndrome, ventricular fibrillation was often triggered by supraventricular arrhythmia.[19,20] Digoxin and verapamil may facilitate the appearance of ventricular fibrillation in these patients. Ventricular fibrillation has been noted to occur shortly after the acute administration of digitalis for treatment of atrial fibrillation.[19]

Ventricular tachyarrhythmias are often the cause of sudden death in patients with severe aortic stenosis. There are but a few reports of aortic stenosis and sudden death during ambulatory monitoring. Of the four cases reported by Olshausen et al.,[21] all died due to ventricular fibrillation.

Sudden cardiac death is the mode of death in approximately 50% of patients with idiopathic dilated and hypertrophic cardiomyopathy. The incidence of sudden death in dilated cardiomyopathy is even greater than in postmyocardial infarction patients.[22] It is likely that in patients with moderate heart failure, ventricular tachyarrhythmia is a major cause of sudden death.[23,24] In contrast, in patients with advanced heart failure, bradyarrhythmias are more common.[25] Right ventricular dysplasia is a special form of dilated cardiomyopathy in which sustained ventricular tachycardia or ventricular fibrillation play an important role. It may represent a major cause of sudden death in young people.[26,27] The precise mechanism of sudden cardiac death in patients with hypertrophic cardiomyopathy is not fully understood.[28,29] Recent clinical observations suggest that both abnormal hemodynamic response and malignant ventricular arrhythmias are the important causes of cardiac arrest in hypertrophic cardiomyopathy.[30] In a pediatric population[31] and in adults with terminal illness,[5] bradyarrhythmias, not tachyarrhythmias, are the main terminal event associated with sudden death. In some cases, sudden cardiac death may be triggered by supraventricular tachyarrhythmias.[32]

Electrocardiographic Characteristics

In more than two-thirds of cases, sinus rhythm is the basic rhythm which characteristically accelerates in the hours prior to the development of ventricular tachyarrhythmia (Fig. 5).[6-9] Olshausen et al.[10] observed that atrial fibrillation was the basic rhythm in 34% of the 61 patients who died suddenly while wearing an ambulatory electrocardiographic recorder. We observed that with tachyarrhythmic deaths, an increase in heart rate occurred within three hours of the event (83 versus 89 beats per minute, $P < 0.05$) (Fig. 5). In the absence of sinus rhythm, rapid atrial fibrillation was the most common rhythm, either chronic or appearing acutely during the recording.

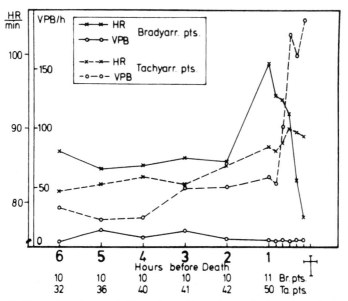

Figure 5. Mean heart rate (HR) and median of ventricular premature beats (VPB) during the last 6 hours before death. The numbers of included brady-arrhythmic (Bradyarr. pts.) and tachyarrhythmic (Tachyarr. pts.) patients are given below the corresponding hour before death (from Olshausen et al.[10]).

ST Changes

Ischemic changes in the ST segment were infrequently observed. We observed ST segment depression only in 12.7% of our cases in which this information was available. When recorded, ST segment depression of greater than 1 mm occurred more frequently than ST elevations. In another study, ST segment changes were observed before sudden death in 16% of patients.[10] Ischemic ST segment changes were more common in patients dying with brady-arrhythmia, compared to ventricular tachyarrhythmias. Gomes et al.[33] found that electrocardiographic changes compatible with silent myocardial ischemia preceded ventricular tachycardia only in 2 of 14 patients (14%) who had a recorded in-hospital episode of ventricular tachycardia or ventricular fibrillation. In contrast, Pepine et al.[34] observed electrocardiographic evidence of ischemia prior to sudden death in 52% of patients. There are only a few instances of sudden death associated with Prinzmetal's variant angina recorded in the literature.[35] However, the association of arrhythmias with ischemic electrocardiographic changes is well known in this syndrome.[36]

The incidence of ischemic ST changes may not reflect the real occurrence of clinical ischemia in ambulatory death. There are several reasons for this. The sampling is biased since it includes only those patients wearing an electrocardiographic monitor and as such, is not a sample of the general population. In addition, there are very few instances of first myocardial infarction recorded as the first manifestation of sudden death since these patients are usually asymptomatic and rarely undergo ambulatory electrocardiographic monitoring. It is also possible that clinical ischemia may exist without detection by conventional electrocardiogram. This is even more likely when recording only one or two leads.[8,14] In addition, ischemia sufficient to cause sudden death may be so subtle that it is not manifested by the recording systems that are currently used.

QT Interval

Measurement of the QT interval has been infrequently recorded before sudden death, due in part to the difficulty of obtaining a precise measurement using the current electrocardiographic leads.[10,12,13,15] We examined the QT interval prior to the fatal arrhythmia and found no significant differences. Measurement of the QT interval in patients taking one or more antiarrhythmic drugs is even more difficult. Consequently we cannot conclude that an increase in the QT interval does not play a role as a triggering mechanism of sudden death. Nevertheless, the QT interval may be a marker of sudden death since its prolongation in surface electrocardiograms has been described in survivors of out-of-hospital ventricular fibrillation.[37]

Frequency of Premature Ventricular Complexes

The number of premature ventricular complexes that appear during ambulatory recording prior to sudden death varies widely. Frequent and complex ventricular premature beats are common in these patients and usually increase before the fatal event.[8,9,14] Lewis[14] reported an increase in the complexity of ventricular arrhythmias in 70% of cases prior to death. Many patients were observed to have frequent, repetitive complex premature ventricular contractions before their cardiac arrest. Nevertheless, the ventricular tachyarrhythmic cardiac arrest can occur without an increase of ectopics in the previous minutes. Olshausen et al.[10] observed an increase in ectopic activity in most patients prior to tachyarrhythmic death. Ventricular premature beat frequency did not change during the six hours before death, but increased abruptly during the last hour (Fig. 5) from 60 to 196 beats per hour. In that study, 14% had greater than 500 ventricular premature beats per hour, and 42% had greater than three triplets per hour (Fig. 6).

Characteristics of Ventricular Tachycardia that Degenerate to Ventricular Fibrillation

The morphology of the initiating ventricular tachycardia may be either monomorphic or polymorphic. Monomorphic ventricular

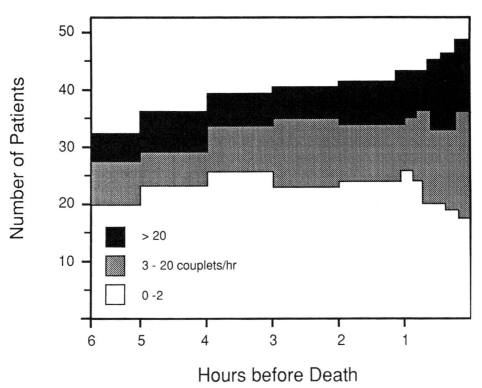

Figure 6. Hourly frequency of runs of ventricular tachycardia during the last hours before death in patients who died suddenly due to ventricular tachyarrhythmias (from Olshausen et al.[10]).

tachycardia occurred in two-thirds of the cases. In some instances, runs of polymorphic ventricular tachycardia were observed to change to monomorphic tachycardia. The duration of QRS complex during ventricular tachycardia was variable but was usually greater than 0.14 seconds, and often increased with the duration of tachycardia. Fatal ventricular tachycardia was usually rapid and as fast as 170 beats per minute.[9] An acceleration of the fatal ventricular tachycardia often occurred from 231 ± 11 to 247 ± 12 beats per minute before ventricular fibrillation.[8] The duration of the ventricular tachycardia preceding ventricular fibrillation varied from a few seconds to several minutes. It was significantly longer in cases of monomorphic ventricular tachycardia compared to polymorphic ventricular tachycardia.

In 25 patients (11%), we observed that ventricular fibrillation appeared immediately after a premature ventricular contraction, while in 102 cases (44%), it was secondary to ventricular flutter or, more commonly, to sustained ventricular tachycardia. In the remaining patients, sustained ventricular tachycardia occurred following a period of asystole. The frequency of ventricular tachycardia before ventricular fibrillation suggests that sudden death could be avoided if the preceding ventricular tachycardia could be interrupted.

The average coupling interval of the first complex of fatal ventricular tachycardia has been observed to be shorter than the shortest coupling interval found during ambulatory recording (442 ± 19 msec).[8] This does not, however, indicate that fatal ventricular tachycardia always begins with an R-on-T phenomenon. The R-on-T phenomenon was principally seen in ventricular fibrillation of abrupt onset and in cases of polymorphic ventricular tachycardia. Olshausen et al.[10] observed the R-on-T phenomenon occurred in 20% of the episodes of fatal ventricular tachycardia. Lewis et al.[14] observed that R-on-T preceded ventricular fibrillation or torsade de pointes in 9 of 12 cases. Adgey et al.[4] studied 48 consecutive patients who developed ventricular fibrillation outside the hospital after the arrival of a mobile coronary unit. An R-on-T extrasystole occurred in 69% of the patients and was the most important factor in the initiation of ventricular fibrillation. In 12%, a late cycle extrasystole or idioventricular rhythm initiated ventricular fibrillation. In contrast to our observations,[6,7] ventricular fibrillation was preceded by typical ventricular tachycardia only in 19% of cases. This difference is probably related to the fact that most of Adgey's patients died secondary to acute myocardial infarction, whereas very few patients in our study had evidence of acute ischemia.

Clinical Characteristics of the Onset of Ventricular Fibrillation

Ventricular fibrillation is the most important single cause of death in acute myocardial infarction occurring outside the hospital and represents approximately 6% to 10% of patients hospitalized for acute myocardial infarction.[1,38] It is probable that acute ischemia explains the episodes of primary ventricular fibrillation rather than sustained ventricular tachycardia. In the latter instance, the trigger is usually a premature ventricular complex. Ventricular fibrillation triggered by R-on-T extrasystole has also been reported in other series of acute infarction.[38]. Our studies of the risk factors for ventricular fibrillation during the early phase of acute myocardial infarction[2] suggest that hypotension (<110 mm Hg), ST segment elevation (>10 mm), and inferior myocardial infarction are all important predictors.[2]

Ventricular tachyarrhythmia is often the cause of sudden death in patients with valvular heart disease. Olshausen et al.[21] reported four patients with aortic valve disease whose deaths occurred while wearing an ambulatory electrocardiographic recording device. Ventricular fibrillation was the mechanism in all cases, three of which were preceded by monomorphic ventricular tachycardia and one by polymorphic ventricular tachycardia initiated by an R-on-T phenomenon. Runs of ventricular tachycardia were observed in three patients and atrial fibrillation was the dominant rhythm in two. None of these patients died during exercise. Stokes-Adams syncope with transitory complete heart block is a common clinical rhythm disorder in aortic stenosis. In pediatric patients, Walsh and Kongrad[31] reported that ventricular tachyarrhythmias occurred only in 22% of sudden deaths (Fig. 7). Ventricular tachyarrhythmias occurred three times more frequently in patients with congenital heart disease than in noncardiac patients who died suddenly (35% versus 11%).[31]

Successful resuscitation of patients is largely a question of the time between the onset of ventricular fibrillation to the administration of defibrillative shock. Milner et al.[39] observed that only 6 of 12 patients who experienced in-hospital cardiac arrest due to ventricu-

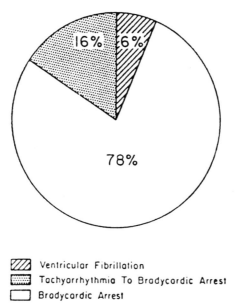

Ventricular Fibrillation
Tachyarrhythmia To Bradycardic Arrest
Bradycardic Arrest

Figure 7. Summary of the terminal cardiac electrical activity in 100 pediatric patients (from Walsh and Krongrad[31]).

lar tachyarrhythmia survived. Survivors did not differ from non-survivors in age, ejection fraction, extension of atherosclerotic lesion, or time until first defibrillation. In contrast, nonsurvivors had a shorter duration of ventricular tachycardia before ventricular fibrillation and a slower ventricular tachycardia rate at the time of cardiac arrest.

In summary, ventricular fibrillation is often secondary to ventricular tachycardia, and is the major mechanism of ambulatory cardiac arrest. The basal heart rate often accelerates before cardiac arrest and ventricular premature beats become more frequent and complex. Changes in the QT interval are inconsistent. The importance of ischemic ST segment abnormalities as a cause of cardiac arrest remains uncertain but is a significant factor in many studies.

Group II: Torsade de Pointes

The definition of the term torsade de pointes remains controversial. We have used the definition of torsade de pointes that corresponds to the patients with the morphology described by

Desertenne[40] (Fig. 8). Using that definition, torsade de pointes is preceded by a long QT interval, a long coupling interval, and a slow basal rate. The term torsade de pointes is used often erroneously in cases of polymorphic ventricular tachycardia, which is a variant of classic ventricular tachycardia. At other times, true torsade de pointes is misconstrued as classic ventricular tachycardia. The recognition of torsade de pointes has increased with the use of ambulatory electrocardiographic monitoring. Nevertheless, its incidence is underestimated due to the lack of uniformity in electrocardiographic terminology, which requires that the QT interval is precisely measured. A coupling interval of 600 milliseconds combined with R-on-T phenomenon is often a predictor of torsade de pointes.

Clinical and Electrocardiographic Characteristics

The 42 cases of torsade de pointes represent 18% of our total series (Table 1). The mean age was 60 years, and 60% of the patients were female. Only 50% had evidence of prior ischemic heart disease. In one series,[8] only one of the 13 patients had coronary heart disease. Proarrhythmia was considered the cause in 69%. Leclercq et al.[8] also observed a female predominance and a low incidence of coronary

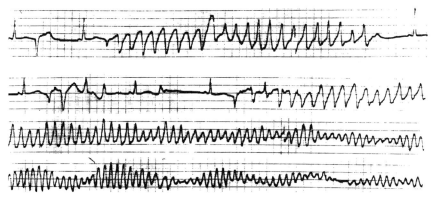

Figure 8. Typical pattern of torsade de pointes in a female treated with quinidine for nonsustained ventricular tachycardia in the absence of heart disease. A long sequence of torsade de pointes includes ventricular fibrillation (from Bayés de Luna et al.[6]).

heart disease. Hypokalemia was also related to occurrence of the arrhythmia. Sixty-one percent of our series were hospitalized for the antiarrhythmic drug adjustment. Patients with a long QT syndrome often experienced torsade de pointes that deteriorated into ventricular fibrillation. In this condition, sudden death is usually induced by physical or mental stress.[41,42] This is in contrast to the usual patients with torsade de pointes in whom sudden death occurs more frequently at rest or during sleep.

Slowing of the basal heart rate frequently occurred prior to the event.[8] The frequent occurrence of bradycardia before the torsade de pointes may explain the nocturnal predominance of this event. By definition, coupling interval prior to torsade de pointes is long, in addition to a long RR cycle. A postextrasystolic pause is frequently observed immediately before the first torsade de pointes. Circulatory collapse is due usually to prolonged torsade de pointes or its degeneration into ventricular fibrillation. Resuscitation of torsade de pointes is usually successful if recognized early and is best treated with ventricular overdrive pacing.

Group III: Bradyarrhythmias

Clinical and Electrocardiographic Characteristics

We observed bradyarrhythmic cardiac arrest in 48 patients, representing 20.6% of the total group. This incidence of bradyarrhythmia is similar to other series.[8,10] The mean age was 70 years and 61% were female. Seventy percent had evidence of coronary heart disease. Other forms of heart disease including pulmonary embolism and dissecting aneurysm were present in 20% of cases. In the remaining patients, evidence of cerebrovascular disease was present. Bradyarrhythmia was usually characterized as an irreversible depression of the sinus rhythm and subsidiary pacemaker automaticity.

Congestive heart failure[9] and evidence of ischemic ST segment changes before sudden death were common. This is in contrast to patients whose cardiac arrest occurred with ventricular tachycardia or ventricular fibrillation. Acute ischemia was observed in 66% of the patients and was associated with electromechanical dissociation in 72%.[8] Antiarrhythmic drug use was less frequent in these patients and proarrhythmia was suspected in very few patients.[8]

Luu et al.[25] studied the rhythms observed at the time of unexpected cardiac arrest in 21 patients with advanced heart failure who were awaiting hospital discharge after transplant evaluation. Only 38% of patients had ventricular tachycardia or ventricular fibrillation at the time of arrest. The remaining patients had severe sinus bradycardia, atrioventricular block, or electromechanical dissociation[25] (Fig. 9).

Advanced atrioventricular block was seen in 5% to 8% of patients with acute myocardial infarction. This may be the cause of sudden death in itself, or it may facilitate the appearance of ventricular arrhythmias.[43] Asystole occurs in 1% to 14% of patients with acute myocardial infarction and is associated with high mortality.[43]

Abrupt depression of sinus automaticity or sinoatrial block was frequent. In many instances, they were related to acute ischemia or electromechanical dissociation (Fig. 10). Atrioventricular block occurred in only 20% of this group. Severe bradycardia and a high degree of atrioventricular block occurred in patients with myocardial infarction.

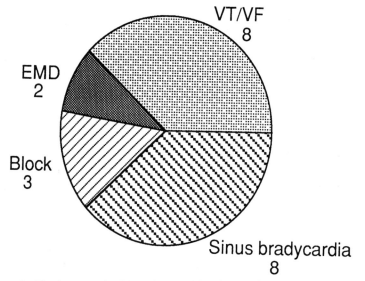

Figure 9. Final events in 21 patients with advanced heart failure who died suddenly. (EMD = electromechanical dissociation; VT–VF = ventricular tachycardia-ventricular fibrillation) (from Luu et al.[25]).

Bradyarrhythmia is the main cause of sudden death in patients with noncardiac terminal illness. In 23 hospitalized terminal patients without apparent cardiac disease, the dominant terminal rhythm was bradyarrhythmia in 83%.[5] The terminal electrical events were due to progressive slowing of the heart rate in 48%, short runs of ventricular tachyarrhythmias progressing to bradycardia and asystole in 13%, progressive slowing associated with runs of ventricular tachyarrhythmia progressing to ventricular fibrillation in 22%, ventricular tachyarrhythmia terminating with bradycardia and asystole in 4%, and ventricular tachyarrhythmias degenerating into ventricular fibrillation in 13%. ST segment elevation was observed in 25% of the terminal events. The mechanism of ST segment elevation in patients dying without apparent heart disease is unclear, although coronary artery spasm or hypoxia leading to epicardial injury may be important factors. In a pediatric population with noncardiac terminal illness, bradyarrhythmia remains the most frequent cause of death[31] (Fig. 7).

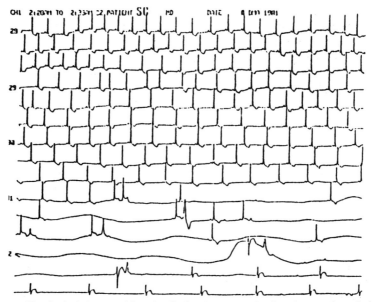

Figure 10. Ambulatory sudden death due to a progressive depression of sinus and subsidiary automatism in a postmyocardial infarction patient in subacute phase. The primary cause of death was cardiac rupture with electromechanical dissociation.

Severe vagal dystonia with cardiac asystole has been described in apparently healthy people who die suddenly.[44] Milstein et al.[44] studied six survivors of suspected asystolic sudden cardiac arrest without structural heart disease, with normal conventional electrophysiological study. During head-up tilt testing, all patients developed syncope associated with a marked decrease in mean arterial pressure and heart rate. Thus, in apparently healthy people, a neurally mediated hypotension-bradycardia syndrome may cause sudden cardiac death.

In summary, most patients with bradyarrhythmic cardiac arrest appear to have severe heart disease. Acute ischemic heart disease is common, as is congestive heart failure. Electromechanical dissociation is often present and resuscitation efforts are generally unsuccessful.

Limitations of Studies of Sudden Death Recorded by Ambulatory Electrocardiography

To collect a sufficient number of patients, a cooperative effort of cardiac centers is required. This dependence on multicenter cooperation results in often incomplete and unreliable data. In addition, these subjects may not be characteristic of the general population and therefore these data may be inappropriate to extrapolate broadly to all patient groups. The patients were usually wearing an ambulatory recorder because they had serious heart disease. Therefore, the findings obtained reflect only the mechanism of ambulatory sudden death in patients with known heart disease or in patients with ventricular arrhythmias, with or without coronary heart disease.

We can, however, draw several conclusions from the results of these studies. Clearly ventricular fibrillation is usually preceded by sustained ventricular tachycardia. Therefore, devices used to treat ventricular fibrillation such as the automatic implanted defibrillator must be able to recognize and treat ventricular tachycardia and prevent ventricular fibrillation. In addition, to prevent sustained ventricular tachycardia, sinus tachycardia, or accelerated heart rate accompanying supraventricular arrhythmia is also important. This is often an expression of increased adrenergic stimulation. Elimination of this trigger factor may help to suppress ventricular tachycardia and fibrillation. It is possible that the increase in heart rate that occurs before ventricular fibrillation can be reduced with β blockers[45] and may explain the beneficial effect of these drugs in the prevention of sudden death. In other situations, arrest may be triggered by a postextrasystolic pause.[8] It is possible that a pacemaker could prevent sudden death in these patients. These two phenomena, sympathetic tone and cardiac pause, are independent but may have an additive or an interactive effect on the occurrence of ventricular tachyarrhythmias.[46]

There is also evidence that cardiac arrest may be due to the proarrhythmic effect of antiarrhythmic drugs, even in patients without heart disease. This was seen particularly in the torsade de pointes group. For this reason, antiarrhythmic agents should be prescribed only when the arrhythmia carries major risk. The potential for proarrhythmic effects of drugs should be examined by electrophysiological study or by ambulatory electrocardiographic recording within a few days of initiating administration. The lack of evidence of proarrhythmia using these two technologies, however, is not a guarantee against subsequent lethal events. The observations in CAST[17,18] indicate that these proarrhythmic events may not be confined just to the initiation of therapy, but occur during the entire course of therapy.

Future Studies

Future studies of the mechanisms of ambulatory cardiac arrest should be prospective and establish a uniform methodology. More definitive studies should include patients with malignant or potentially malignant ventricular arrhythmias. The recording of the function of implantable cardioverter defibrillators will also provide useful information regarding final events.

An attempt also should be made to improve the accuracy of ambulatory electrocardiographic recorders in order to identify ischemia, using instruments equipped with three or more leads. The study of the dynamic changes in the QT interval may also provide a fruitful area of research.[47] In order to achieve this, the recording quality of the devices must be improved to provide consistently accurate and automatic measurement of the QT interval. Ideally, the ambulatory electrocardiographic recorder should display a QT trend to determine whether the dynamic behavior of the QT interval throughout the recording is a marker for malignant ventricular arrhythmias. Our preliminary studies with manual measurement suggest that QT variability is an important factor in the development of ventricular arrhythmias.[47] Recent studies with automatic measurement support these observations.[48] An automatic readout of occurrence of the R-on-T phenomenon may also prove helpful. Measurement of heart rate variability, an important predictor of sudden death, can also provide information regarding sinus automaticity and sympathetic responsiveness of the atrial pacemaker. However, a recent study has not demonstrated a decrease in heart rate variability occurring before sudden death.

Many of these technological developments are in progress and have already provided important information about the mechanism of sudden death. Future developments hold promise for even greater understanding of the unique phenomenon of cardiac arrest.

References

1. Lie KJ, Wellens HJJ, Dorsnar E, et al. Observations on patients with primary ventricular fibrillation complicating acute myocardial infarction. *Circulation* 1975;52:755.
2. Fiol M, Marrugat J, Bayés de Luna A, et al. Ventricular fibrillation predictors in acute myocardial infarction. *Am J Cardiol* 1993:71:117.
3. Quale J, Kimmelstiel C, Schrem S, et al. Identification of risk factors for development of acute myocardial infarction or life-threatening ventricular arrhythmia in unstable angina pectoris. *Am J Cardiol* 1987;59:703.
4. Adgey AA, Devlin JE, Webb SW, et al. Initiation of ventricular fibrillation outside hospital in patients with acute ischemic heart disease. *Br Heart J* 1982;47:55.
5. Wang F, Lien W, Fong T, et al. Terminal cardiac electrical activity in adults who die without apparent cardiac disease. *Am J Cardiol* 1986; 58:491.
6. Bayés de Luna A, Coumel PH, Leclercq JF. Ambulatory sudden death: Mechanisms of production of fatal arrhythmia on the basis of data from 157 cases. *Am Heart J* 1989;117:151.
7. Bayés de Luna A, Guindo J, Rivera J. Ambulatory sudden death in patients wearing Holter devices. *J Ambulat Monitoring* 1989;2:3.
8. Leclercq JF, Coumel P, Maison-Blanche P, et al. Mise en evidence des mecanismes determinants de la mort subite. Enquete cooperative portanat sur 69 cas en registres para la methode de Holter. *Arch Mal Coeur* 1986;79:1024.
9. Kempf FC, Josephson ME. Cardiac arrest recorded on ambulatory electrocardiograms. *Am J Cardiol* 1984;53:1577.
10. Olshausen KV, Witt T, Pop T, et al. Sudden death while wearing a Holter monitor. *Am J Cardiol* 1991;67:381.
11. Pepine C, Morganroth J, McDonald JT, et al. Sudden death during ambulatory ECG monitoring. *Am J Cardiol* 1991;68:785.

12. Roelandt J, Klootwijk P, Lubsen J, et al. Sudden death during long-term ambulatory monitoring. *Eur Heart J* 1984;5:7.
13. Pratt C, Francis MJ, Luck JC, et al. Analysis of ambulatory electrocardiograms in 15 patients during spontaneous ventricular fibrillation with special reference to preceding arrhythmic events. *J Am Coll Cardiol* 1983;2:789.
14. Lewis BH, Antman EM, Graboys TB. Detailed analysis of 24-hour ambulatory ECG recordings during ventricular fibrillation or torsade de pointes. *J Am Coll Cardiol* 1983;2:426.
15. Denes P, Gabster A, Huang SK. Clinical, electrocardiographic and follow-up observations in patients having VF during Holter. *Am J Cardiol* 1981;48:9.
16. Panidis IP, Morganroth J. Sudden death in hospitalized patients: Cardiac rhythm disturbances detected by ambulatory electrocardiographic monitoring. *J Am Coll Cardiol* 1983;2:798.
17. CAST Investigators. Preliminary report: Effect of encainide and flecainide on mortality in a randomized trial of arrhythmia suppression after myocardial infarction. *N Engl J Med* 1989;321:406.
18. CAST II Investigators. Effect of the arrhythmic agent moricizine on survival after myocardial infarction. *N Engl J Med* 1992;327:227.
19. Klein GJ, Bashore TM, Sellers TD, et al. Ventricular fibrillation in the Wolff-Parkinson-White syndrome. *N Engl J Med* 1979;301:1080.
20. Torner-Montoya P, Brugada P, Smeets J, et al. Ventricular fibrillation in the Wolff-Parkinson-White syndrome. *Eur Heart J* 1991;12:144.
21. Olshausen KV, Witt T, Schmidt, et al. Ventricular tachycardia as a cause of sudden death in patients with aortic valve disease. *Am J Cardiol* 1987;50:1214.
22. Olshausen KV, Schafer A, Mehmel HC, et al. Ventricular arrhythmias in idiopathic dilated cardiomyopathy. *Br Heart J* 1984;51:195.
23. Holmes J, Kubo SH, Cody RJ, et al. Arrhythmias in ischemic and nonischemic dilated cardiomyopathy: Prediction of mortality by ambulatory electrocardiography. *Am J Cardiol* 1985;55:146.
24. Kjekshus J. Arrhythmias and mortality in congestive heart failure. *Am J Cardiol* 1990;65:42-I.
25. Luu M, Stevenson WG, Stevenson LW, et al. Diverse mechanisms of unexpected cardiac arrest in advanced heart failure. *Circulation* 1989; 80:1675.
26. Marcus FI, Fontaine GH, Guiraudon G, et al. Right ventricular dysplasia: A report in 24 adult cases. *Circulation* 1982;65:384.
27. Thiene G, Nava A, Corrado D, et al. Right ventricular cardiomyopathy and sudden death in young people. *N Engl J Med* 1988;318:129.
28. Nicod P, Polikar R, Peterson KL. Hypertrophic cardiomyopathy and sudden death. *N Eng J Med* 1987;316:780.
29. Maron BJ, Roberts WC, Epstein SE. Sudden death in hypertrophic cardiomyopathy: A profile of 78 patients. *Circulation* 1982;65:1388.
30. McKenna WJN, Camm AJ. Sudden death in hypertrophic cardiomyopathy: Assessment of patients at high risk. *Circulation* 1989;80:1489.
31. Walsh CK, Krongrad E. Terminal cardiac electrical activity in pediatric patients. *Am J Cardiol* 1983;51:557.

32. Wang Y, Scheinman MM, Chien WW, et al. Patients with supraventricular tachycardia presenting with aborted sudden cardiac death: Incidence, mechanism and long-term follow-up. *J Am Coll Cardiol* 1991; 18:1711.

33. Gomes JA, Alexopoulos D, Winters SL, et al. The role of silent ischemia, the arrhythmic substrate and the short-long sequence in the genesis of sudden cardiac death. *J Am Coll Cardiol* 1989;14:1618.

34. Pepine CJ, Morganroth J, McDonald JT, et al. Sudden death during ambulatory electrocardiographic monitoring. *Am J Cardiol* 1991; 68:785.

35. Myerburg RJ, Kessler KM, Mallon SM, et al. Life-threatening ventricular arrhythmias in patients with silent myocardial ischemia due to coronary artery spasm. *N Engl J Med* 1992;326:1451.

36. Bayés deLuna A, Buetikofer J, Lesser J, et al. Holter ECG study of the electrocardiographic phenomena in Prinzmetal angina attacks with emphasis on the study of ventricular arrthythmias. *J Electrocard* 1985;18:267.

37. Haynes RE, Hallstrom AP, Cobb LA. Repolarizations abnormalities in survivors of out-of-hospital ventricular fibrillation. *Circulation* 1978;57:654.

38. El-Sherif N, Myerburg RJ, Scherlang BJ, et al. Electrocardiographic antecedents of primary ventricular fibrillation. *Br Heart J* 1976;38:415.

39. Milner PJ, Platia EV, Reid PR, et al. Ambulatory electrocardiographic recordings at the time of fatal cardiac arrest. *Am J Cardiol* 1985;56:588.

40. Dessertenne F. La tachycardia ventriculaire a deux toyers opposes variables. *Arch Mal Coeur* 1966;59:263.

41. Schwartz PJ, Locati E. The idiopathic long QT syndrome: Pathogenic mechanisms and therapy. *Eur Heart J* 1985;6:103.

42. Surawicz B, Knoebel SB. Long QT: Good, bad or indifferent? *J Am Coll Cardiol* 1984;4:398.

43. Alpert JS. Conduction disturbances. In: Gersh BJ, Rahimtoola SH, eds. *Acute Myocardial Infarction.* New York: Elsevier; 1991:249.

44. Milstein S, Buetikofer J, Lesser J, et al. Cardiac asystole: A manifestation of neurally mediated hypotension-bradycardia. *J Am Coll Cardiol* 1989;14:1626.

45. Coumel P, Leclercq JF, Zimmermann M. The clinical use of β-blockers in the prevention of sudden death. *Eur Heart J* 1986;7(Suppl A):187.

46. Leclercq JF, Maison-Blanche P, Cuchemezand B, et al. Respective role of sympathetic tone and of cardiac pauses in the genesis of 62 cases of ventricular fibrillation recorded during Holter monitoring. *Eur Heart J* 1988;9:1276.

47. Homs E, Viñolas X, Guindo J, et al. Automatic QTc lengthening measurement in Holter ECG as a marker of life-threatening arrthythmias in postmyocardial infarction patients. *J Am Coll Cardiol* 1993;21:274A. Abstract.

48. Marti V, Guindo J, Homs E, et al. Peaks of QTc lengthening measured in Holter recordings as a marker of life-threatening arrhythmias in postmyocardial infarction patients. *Am Heart J* 1992;124:234.

Chapter IV

Mechanisms and Pathology of Sudden Death

The mechanism by which sudden cardiac death occurs continues to be an enigma. For the most part, therapy has been empiric, based on superficial observations related to the presentation of sudden death event. The greater understanding of the complexity of ischemia and the availability of new pharmacologic agents has expanded our knowledge of the mechanism by which the electrical integrity of the heart is lost.

The quest for the mechanism of sudden death long preceded 18th century Pope Clement XI's instruction to his court physician, Lancisi, to investigate the increased number of sudden deaths occurring in Rome.[1] After an exhaustive analysis, Lancisi concluded that a single cause could not be identified. Contrary to his longstanding conclusions, the era is now ending in which a single cause—the ventricular contraction—was presumed to be the major cause of sudden death. The results of the Cardiac Arrhythmia Suppression Trial (CAST) provide a watershed in our understanding of the mechanisms and prevention of sudden death.[2] They also encourage a reassessment of our current attitude in regard to this problem. It had been proposed that the eradication of ventricular ectopy in patients with coronary heart disease could prevent sudden death.[3] The CAST observations indicate that this eradication or suppression of ventricular ectopy, at least with three commonly used drugs, actually results in an increased mortality rate. Although disappointing in some respects, these observations now provide a long overdue opportunity to examine other mechanisms of sudden death in coronary heart disease.

From: S. Goldstein, A. Bayés-de-Luna, J. Guindo-Soldevila: *Sudden Cardiac Death*. Armonk, NY: Futura Publishing Co., Inc., © 1994.

Definition of Sudden Death

Investigation into the mechanism of sudden death requires a definition of the event, a definition that has proved elusive. Lancisi divided sudden death in three parts:[1]

> Indeed this absolutely complete cessation of animal movements and the departure of a soul from a body even though it happens at all times more swiftly than itself, is nevertheless divided for the sake of common parlance and for greater clarity of teaching into natural, untimely and violent death, and these again into slowly and sudden deaths, and to those that as are foreseen and 'forcefelt' and finally into such as are unforeseen, unperceptible and unexpected.

The need for a definition has been predicated on the hypothesis that there are both arrhythmic and nonarrhythmic mechanisms of cardiac arrest which require different therapeutic approaches. The choice of antiarrhythmic or anti-ischemic drugs would be based upon the presumed mechanism in a given patient. In light of current events, such a definition may at least be unnecessary. Simplistic definitions dependent on events occurring within one hour or less[4] have been supplemented by more mechanistically based definitions that depend on the clinical presentation of the event. The attempt to define mechanical and arrhythmic presentation of sudden death is fraught with difficulty since the occurrence of either event can lead to the other. Because of these difficulties, definitions that include both time and clinical setting have been proposed. The Cardiac Arrhythmia Pilot Study, using a time- and etiology-based assessment, concluded that sudden death usually equates to arrhythmic death.[5] Using this methodology, approximately 25% of the arrhythmic deaths were associated with myocardial ischemia or infarction. Using the Hinkle-Thaler classification system,[6] Marcus et al.[7] observed that 58% of the presumed arrhythmic sudden deaths were preceded by symptoms of myocardial ischemia. Not only is it difficult to separate ischemia from the arrhythmic event, clearly that mechanical dysfunction can occur rapidly, leading to ventricular failure in minutes. In addition, prolonged periods of seemingly life-threatening arrhythmias, such as ventricular tachycardia, can manifest as symptoms of left ventricular failure.

Ischemic heart disease in the western world remains the major cause of sudden death and total mortality, and this predominance is confirmed by many investigators.[8] Evidently sudden death due to ischemic heart disease is the usual mechanism of death in patients over the age of 35. In a study of sudden death occurring in the United States conducted in 1985, 56% of the deaths due to ischemic heart disease were out-of-hospital deaths or had occurred in the emergency room.[9] There has been very little change in the overall occurrence of sudden death if one defines sudden death as dying out-of-hospital or in the emergency room. There has been, however, a trend toward increased emergency room deaths and a decreasing number of out-of-hospital deaths as patients are educated about early response to symptoms. In our study[10] of resuscitated out-of-hospital victims of cardiac arrest, ischemia occurred in approximately two-thirds of the victims (Fig. 1). Angiographic findings in patients resuscitated from out-of-hospital cardiac arrest reveal that 94% of the patients had severe stenosis in one or more of their major coronary arteries and

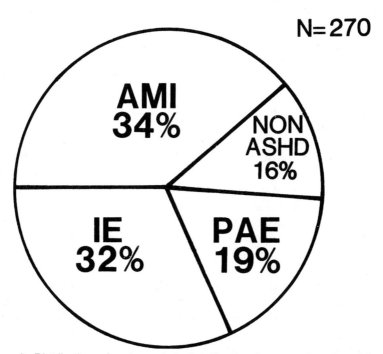

Figure 1. Distribution of entry event classification in resuscitated sudden death victims. AMI = acute myocardial infarction; IE = ischemic event; PAE = primary arrhythmic event; NON ASHD = deaths unrelated to arteriosclerotic heart disease.

most of the patients had extensive ventricular wall contraction abnormalities.[11] It is therefore clear that coronary heart disease is the common denominator of most patients dying suddenly. The mechanism, however, by which the event occurs remains controversial. Whether the development of ventricular ectopy and its degeneration into ventricular fibrillation is the primary mechanism of the event, or whether arrhythmic degeneration is a result of acute ischemia, remains an issue and has significant therapeutic implications.

Ventricular Arrhythmia and Antiarrhythmic Therapy

Strong evidence exists that frequent and complex ventricular ectopy in patients with coronary heart disease is an important predictor of sudden death,[12,13] particularly in the postinfarction population.[14] Ventricular ectopy, however, in the absence of heart disease has no predictive importance.[15] The specificity of ventricular ectopy for mortality, even in the setting of coronary heart disease, varies widely in relation to the extent of left ventricular function. High-frequency ventricular ectopy occurs in about 10% of patients with preserved ventricular function and is associated with a two- to three-fold increase in mortality.[16] As the ejection fraction falls, ventricular ectopy becomes a more common phenomenon. In the setting of advanced ventricular dysfunction, frequent multiple and multiform ventricular premature beats occur in almost 50% of the patients and are poor predictors of total and sudden death.[17] In these disparate settings, the role of suppression of ventricular ectopy is not clear, and a unifying hypothesis is lacking.

The importance of ventricular ectopy as a predictor of both total and sudden death mortality has led to a variety of investigations into the use of antiarrhythmic agents in coronary heart disease. Although limited by relatively small size, none of these investigations, however, demonstrated efficacy[18–20] (see Chapter XVII). These investigations have taken a number of different forms, from the treatment of all patients with ischemic heart disease, regardless of the presence of ventricular ectopy, to the more recent approach of suppression of high-frequency ventricular ectopy in postmyocardial infarction patients. The International Mexiletine and Placebo Arrhythmia Control Trial (IMPACT) study[21] is an example of the former approach and CAST[2] an example of the latter strategy. In the IMPACT Study, mexiletine randomly administered to postinfarction patients showed a modest decrease in ventricular ectopy and a trend toward a higher mortality in the mexiletine group. The failure to achieve a benefit was attributed both to the lack of potency of mexiletine and to its potential adverse effect on patients without ectopy. CAST, on the other hand, compared encainide, flecainide, and moricizine to a placebo after ventricular ectopic beat suppression by one of the active agents was demonstrated using Holter recording. The encainide-flecainide arm of the study was prematurely ended due to a threefold increase in mortality in patients assigned to active therapy in spite of an 80% suppression of ventricular ectopic beat.[2] The extension of CAST examined the effect of moricizine alone on sudden death mortality.[22] In that part of the study, moricizine also demonstrated a lack of benefit and an increased mortality. We observed that the empiric use of both quinidine and procainamide was associated with an adverse effect on mortality in high-risk patients[23] (Fig. 2).

With the failure of arrhythmia suppression guided by ambulatory monitoring, more physiological approaches were developed to examine the appropriate use of antiarrhythmic agents.[24] These ap-

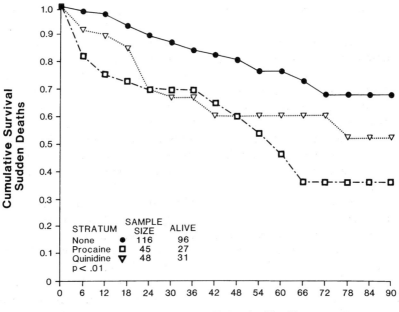

Figure 2. Cumulative sudden death survival for the study population divided by those taking no medication, procainamide, and quinidine after out-of-hospital rescuscitation (from Mossvi et al.[23]).

proaches are based on more specific physiological effects of the drugs on the myocardium. Numerous studies examined the use of programmed ventricular stimulation techniques to guide arrhythmia suppression. Patients presumed to be at high risk of sudden death, such as those resuscitated from a previous cardiac arrest, were examined using this technique. Suppression of arrhythmia induction using stimulation techniques was used as evidence of drug efficacy.[25] It has therefore been deemed unethical to withhold that antiarrhythmic drug from the patient once suppression is demonstrated. One randomized placebo control study, however, examined the benefit of class I agents on mortality in postinfarction patients in whom inducible ventricular tachycardia by programmed stimulation was demonstrated.[26] After demonstrating inducibility, patients were randomized as to quinidine, mexiletine, and dysopyramide administration at doses determined to achieve "therapeutic" serum levels. No benefit was observed in the patients randomized to the active treatment group when compared to the placebo controls. Investigations comparing drug therapy guided by ambulatory monitoring to electrophysiological stimulation failed to show any benefit of one technique over the other (see Chapter XVII). These observations indicate that ventricular ectopic beat suppression alone can no longer be viewed as a surrogate for improved survival and urge a more imaginative assessment of antiarrhythmic therapy.

Most clinical studies examine the efficacy of antiarrhythmic agents on spontaneous arrhythmias in a relatively stable ischemia-free state. It is possible that drugs that suppress arrhythmias in the nonischemic state may become proarrhythmic in the setting of ischemia. The failure of the encainide-flecainide arm of CAST may be explained by such a mechanism. The interrelationship between ischemia and arrhythmogenesis in man was reported by Morady and associates[27] during programmed stimulation. They demonstrated that myocardial ischemia evidenced by transmyocardial lactate production was a requirement for electrophysiological induction of ventricular tachycardia in some survivors of cardiac arrest.

In an animal model, lidocaine and mexiletine suppressed ventricular ectopy in the ischemia-free state but had little or no antiarrhythmic effect in the setting of ischemia coupled with sympathetic stimulation.[28] In contrast, propranolol and amiodarone were both effective in the ischemic and nonischemic setting. Models such as these may provide a different and more comprehensive approach to the investigation of antiarrhythmic therapy.[29] It is possible that pleuripotential drugs like propranolol and amiodarone may have a more important role in arrhythmia therapy.

The importance of arrhythmia control in general, however, is supported by the success of the automatic implantable cardiac defibrillator. Although not as yet investigated in a randomized controlled trial, the device appears to be effective in the prevention of arrhythmic deaths in high-risk patients.[30] It should not be presumed, however, that this supports the primacy of arrhythmia suppression in the prevention of sudden death. It is merely an acceptance that ventricular fibrillation is one of the major final common pathways to sudden death. Although we have been aware for almost three decades of the benefit of early external defibrillation in patients with acute myocardial infarction, asystole remains an important consideration. Newer automatic devices incorporate pacemaker function (see Chapter XVIII).

Myocardial Ischemia

Although sudden death is intimately related to ischemia, the linkage has been difficult to document. The observations by Spain[31] and Roberts[32] suggested that coronary occlusion and infarction were not important factors in sudden death. Our initial investigations of out-of-hospital resuscitated cardiac arrest victims, however, implied a strong role for ischemia and infarction in the pathophysiology of sudden cardiac arrest.[10] This was supported by other studies of resuscitated sudden death victims.[33,34] The expansion of our understanding of the pathology of sudden death was in part created by the work of Haerem[35] and by Frink and associates.[36] Both studies demonstrated the presence of platelet aggregates in individuals dying suddenly of coronary heart disease, many of whom failed to show any acute lesions of epicardial vessels. Patients who died suddenly had the greatest number of platelet aggregates when compared to patients with chronic coronary heart disease. Mural coronary thrombi were proposed as a source for fragmentation and dispersion of platelet aggregates. It remained for Davies and Thomas[37] to describe the relationship of coronary pathology to sudden death. Their demonstration[37] of atherosclerotic plaque fissuring, coronary mural thrombi, platelet aggregates, and microinfarction in patients dying suddenly with coronary heart disease established that link (Table 1). They also observed that intramyocardial platelet aggregation was common in patients dying suddenly of unstable angina[38,39] (Figs. 3, 4). Intravascular masses of platelets could be found in 30% of these patients. These masses were seen in small arteries and capillaries downstream from fissured atheromatous plaques with exposed mural thrombi. Approximately 40% of these patients experienced chest or arm pain in the two weeks before their death. Davies et al.[38,39] suggested that the expression of ischemia, infarction, and sudden death is a result of an interaction between plaque fissure and thrombus formation (Fig. 5). In 168 patients dying suddenly of coronary heart disease, 53.5% had mural intraluminal coronary thrombi and 29.8% had occlusive intraluminal thrombi. The importance of these observations, however, has been challenged by Kragel et al.,[40] who examined coronary lesions in patients dying from major epicardial coronary artery disease and unstable angina pectoris who experienced both sudden death and acute myocardial infarction. They observed a similar frequency in both thrombus formation and plaque hemorrhage in both groups of patients. The type of thrombus and the amount of luminal obstruction by the thrombus was similar in both groups. An intraluminal thrombus was present in 29% of both unstable angina patients and those dying suddenly, compared to 69% in patients who had an acute myocardial infarction. The platelet

Table 1

Distribution of Vascular Events in Sudden Ischemic Death

	Atheroma-Basal Control	Related Control	Test	Total
No acute arterial lesion	63(91.3%)	47(78.3%)	32(19%)	142
Plaque fissure alone	6(8.7%)	10(16.7%)	13(7.7%)	29
Mural thrombus	0	3(5%)	73(43.5%)	76
Occlusive thrombus	0	0	50(29.8%)	50
Total	69(100%)	60(100%)	168(100%)	297

Basal control = nonatheroma deaths; atheroma-related control = nonsudden atheromatous deaths; Test = deaths with 6 hours of symptomatic onset with evidence of coronary heart disease.
(Davies MJ, Bland JM, Hangartner RW, Angelini A, Thomas AC Factors influencing the presence or absence of acute coronary artery thrombi in sudden ischaemic death. *Eur Heart J* 1989;10:203–208.)

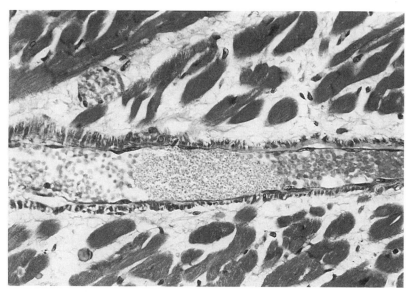

Figure 3. Thrombus localized in small artery of patient dying suddenly with unstable angina (from Davies et al.[38]).

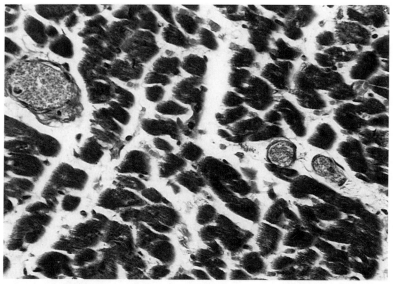

Figure 4. Thrombus in capillary in patient with unstable angina dying suddenly (from Davies et al.[38]).

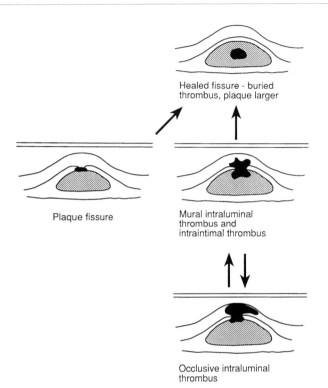

Healed fissure - buried
thrombus, plaque larger

Plaque fissure

Mural intraluminal
thrombus and
intraintimal thrombus

Occlusive intraluminal
thrombus

Figure 5. Plaque fissuring. The causes of acute myocardial infarction, sudden ischemic death, and crescendo angina (from Davies et al. *Br Heart J* 1985;53:363–373).

thrombi were observed in patients dying suddenly or in the setting of unstable angina. In patients dying of acute infarction, the thrombus was made up predominantly of fibrin. The occurrence of plaque rupture was also similar in the three groups. Plaque hemorrhage was significantly less in patients with unstable angina and sudden death, 64% and 38%, respectively, compared to 90% of the patients with acute myocardial infarction. Figure 6 shows the theoretical progression of coronary heart disease, based on the observations of Kragel et al.,[40] in patients with acute myocardial infarction, sudden cardiac death, and unstable angina. In all three groups, the mean percent of collagen deposition increases, with an increasing degree of luminal narrowing. Severely narrowed arteries associated with acute myocardial infarction usually demonstrate a plaque rupture with occlusive thrombus, whereas nonocclusive thrombus formation

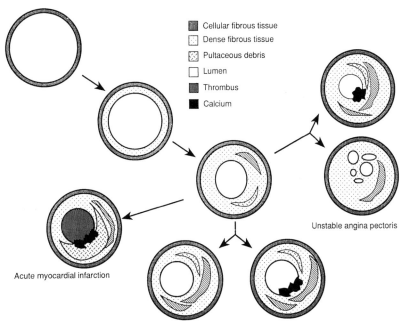

Figure 6. Diagram of coronary artery plaque morphology in patients with fatal coronary artery disease due to acute myocardial infarction, sudden coronary death without transmural left ventricular necrosis or unstable angina pectoris without transmural left ventricular necrosis. In all three groups, the mean percent of cellular fibrous tissue decreases with increasing degrees of luminal narrowing, and the mean percent of dense fibrous tissue, calcific deposits, and pultacous debris rich in extracellular lipid increases. Severely narrowed segments in the group with acute myocardial infarction contain more pultaceous debris and are characterized by plaque rupture with associated hemorrhage and occlusive intraluminal thrombus. Severely narrowed segments in the group with unstable angina pectoris are characterized by the presence of multiluminal channels. Nonocclusive thrombus and plaque hemorrhage with or without plaque rupture can be seen in all three groups (from Kragel et al.[40]).

and plaque hemorrhage were usually seen in both unstable angina and sudden death.

Triggering events for the initiation of these pathological processes have come under recent investigation. Muller et al. called attention to the importance of circadian rhythm as a mechanism for the precipitation of acute ischemic events, including acute myocardial infarction[41] and sudden death[42] (Fig. 7). They observed an association between morning ischemic events to the sudden morning circadian increase in serum norepinephrine, heart rate, blood pressure, platelet activation,[43] and decreased fibrinolytic activity.[44] It is possible that triggering phenomena such as these seen in the setting of circadian rhythmicity may provide an explanation of the timing of an ischemic event.

Clinical trials of many drugs aimed at modulating ischemia and preserving the integrity of coronary blood flow support the ischemia hypothesis. The restoration or improvement of coronary blood flow by coronary bypass surgery was observed to have a special effect on sudden death in the Coronary Artery Surgery Study[45] (see Chapter XVIII). The ability of platelet-active agents such as aspirin to decrease sudden death in patients with unstable angina has been reported.[46] Aspirin therapy has also been estimated to reduce the risk of vascular death by 13% and nonfatal reinfarction by 31%[47] (see Chapter XVII).

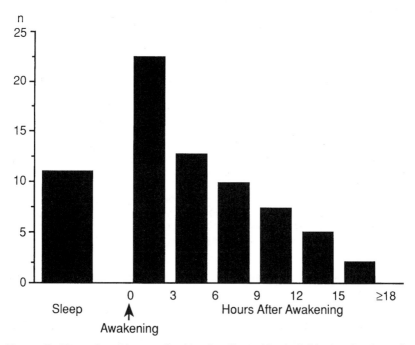

Figure 7. Time of sudden cardiac death adjusted for individual wake times (n = 84) showing a significantly increased relative risk of 2.6 (95% confidence interval 1.6, 4.2) during the initial 3 hours after awakening compared with other times of day (from Willich et al. *Am J Cardiol* 1992;70:65–68.)

β-adrenergic blocking agents have also been shown to decrease both total and sudden death mortality[48,49] (see Chapter XVII). Propranolol administered to high-risk postmyocardial infarction patients with ventricular fibrillation, ventricular tachycardia, and high-frequency ventricular premature beats resulted in a decrease in sudden death.[50] Muller et al.[51] observed a salutary effect on the early morning occurrence of myocardial infarction in patients receiving β-adrenergic blocking agents. These observations were also supported by the effects of propranolol on the occurrence of early morning sudden death in the β-Blocker Heart Attack Trial.[52] The well-known ability of β-blockers to limit ischemia has been ascribed to their negative chronotropic and inotropic mechanism. In ischemic animal studies, however, a direct effect of propranolol was observed on mitochondrial salvage and preservation at ATP content.[53] In addition, β-blockers increase the ventricular fibrillation threshold in ischemic animals[54] and decrease the frequency of ventricular ectopy in postmyocardial infarction patients.[16] It has been suggested by some investigators that lipophilic β-blockers are more effective in preventing sudden death since they enter the central nervous system tissue more easily. This has been used to support the hypothesis that β-blockers exert their effect by altering the central nervous system control of the myocardial arrhythmic integrity. The specific mechanism by which β-blockers prevents sudden death, however, remains uncertain. Their efficacy, however, is supported by an expanding volume of basic and clinical investigations.

Ventricular Dysfunction

Sudden death in patients with advanced left ventricular dysfunction and heart failure has a more complex genesis than in those patients dying with acute ischemia or infarctions (see Chapter X). The scarred ventricle with its heterogeneity of both depolarization and repolarization is an ideal setting in which ventricular arrhythmias can occur.[55] The increase in serum catecholamine levels and other unknown metabolic substances that occur in heart failure may adversely alter the function and electrical integrity of the heart.[56] A relationship does exist between ventricular arrhythmias, left ventricular dysfunction, and sympathetic activation. In patients with left ventricular dysfunction, an examination of norepinephrine turnover was carried out in patients who had been resuscitated from out-of-hospital cardiac arrest.[57] The rate of cardiac norepinephrine spillover had a fivefold increase in resuscitated sudden death patients when compared to subjects who had not experienced sudden death (Fig. 8). This disproportionate increase in norepinephrine spillover suggests a selective activation of cardiac sympathetic outflow associated with reduced left ventricular function. Depressed left ventricular function is closely related to reflex cardiac sympathetic activation and together these two processes can provide the environment for the development of ventricular arrhythmia and cardiac arrest. Increased serum norepinephrine concentration in patients with worsening congestive heart failure before their death was observed by Kao and associates[58] (Fig. 9). This antecedent increase in

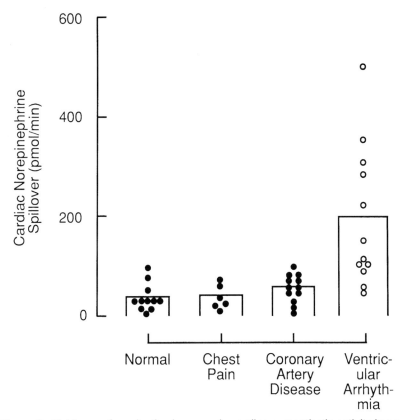

Figure 8. Evidence of a selective increase in cardiac sympathetic activity in patients with sustained ventricular arrthythmias (from Meredith et al.[57]).

serum norepinephrine further suggests a mechanistic relationship between ventricular dysfunction, norepinephrine sympathetic activation, ventricular arrhythmias, and cardiac arrest (see Chapter II).

A study of patients with advanced heart failure using the vasodilators hydralazine and isosorbide dinitrate reported a decrease in total mortality[59] (see Chapter XVII). A subsequent comparison of this drug combination to the ACE inhibitor, enalapril, suggested a decrease in sudden death mortality in the enalapril-treated patients.[60] In the Cooperative North Scandinavian Enalapril Survival Study (CONSENSUS) trial,[61] mostly of hospitalized patients, enalapril demonstrated a decrease in total mortality with no significant effect on sudden death. In the Studies of Left Ventricular Dysfunction (SOLVD),[62] enalapril demonstrated an overall decrease in mortality, but had no effect on sudden death mortality. Angiotensin-converting enzyme inhibitors have been shown to have a salutary effect on ventricular ectopy, norepinephrine, and potassium concentrations in patients with severe heart failure.[63] Animal studies indicate that these drugs can prevent ventricular dysfunction by a direct action on tissue conversion of angiotensin I to angiotensin II.[64,65] The efficacy of angiotensin-converting enzyme inhibitors on sudden death re-

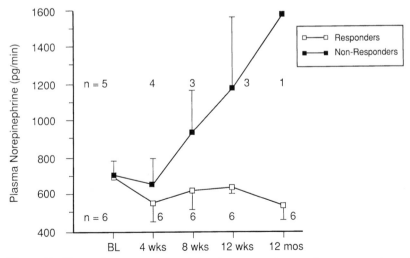

Figure 9. Mean plasma norepinephrine for responders and nonresponders at baseline and during follow-up. In nonresponders, mean plasma norepinephrine at last available follow-up (mean = 4.2 months) was significantly higher than for responders at 12-month follow-up ($P = 0.02$) (from Kao et al.[58]).

mains uncertain, although their ability to decrease total mortality in patients with symptomatic heart failure and asymptomatic left ventricular dysfunction (see Chapter XVII) is well established.

β-adrenergic blocking agents, because they cause down-regulation of myocardial β-adrenergic receptors in the failing heart, have also been examined in the treatment of heart failure.[66,67] Initial studies demonstrated that the use of propranolol in high-risk postmyocardial infarction patients characterized by both heart failure and high-frequency arrhythmias resulted in a beneficial effect on sudden cardiac death.[50] A retrospective analysis of the β-Blocker Heart Attack Trial also suggests that in patients with a history of heart failure, propranolol therapy resulted in a decrease in the incidence of sudden death[68] (see Chapter XVII).

In view of these observations, the uncertain benefit of antiarrhythmic therapy and the observed benefits of interventions directed at limiting ischemia and improving ventricular function, a reconsideration of the mechanisms and prevention of sudden death, without the constraints of previous paradigms is required. It is time to examine the interaction between ventricular ectopy, myocardial ischemia and infarction, the failing left ventricle, and sudden cardiac death (see Chapter II). Examination of these interrelated disorders may lead to a better understanding of both the maintenance and the disintegration of the heart's electrical integrity. As we continue to consider the role of antiarrhythmic therapy in sudden death, we must also investigate the importance of ischemia on the action of these agents. Clearly it is critical to the development of ventricular fibrillation. In the scarred and decompensated left ventricle, however, the myocardial substrate for ventricular fibrillation exists and the role of ischemia is less apparent and may be more subtle. The observations gained from pharmacological intervention in patients with ischemic disease can provide us with probes into the mechanisms by which sudden death occurs. The abyss between our understanding of physiological mechanisms of sudden death and pharmacological interventions is considerable. A greater understanding of the mechanisms by which sudden death occurs is required before we can fully develop pharmacological interventions.

References

1. Lancisi GM. *De Subitaneis Mortibus.* Rome: Buagni; 1706.
2. Cardiac Arrhythmia Suppression Trial (CAST) Investigators. Preliminary Report: Effect of encainide and flecainide on mortality in a ran-

domized trial of arrhythmia suppression after myocardial infarction. *New Engl J Med* 1989;321:406.

3. Lown B. Sudden cardiac death: The major challenge confronting contemporary cardiology. *Am J Cardiol* 1979;43:313.

4. Goldstein S. The necessity of a uniform definition of sudden coronary death: witnessed death within 1 hour of the onset of acute symptoms. *Am Heart J* 1982;103.

5. Greene HL, Richardson DW, Barker AH, et al. and the CAPS Investigators. Classification of deaths after myocardial infarction as arrhythmic or nonarrhythmic (The Cardiac Arrhythmia Pilot Study). *Am J Cardiol* 1989;63:1.

6. Hinkle LE, Thaler HT. Clinical classification of cardiac deaths. *Circulation* 1982;65:457.

7. Marcus FI, Cobb LA, Edwards JE, et al. and the Multicenter Post Infarction Research Group. Mechanism of death and prevalence of myocardial ischemic symptoms in the terminal event after acute myocardial infarction. *Am J Cardiol* 1988;61:8.

8. Gillum RF. Sudden coronary death in the United States—1980–1985. *Circulation* 1989;79:756.

9. Drory Y, Turetz Y, Hiss Y, et al. Sudden unexpected death in persons < 40 years of age. *Am J Cardiol* 1991;68:1388.

10. Goldstein S, Landis JR, Leighton R, et al. Characteristics of the resuscitated out-of-hospital cardiac arrest victim with coronary heart disease. *Circulation* 1981;64:977.

11. Weaver WD, Lorch GS, Alvarez HA, et al. Angiographic findings and prognostic indicators in patients resuscitated from sudden cardiac death. *Circulation* 1976;54:895.

12. Ruberman W, Weinblatt E, Goldberg JD, et al. Ventricular premature beats and mortality after myocardial infarction. *N Engl J Med* 1977;297:750.

13. Temesy-Armos PN, Vanderbrug Medendorp S, Goldstein S, et al. Predictive value of ventricular arrhythmias in resuscitated out-of-hospital cardiac arrest victims. *Eur Heart J* 1988;9:625.

14. Bigger JT Jr, Fleiss JL, Kleiger R, et al. and the Multicenter Post-Infarction Research Group. The relationships among ventricular arrhythmias, left ventricular dysfunction and mortality in the 2 years after myocardial infarction. *Circulation* 1984;69:250.

15. Crow R, Prineas R, Blackburn H. The prognostic significance of ventricular ectopic beats among the apparently healthy. *Am Heart J* 1981;101:244.

16. Friedman LM, Byington RP, Capone RJ, et al., Writing Group for the β-Blocker Heart Attack Trial Research Group. Effect of propranolol in patients with myocardial infarction and ventricular arrhythmia. *J Am Coll Cardiol* 1986;7:1.

17. Wilson JR, Schwartz S, St. John Sutton M, et al. Prognosis in severe heart failure: relation to hemodynamic measurements and ventricular ectopic activity. *J Am Coll Cardiol* 1983;2:403.

18. Ryden L, Arnman K, Conradson TB, et al. Prophylaxis of ventricular tachyarrhythmias with intravenous and oral tocainide in patients with and recovering from acute myocardial infarction. *Am Heart J* 1980;100:1006.

19. Bastian BC, Macfarlane PW, McLauchlan JH, et al. A prospective randomized trial of tocainide in patients following myocardial infarction. *Am Heart J* 1980;100:1017.
20. Hugenholtz PG, Hagemeijer F, Lubsen J, et al. One-year follow-up in patients with persistent ventricular arrhythmias after myocardial infarction treated with aprindine or placebo. In: Sandoe E, Julian DG, Pell JW, eds. *Management of Ventricular Tachycardia: Role of Mexiletine.* Amsterdam: Excerpta Medica; 1978;572–578.
21. IMPACT Research Group. International mexiletine and placebo antiarrhythmic coronary trial: I. Report on arrhythmia and other findings. *J Am Coll Cardiol* 1984;4:1148.
22. The Cardiac Arrhythmia Suppression Trial (CAST) II Investigators. Effect of the antiarrhythmic agent moricizine on survival after myocardial infarction. *N Engl J Med* 1991;327:227.
23. Moosvi AR, Goldstein S, Vanderbrug Medendorp S, et al. Effect of empiric antiarrhythmic therapy in resuscitated out-of-hospital cardiac arrest victims with coronary artery disease. *Am J Cardiol* 1990;65:1192.
24. Task Force of the Working Group on Arrhythmias of the European Society of Cardiology. The Sicilian gambit: A new approach to the classification of antiarrhythmic drugs based on their actions on arrhythmogenic mechanisms. *Circulation* 1991;84:1831.
25. Ruskin JN, DiMarco JP, Garan H. Out-of-hospital cardiac arrest: Electrophysiologic observations and selection of long-term antiarrhythmic therapy. *N Engl J Med* 1980;303:607.
26. Denniss AR, Ross DL, Cody DV, et al. Randomized controlled trial of prophylactic antiarrhythmic therapy in patients with inducible ventricular tachyarrhythmias after recent myocardial infarction. *Eur Heart J* 1988;9:746.
27. Morady F, DiCarlo LA, Krol RB, et al. Role of myocardial ischemia during programmed stimulation in survivors of cardiac arrest with coronary artery disease. *J Am Coll Cardiol* 1987;9:1004.
28. Schwartz MD, Vanoli E, Zaza A, et al. The effect of antiarrhythmic drugs on life-threatening arrhythmias induced by the interaction between acute myocardial ischemia and sympathetic hyperactivity. *Am Heart J* 1985;109:937.
29. Lynch JJ, Lucchesi BR. How are animal models best used for the study of antiarrhythmic drugs? In: Hearse D, Manning A, Janse M, eds. *Life-Threatening Arrhythmias During Ischemia and Infarction.* New York: Raven Press; 1987:169–196.
30. Tchou PJ, Kadri N, Anderson J, et al. Automatic implantable cardioverter defibrillators and survival of patients with left ventricular dysfunction and malignant ventricular arrhythmias. *Ann Intern Med* 1988;109:529.
31. Spain DM, Bradess VA. The relationship of coronary thrombosis to coronary atherosclerosis and ischemic heart disease (a necropsy study covering a period of 25 years). *Am J Med Sci* 1960;240:701.
32. Roberts WC. Coronary thrombosis and fatal myocardial ischemia. *Circulation* 1974;49:1. Editorial.

33. Liberthson RR, Nagel EL, Hirschman JC, et al. Pathophysiologic observations in prehospital ventricular fibrillation and sudden cardiac death. *Circulation* 1974;49:790.

34. Baum RS, Alvarez H, Cobb LA. Survival after resuscitation from out-of-hospital ventricular fibrillation. *Circulation* 1974;50:1231.

35. Haerem JW. Platelet aggregates in intramyocardial vessels of patients dying suddenly and unexpectedly of coronary artery disease. *Atherosclerosis* 1972;15:199.

36. Frink RJ, Trowbridge JO, Rooney PA. Nonobstructive coronary thrombosis in sudden cardiac death. *Am J Cardiol* 1978;42:48.

37. Davies MJ, Thomas A. Thrombosis and acute coronary artery lesions in sudden cardiac ischemic death. *N Engl J Med* 1984;310:1137.

38. Davies MJ, Thomas AC, Knapman PA, et al. Intramyocardial platelet aggregation in patients with unstable angina suffering sudden ischemic cardiac death. *Circulation* 1986;73:418.

39. Roberts WC, Potkin BN, Solus DE, et al. Mode of death, frequency of healed and acute myocardial infarction, number of major epicardial coronary arteries severely narrowed by atherosclerotic plaque, and heart weight in fatal atherosclerotic coronary artery disease: Analysis of 889 patients studied at necropsy. *J Am Coll Cardiol* 1990;15:196.

40. Kragel AH, Gertz SD, Roberts WC. Morphologic comparison of frequency and types of acute lesions in the major epicardial coronary arteries in unstable angina pectoris, sudden coronary death and acute myocardial infarction. *J Am Coll Cardiol* 1991;18:801.

41. Muller JE, Tofler GH, Stone PH. Circadian variation and triggers of onset of acute cardiovascular disease. *Circulation* 1989;79:733.

42. Muller JE, Ludmer PL, Willich SN, et al. Circadian variation in the frequency of sudden cardiac death. *Circulation* 1987;75:131.

43. Tofler GH, Brezinski D, Schafer AI, et al. Concurrent morning increase in platelet aggregability and the risk of myocardial infarction and sudden cardiac death. *N Engl J Med* 1987;316:1514.

44. Rosing DR, Brakman P, Redwood DR, et al. Blood fibrinolytic activity in man: Diurnal variation and the response to varying intensities of exercise. *Circ Res* 1970;27:171.

45. Holmes DR Jr, Davis K, Gersh BJ, et al. and participants in the Coronary Artery Surgery Study (CASS). Risk factor profiles of patients with sudden cardiac death and death from other cardiac causes: A report from the Coronary Artery Surgery Study. *J Am Coll Cardiol* 1989;13:524.

46. Lewis HD, Davis JW, Archibald DG, et al. Protective effects of aspirin against acute myocardial infarction and death in men with unstable angina. *N Engl J Med* 1983;309:396.

47. Antiplatelet Trialists' Collaboration. Secondary prevention of vascular disease by prolonged antiplatelet treatment. *Br Med J* 1988;296:320.

48. β-Blocker Heart Attack Trial Research Group. A randomized trial of propranolol in patients with acute myocardial infarction. I. Mortality Results. *JAMA* 1982;247:1707.

49. Lund-Johansen P, Norwegian Multicenter Group. The Norwegian Multicenter Study on timolol after myocardial infarction. Part II. Effect in different risk groups, causes of death, heart arrest, reinfarctions,

rehospitalizations and adverse experiences. *Acta Med Scand* 1981; 651:243.

50. Hansteen V, Moinichen E, Lorentsen E, et al. One year's treatment with propranolol after myocardial infarction: Preliminary report of Norwegian multicentre trial. *Br Med J* 1982;284:155.

51. Muller JE, Stone PH, Turi ZG, et al., and the MILIS Study Group. Circadian variation in the frequency of onset of acute myocardial infarction. *N Engl J Med* 1985;313:1315.

52. Peters RW, Muller JE, Goldstein S, et al., for the BHAT Study Group. Propranolol and the morning increase in the frequency of sudden cardiac death (BHAT Study). *Am J Cardiol* 1989;63:1518.

53. Kloner RA, Fishbein MC, Braunwald E, et al. Effect of propranolol on mitochondrial morphology during acute myocardial ischemia. *Am J Cardiol* 1978;41:880.

54. Anderson JL, Rodier HE, Green LS. Comparative effects of β-adrenergic blocking drugs on experimental ventricular fibrillation threshold. *Am J Cardiol* 1983;51:1196.

55. Downar E, Harris L, Mickleborough LL, et al. Endocardial mapping of ventricular tachycardia in the intact human ventricle: Evidence for reentrant mechanisms. *J Am Coll Cardiol* 1988;11:783.

56. Packer M. Neurohormonal interactions and adaptations in congestive heart failure. *Circulation* 1988;77:721.

57. Meredith IT, Broughton A, Jennings GL, et al. Evidence of a selective increase in cardiac sympathetic activity in patients with sustained ventricular arrhythmias. *N Engl J Med* 1991;325:618.

58. Kao W, Gheorghiade M, Hall V, et al. Relationship of plasma norepinephrine to clinical status during long-term medical therapy in patients with dilated cardiomyopathy. *Clin Res* 1988;36:822A. Abstract.

59. Cohn JN, Archibald DG, Ziesche S, et al. Effect of vasodilator therapy on mortality in chronic congestive heart failure. *N Engl J Med* 1986;314:1547.

60. Cohn JN, Johnson G, Ziesche S, et al. A comparison of enalapril with hydralazine-isosorbide dinitrate in the treatment of chronic congestive heart failure. *N Engl J Med* 1991;325:303.

61. The CONSENSUS Trial Study Group. Effects of enalapril on mortality in severe congestive heart failure. *N Engl J Med* 1987;316:1429.

62. The SOLVD Investigators. Effect of enalapril on survival in patients with reduced left ventricular ejection fractions and congestive heart failure. *N Engl J Med* 1991;325:293.

63. Cleland JGF, Dargie HJ, Hodsman GP, et al. Captopril in heart failure: A double blind controlled trial. *Br Heart J* 1984;52:530.

64. Linz W, Scholkens BA, Han YF. Beneficial effects of the converting enzyme inhibitor, ramipril, in ischemic rat hearts. *J Cardiovasc Pharmacol* 1986;8:S91.

65. Westlin W, Mullane K. Does captopril attenuate reperfusion-induced myocardial dysfunction by scavenging free radicals? *Circulation* 1988;77:30.

66. Waagstein F, Caidahl K, Wallentin I, Bergh C-H, Hjalmarson A. Long-term β-blockade in dilated cardiomyopathy. *Circulation* 1989;80:551.

67. Bristow MR, Ginsburg R, Umans V, et al. β_1- and β_2-adrenergic-receptor subpopulations in nonfailing and failing human ventricular myocardium: Coupling of both receptor subtypes to muscle contraction and selective β_1-receptor down-regulation in heart failure. *Circ Res* 1986;59:297.
68. Chadda K, Goldstein S, Byington R, et al. Effect of propranolol after acute myocardial infarction in patients with congestive heart failure. *Circulation* 1986;73:511.

Chapter V

Risk Factors and the Environment

General Incidence

The incidence of sudden cardiac death varies considerably from country to country[1] with relation to the prevalence of coronary artery disease. Since coronary heart disease is characteristic of industrialized societies and an aging population, the prevalence of sudden cardiac death is greater in the western world than in the rest of the world. According to the World Health Organization (WHO), the incidence of sudden cardiac death in industrialized areas varies between 19 and 159 per 100,000 inhabitants per year among men between ages of 35 and 64. In the United States, the incidence fluctuation is approximately 400,000 annually. Sudden cardiac death represents 12% to 32% of total natural deaths.[2] In one of the first epidemiologic studies of sudden death carried out by Kuller et al.,[3] cardiac mortality represented 75% of total deaths, 32% of which were sudden deaths. These were defined as unexpected death within the first 24 hours of symptoms. The Framingham study,[4] using a one-hour interval from the onset of symptoms, observed a 13% incidence of sudden death. In the combined Albany-Framingham prospective study,[5] in 4120 males between 45 and 74 years, 234 deaths of coronary origin occurred in the 16 years covered by the study. One hundred and nine deaths (47%) occurred in the first hour after the onset of symptoms. In Spain, Cosin et al. observed a sudden death mortality of 39 per 100,000 inhabitants per year, representing less than 10% of the total number of deaths.[6] The World Health Organization initiated

From: S. Goldstein, A. Bayés-de-Luna, J. Guindo-Soldevila: *Sudden Cardiac Death*. Armonk, NY: Futura Publishing Co., Inc., © 1994.

the MONICA study in 1982 to examine the incidence of sudden death and coronary heart disease throughout the world.[7]

In the United States and other industrialized countries, the incidence of sudden cardiac death is lessening due to the overall decrease in coronary heart disease mortality.[8,9] This decrease has been attributed to improved medical therapy and more effective systems for resuscitating victims of out-of-hospital cardiac arrest. In spite of this, the incidence of sudden cardiac death remains high and is still a major challenge confronting contemporary cardiology.

Timing of Sudden Death

A number of studies have shown that sudden cardiac death displayed a prominent circadian pattern, with a primary peak occurring between 7 AM and 11 AM[10] (see Chapter IV). In Framingham,[10] the risk of sudden cardiac death is approximately 70% greater from 7 AM to 9 AM than during the rest of the day. A circadian variation of sudden cardiac death, similar to that of the occurrence of nonfatal myocardial infarction and episodes of myocardial ischemia, was observed. Similar observations were made in the Spanish Trial on Sudden Death[6] (Fig.1). In contrast, however, during Holter recording,[11] a circadian relationship to sudden death due to ventricular fibrillation was not observed. Torsade de pointes, however, did occur with a nocturnal predominance, perhaps related to the slow heart rate during the night.

Unmodifiable Risk Factors and the Environment

Age

There are two peaks of sudden death incidence concerning age: the first from birth to six months (sudden infant death syndrome) and the second from 45 to 75 years. The incidence of sudden infant death[12] peaks between the second and fourth months (see Chapter XV) and is uncommon after the sixth month. It is of interest that during the first two weeks of life, when mortality is higher due to other causes, sudden infant death is rarely seen. The epidemiologic studies carried out by the University of Pittsburgh[13] in children and ado-

TIME OF DEATH
SSD/NSD

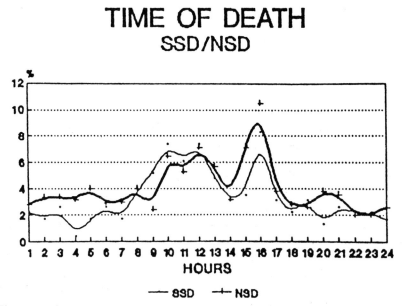

Figure 1. Circadian variation of sudden cardiac death in the Spanish Trial on Sudden Death. SSD = sudden death; NSD = nonsudden death (from Cosin et al.[6]).

lescents (1 to 21 years) observed a prevalence of sudden death of 5 per 100,000 per year, or 22% of nontraumatic deaths. During this age span, the maximum peaks were between the first and fourth year of life, due mainly to infection or unknown causes. In the 14- to 21-year-old group, the maximum peaks were due to cardiovascular causes, epilepsy, intracranial hemorrhage, and bronchial asthma.

In adults, sudden death is closely linked to the presence of coronary heart disease. In coronary heart disease, the highest proportion of sudden deaths are seen in young adults and declines progressively with age. Kuller et al.[14] observed that, at 20 to 29 years of age, 31% of deaths were sudden. In known coronary heart disease, 76% died suddenly. In Framingham,[15] sudden death declined to 62% in patients between 45 and 54 years old with coronary heart disease and fell progressively to 42% in the 65- to 74-year-old group. In the Spanish Trial on Sudden Death, the mean age of sudden death was 65 years for males and 74 for females.[6]

Although the incidence of sudden death parallels the incidence of coronary heart disease and increases with age, the proportion of those who die suddenly are higher in younger patients. This differential effect of age may be due to older patients having more advanced coronary heart disease, and therefore the incidence of death due to heart failure is greater.

Gender

Sudden death is more common in males than in females[15,16] by a ratio of 3 to 1. This is due to the lower prevalence of coronary heart disease in premenopausal women. During the 26 years of the Framingham study, sudden deaths occurred in 6.2% of the men and in 1.7% of the women. Similar results were found in other studies,[16] including the Spanish Trial on Sudden Death,[6] where the study mortality rate was 63 per 100,000 per year for males and 19.5 per 100,000 per year for females (a ratio of 3 to 1).

Females attained a comparable incidence of sudden death, 20 years older than men. However, more females than males die suddenly without clinical evidence of coronary heart disease. While 53% of males dying suddenly had a history of coronary heart disease, only 32% of females had a history of coronary heart disease. In females with known coronary heart disease, only the hematocrit had a high predictive value for sudden death. At all levels of multivariate risk, females present only one-third the incidence of sudden death compared to males. Since the frequency of sudden death is much higher in postmenopausal women compared to premenopausal women of the same age, it is likely that a hormonal factor influences the result.[17]

Familial Factors

Hereditary genetic factors are important in less common causes of sudden death, such as in the Jervell and Lange-Nielsen syndrome, a recessive autosomal genetic disease, and the Romano-Ward syndrome, an autosomal dominant disease.[18] In 1991, Keating et al.[19] reported a genetic linkage between the long QT syndrome and a DNA marker at the locus of the H-*ras*-1 gene on the short arm of chromosome 11 in a large, multigenerational Utah family. Hypertrophic cardiomyopathy, an important cause of sudden death in young people, particularly athletes and females, also has a genetic predisposition.[20] Arrhythmogenic right ventricle dysplasia[21] and mitral valve prolapse,[22] in which the familial history of syncope or sudden death are clear risk markers, also have genetic predisposition. In addition, familial cases of sudden death in infancy and adolescence have been described, although without evidence of a hereditary pattern.

Race

There is no clear relationship between sudden death and race. The lower incidence of sudden death in Japan is due mainly to cultural factors such as diet. Despite the fact that Japanese Americans have a higher incidence of coronary heart disease and therefore sudden death than those living in Japan, it does not reach the incidence of the United States white population.[23] This suggests a possible relationship between racial and cultural factors.

Water Quality

The quality of the water supply has also been thought to affect the incidence of ischemic heart disease and sudden death within an otherwise similar population. Hard water is considered to be protective, while soft water contributes to mortality of ischemic heart disease[24] (Fig. 2). One of the key determinants in the higher mortality of people living in soft water areas may be related to a magnesium deficiency.

Coronary Risk Factors

Risk factors have different importance in males and females. In males without known coronary heart disease, age, hypercholesterolemia, smoking habits, obesity, arterial hypertension, and left ventricular enlargement are predictors of sudden death. In the presence of coronary heart disease, the only risk factor with positive predictive value is the electrocardiographic presence of left ventricular hypertrophy and intraventricular conduction defect. In females without evidence of coronary heart disease, the factors associated with a higher incidence of sudden death are age, vital capacity, hematocrit, hypercholesterolemia, and glucose intolerance.[25]

Hypertension increases the risk of coronary heart disease, whether diastolic or systolic, fixed or labile, and is independent of age

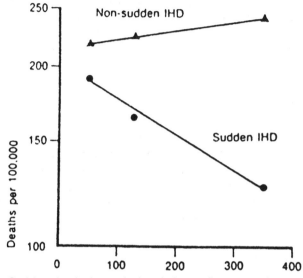

Figure 2. Sudden death due to ischemic heart disease and water hardness. IHD = ischemic heart disease (from Anderson TW[24]).

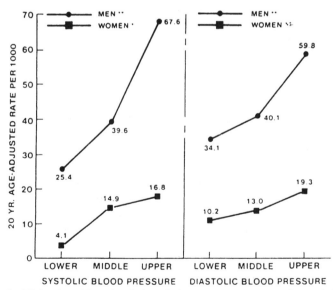

Figure 3. Risk of sudden death in relation to average systolic and diastolic blood pressure (from Kannel et al.[26]).

and sex.[25] Arterial hypertension also significantly increases the risk of sudden death[26] (Fig. 3). While the risk of sudden death doubles with mild to moderate blood pressure elevation (140–160/90–94), it increases even more with severe arterial hypertension.[26] Some antihypertensive therapy is also associated with an increased risk of sudden death. This may reflect the severity of hypertension of patients treated with drugs, rather than the harmful effect of the antihypertensive drugs themselves. In the Spanish Trial on Sudden Death, hypertension was the most significant predictor of sudden death in both sexes ($P < 0.001$).[6]

The Spanish Trial on Sudden Death[6] reported that hypercholesterolemia was significantly related to sudden cardiac death, while in the Framingham study,[26] it was not a factor. When age groups were analyzed separately, cholesterol levels in young adults increased the incidence of sudden death. Although at first it might be thought that the importance of cholesterol in atherogenesis would decline with age, Schatzkin et al.[4] suggest that change is due fundamentally to the premature death from coronary disease in many patients with high cholesterol. With aging, hypercholesterolemia loses statistical significance. Another possible explanation is that until now only total cholesterol levels have been analyzed. It is possible that future analysis of LDL and HDL fractions will clarify the relationship between hyperlipidemia and sudden death.[26] After myocardial infarction, hypercholesterolemia was associated significantly with an increase in both total and sudden cardiac death.[27]

Cigarette smoking greatly increases the risk of sudden death in males.[28-36] It is surprising that the effect of smoking on sudden death observed in males is not evident in females.[26] Although several studies demonstrate the important association between smoking and coronary heart disease,[35] the adverse effects of smoking seem transitory, nonaccumulative, and reversible.[26] Independent of the duration of smoking, in Framingham, those who gave up smoking had a rapid decline in their risk of sudden death to half that of patients who continued smoking.[26] Hallstrom et al.[28] observed that, after three years of follow-up, patients resuscitated after an out-of-hospital heart attack had a higher incidence of recurrent sudden death if they continued smoking (27% versus 19%). Similarly, in the β-Blocker Heart Attack Trial, Jafri et al. demonstrated that persistence in smoking after a myocardial infarction doubled the risk for subsequent events, including sudden death.[36]

Diabetes has been observed to double the total mortality of coronary heart disease.[37] Its impact is greater in females than in males. It also varies substantially according to other risk factors. Diabetes has a direct myocardial effect, predisposing to heart failure, and acting on coagulation to reduce fibrinolytic activity by raising the levels of fibrinogen and coagulation factors VII and VIII.[38] Glucose intolerance and diabetes increase the risk of sudden death in females. Glycosuria increases the incidence of sudden death in both sexes, although more importantly in females.[15,16]

Obesity increases the risk of coronary heart disease and is often associated with other risk factors, including hypertension, glucose intolerance, and a sedentary lifestyle. Consequently it is not surprising that obesity is associated with an increased risk of sudden death. The proportion of sudden deaths due to coronary heart disease also increased with obesity and appear independent of other risks of coronary heart disease.[15]

Hematocrit is also associated with a greater risk of sudden death in females, but not in males.[25] The mechanism by which hematocrit produces this effect is not clear, although a link between blood viscosity and hypercoagulability has been implicated.

Sedentary lifestyle is thought to have an adverse effect on the cardiovascular system and increases the level of the other coronary risk factors. The epidemiologic studies of Froelicher and Brown[39] suggest that physical exercise protects against coronary heart disease. This advantage is present only in males and is slight in comparison to the principal coronary risk factors.

The role of exercise on the incidence of sudden death is even more speculative. Paffenbarger et al.[40] suggest that physical activity reduces cardiac mortality, especially sudden death, in the 35- to 54-year-old population. If sedentary lifestyle, heavy smoking, and arterial hypertension were combined, the risk of sudden death is increased twentyfold. In a retrospective study of 163 cases of out-of-hospital sudden death, Siscovick et al.[41] concluded that intense physical exercise is protective of the occurrence of sudden death. The observed risk of sudden death was 55% to 65% less in physically active individuals. In contrast, Kannel and Sortie[42] found little relation between physical exercise and the risk of sudden death. Current evidence indicates that while a sedentary lifestyle contributes to mortality, its effect is slight in comparison to other risk factors. In contrast, Friedman et al.[43] reported a number of cases of sudden death occurring during moderate or strenuous exercise. They suggested that while physical activity can reduce the incidence of coronary attacks and mortality due to coronary heart disease, exercise can occasionally trigger sudden death.

Electrocardiographic Changes

The presence of electrocardiographic signs of left ventricular enlargement, intraventricular conduction disorders, and nonspecific repolarization changes are associated with an increase in sudden death[26] (Fig. 4). The incidence of sudden death in patients with left ventricular enlargement or intraventricular conduction delay is comparable to that of patients with symptomatic coronary heart disease.[26] Their importance increases in the presence of known coronary artery disease.

Premature ventricular contractions in patients who have suffered a myocardial infarction are clearly associated with an increased incidence of sudden death (see Chapter VII). This is especially true when they are frequent and complex[44-47] and are associated with ventricular dysfunction. Rubermann et al.[44] found that the R-on-T, polymorphic ventricular premature contractions, and salvos of ventricular tachycardia are associated with an increase in total and

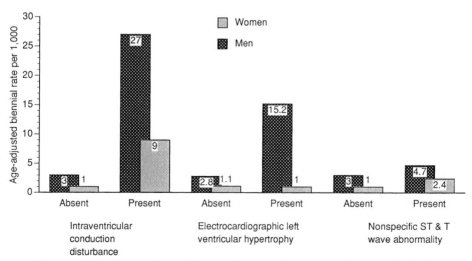

Figure 4. Electrocardiographic alterations and risk of sudden death in the Framingham study (from Kannel et al.[26]).

sudden deaths. Moss et al.[45] observed that only ventricular premature beat bigeminy and polymorphism are markers of sudden death. Bigger also demonstrated that total and sudden death is related to the frequency of premature impulses.[46] When the rate rises from one to ten per hour, mortality increases significantly. The BHAT confirmed that premature ventricular complexes are an independent risk marker of sudden death.[47] In contrast, exercise-induced arrhythmias apparently have no predictive value.[48] Localization of the infarction is also related to prognosis. There is a greater total mortality after anterior myocardial infarction than after inferior myocardial infarction, even when corrected for infarct size.[49] Patients with non-Q wave myocardial infarctions have a natural history clearly different from that of patients with Q wave infarctions. Acute mortality in patients with non-Q wave infarcts is approximately half that of the patients with Q wave infarcts. Non-Q wave infarctions, however, have a higher risk of reinfarction and an accelerated late mortality rate.[50] Patients whose electrocardiogram demonstrates persistent advanced heart block or new intraventricular conduction abnormalities during an acute myocardial infarction also have an increase in mortality rate.[51] Other electrocardiographic parameters associated with increased total mortality are persistent ST segment alterations and Q waves in multiple leads.[52] Ventricular late potentials are associated with a high risk of malignant ventricular arrhythmias and sudden death in postmyocardial infarction patients.[53] Although their sensitivity is high, their specificity and predictive accuracy for the development of malignant ventricular arrhythmias or sudden cardiac death are relatively low.

Multivariate Risk

Multivariate logistic analysis in the Framingham study,[26] including all coronary risk factors, indicates that in males, age, systolic pressure, cigarette smoking, and relative body weight are all independently related to the incidence of sudden death. In females, aside from age, only hypercholesterolemia and vital capacity are associated independently with an increased risk of sudden death (Fig. 5). Using these parameters, there is a wide variation in the risk of sudden death (Table 1). Forty-two percent of sudden deaths in males and 53% in females occur in the tenth of the population in the top decile of multivariate risk (Table 1).

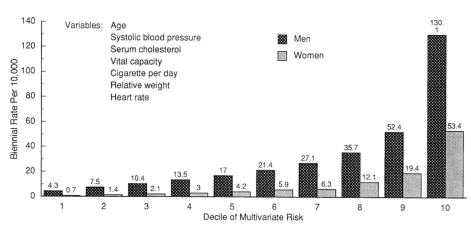

Figure 5. Risk of sudden death according to the multivariate risk decile (from Kannel WB[26]).

Table 1

Risk of Sudden Death According to the Multivariate Risk Decile*

	Probability of Sudden Death per 1000	
*Multivariate Risk Decile***	*Men*	*Women*
1	0.43	0.07
2	0.75	0.14
3	1.04	0.21
4	1.35	0.30
5	1.70	0.42
6	2.14	0.59
7	2.71	0.83
8	3.57	1.21
9	5.24	1.94
10	13.01	5.34
Percentage of cases in the upper decile	42%	52%

*Based on data from the Framingham study.[25]
**The risk variables include age, ECG alterations, systolic blood pressure, hypercholesterol, vital capacity, smoking habit, weight, and heart rate.

Clinical Implications

It is important to conceptualize sudden cardiac death as a manifestation of coronary heart disease which occurs as a consequence of a variety of risk factors and living habits. Marginal changes in blood pressure, cholesterol and cigarette smoking may not be important in themselves, but can summate to cause sufficient ischemia to precipitate sudden death.

References

1. WHO. Sudden cardiac death. Geneva: WHO Technical Report 1985;726.
2. Myerburg R J, Castellanos A. Cardiac arrest and sudden cardiac death. In: Braunwald E. *Heart Disease: A Textbook of Cardiovascular Medicine.* Philadelphia: Saunders; 1992;756.
3. Kuller L, Lilienfeld A, Fisher R. An epidemiological study of sudden and unexpected deaths in adults. *Medicine* 1967;46:341.
4. Schatzkin A, Cupples LA, Heeren T, et al. The epidemiology of sudden unexpected death: Risk factors for men and women in the Framingham Heart Study. *Am Heart J* 1984;107:1300.
5. Doyle JT, Kannel WB, NcNamara PM, et al. Factors related to suddenness of death from coronary disease: Combined Albany-Framingham studies. *Am J Cardiol* 1976;37:1073.
6. Cosín J. Out-of-hospital sudden death in Spain. In: Bayés de Luna A, Brugada P, Cosin J, Navarro Lopez F, eds. *Sudden Cardiac Death.* Dordrecht, The Netherlands: Kluwer Academic Publishers; 1991:19.
7. Gillum RF. Sudden coronary death in the United States 1980–1985. *Circulation* 1989;79:756.
8. Goldberg R J. Declining out-of-hospital sudden coronary death rates: Additional pieces of the epidemiologic puzzle. *Circulation* 1989;79:1369.
9. Tunstall Pedoe H. Actual tendencies of cardiovascular diseases and risk factors: MONICA study of WHO. Geneva: WHO Technical Report 1985;39:5.
10. Willich SN, Levy D, Rocco MB, et al. Circadian variation in the incidence of sudden cardiac death in the Framingham Heart Study Population. *Am J Cardiol* 1987;60:801.
11. Bayés de Luna A, Coumel Ph, Leclercq JF. Ambulatory sudden death: Mechanisms of production of fatal arrhythmia on the basis of data from 157 cases. *Am Heart J* 1989;117:151.
12. Peterson DR. Evolution of the epidemiology of sudden infant death syndrome. *Epidemiologic Rev* 1980;2:97.
13. Neuspiel DR, Kuller LH. Sudden and unexpected natural death in childhood and adolescence. *JAMA* 1985;254:1321.
14. Kuller L, Lilienfeld A, Fischer R. Sudden and unexpected deaths in young adults: An epidemiologic study. *JAMA* 1966;198:158.
15. Kannel WB, Thomas HE. Sudden coronary death: The Framingham study. *Ann NY Acad Sci* 1982;382:3.

16. Baroldi G, Falzi G, Mariani F. Sudden coronary death: A postmortem study in 208 selected cases compared to 97 "control" subjects. *Am Heart J* 1979;98:20.
17. Jick H, Dinan B, Herman R, et al. Myocardial infarction and other vascular diseases in young women: Role of estrogens and other factors. *JAMA* 1978;240:2548.
18. Pyeritz RE. Genetics and cardiovascular disease. In: Braunwald E. *Heart Disease: A Textbook of Cardiovascular Medicine.* Philadelphia: WB Saunders; 1992:1622.
19. Keating M, Atkinson D, Dunn C, et al. Linkage of a cardiac arrhythmia, the long QT syndrome, and the Harvey-ras-1 gene. *Science* 1991;252:704.
20. Maron BJ, Lipson LC, Roberts WC, et al. "Malignant" hypertrophic cardiomyopathy: Identification of a subgroup of families with unusually frequent premature death. *Am J Cardiol* 1978;41:1133.
21. Rizzon P, Breithardt G, Chiddo A. Arrhythmogenic right ventricle. *Eur Heart J* 1989;10(suppl D):1.
22. Kligfield P, Levy D, Devereux RB, et al. Arrhythmias and sudden death in mitral valve prolapse. *Am Heart J* 1987;113:1298.
23. McGill HC. *The Geographic Pathology of Atherosclerosis.* Baltimore: Williams and Wilkins, 1968.
24. Anderson TW, LeRiche WH, Hewitt D, Neri LC. Magnesium water hardness and heart disease. In: Cantin and Seelig, eds. *Magnesium in Health and Disease.* New York: SP Med Science Books; 1980;565.
25. Kannel WB, McGee DL. Modifiable risk factors for sudden coronary death. In: Morganroth J, Horowitz LN, eds. *Sudden Cardiac Death.* Orlando, FL: Grune and Stratton, 1985.
26. Kannel WB, McGee DL, Scharzkin A. An epidemiological perspective of sudden death: 26-year follow-up in the Framingham Study. *Drugs* 1984;28(suppl 1):1.
27. Coronary Drug Project Research Group. Natural history of myocardial infarction in the Coronary Drug Project: Long-term prognostic importance of serum lipid levels. *Am J Cardiol* 1978;42:489.
28. Hallstrom AP, Cobg LA, Ray R. Smoking as a risk factor for recurrence of sudden cardiac arrest. *N Engl J Med* 1986;314:271.
29. Hawkins RI. Smoking, platelets and thrombosis. *Nature* 1972;236:450.
30. Kershbaum A, Bellet S, Dickstein ER, et al. Effect of cigarette smoking and nicotine on serum free fatty acids: Based on a study in the human subject and the experimental animal. *Circ Res* 1981;9:631.
31. Kannel WB. Update on the role of cigarette smoking in coronary artery disease. *Am Heart J* 1981;101:328.
32. DeBias DA, Banerjee CM, Birkhead NC, et al. Effects of carbon monoxide inhalation on ventricular fibrillation. *Arch Environ Health* 1976;31:42.
33. Aronow WS. Carbon monoxide and cardiovascular disease. In: Wynder EL, Hoffmann D, Gori GB, eds. *Proceedings of the Third World Conference on Smoking and Health.* Washington, DC: US Dept of Health, Education, and Welfare publication NIH 76–1221.
34. Siggaard-Andersen J, Petersen FB, Hansen TI, et al. Plasma volume and vascular permeability during hypoxia and carbon monoxide exposure. *Scand J Clin Lab Invest* 1968;103:39.

35. Mulcahy R. Influence of cigarette smoking on morbidity and mortality after myocardial infarction. *Br Heart J* 1983;49:410.
36. Jafri SM, Tilley BC, Peters R, et al. Effects of cigarette smoking and propranolol in survivors of acute myocardial infarction. *Am J Cardiol* 1990;65:271.
37. Kannel WB, Schatzkin A. Sudden death: Lessons from subsets in population studies. *J Am Coll Cardiol* 1985;5:141B.
38. Chakabarti R, Meade TW, WHO Multinational Group. Clotting factors, platelet function and fibrinolytic activity in diabetics and in a comparison group. *Diabetologia* 1976;12:383.
39. Froelicher VF, Brown P. Exercise and coronary heart disease. *J Cardiac Rehab* 1981;1:227.
40. Paffenbarger RS, Hale WE, Brand RJ, et al. Work-energy level, personal characteristics, and fatal heart attack: A birth-cohort effect. *Am J Epidemiol* 1977;105:200.
41. Siscovick DS, Weiss NS, Hallstrom AP, et al. Physical activity and primary cardiac arrest. *JAMA* 1982;248:3113.
42. Kannel WB, Sortie P. Some health benefits of physical activity: The Framingham study. *Arch Intern Med* 1979;139:857.
43. Friedman M, Manwaring JH, Rosenman RH, et al. Instantaneous and sudden deaths: Clinical and pathological differentiation in coronary artery disease. *JAMA* 1973;225:1329.
44. Ruberman W, Weinblatt E, Goldberg JD, et al. Ventricular premature beats and mortality after myocardial infarction. *N Engl J Med* 1977;297:750.
45. Moss AJ, Davis HT, DeCamilla J, et al. Ventricular ectopic beats and their relation to sudden and nonsudden cardiac death after myocardial infarction. *Circulation* 1979;60:998.
46. Bigger JT, Fleiss JL, Kleiger R, et al. The relationships among ventricular arrhythmias, left ventricular dysfunction and mortalilty in the 2 years after myocardial infarction. *Circulation* 1984;69:250.
47. Kostis JB, Byington R, Friedman LM, et al. (BHAT Study Group.) Prognostic significance of ventricular ectopic activity in survivors of acute myocardial infarction. *J Am Coll Cardiol* 1987;10:231–242.
48. Fintel DJ, Platia EV. Exercise testing and cardiac arrhythmias. In: Platia EV, ed. *Management of Cardiac Arrhythmias.* Philadelphia,: JB Lippincott; 1987.
49. Hands ME, Lloyd BL, Robinson JS, et al. Prognostic significance of electrocardiographic site of infarction after correction for enzymatic size of infarction. *Circulation* 1986;73:885.
50. Benhorin J, Moss A, Oakes D, et al. The prognostic significance of first myocardial infarction type (Q wave versus non-Q wave) and Q wave location. *J Am Coll Cardiol* 1990;15:1201.
51. Lie KI, Liem KL, Schrlenburgh RM, et al. Early identification of patients developing late in-hospital ventricular fibrillation after discharge from the coronary unit: A 5.5 year retrospective and prospective study of 1987 patients. *Am J Cardiol* 1978;41:674.
52. Chiang BN, Perlman LV, Fulton M, et al. Predisposing factors in sudden cardiac death in Tecumseh, Michigan: A prospective study. *Circulation* 1970;41:31.
53. El-Sherif N, Turitto G. High-resolution electrocardiography. Armonk: Futura Publishing Company; 1992.

Chapter VI

Neurophysiological and Psychological Aspects of Sudden Death

Intertwined in the studies of sudden death is the tantalizing question of the causal relationship of neurophysiological and emotional triggers. Death coming suddenly during grief or joy, sadness or disappointment, frustration or anger, is the focal point of many anecdotes that run the gamut from laboratory research to newspaper articles and folktales. Yet through these anecdotes runs a thread of reality, if not science, that makes the relationship of these factors seem plausible. Investigations in this area extend from voodoo death to psychological predictors of sudden death.

Engel,[1] in a review of largely anecdotal material and firsthand accounts, paints a colorful design from which certain apparent shapes can be defined that become common denominators of sudden death when viewed retrospectively. He points out that causal relationship between emotions and sudden death has been recounted throughout history. The Bible tells us that when Ananias was charged by Peter,

> "You have not lied to man but to God," he fell down dead; so did Sapphira, his wife, when told that "the feet of them which have buried thy husband are at the door and shall carry thee out" (5 Acts 3:6). Emperor Nerva is said to have died of "a violent excess of anger" against a senator who offended him, as did Valentinian while "reproaching with great passion" the deputies of a German tribe. Pope Innocent IV succumbed suddenly to the "morbid effects of grief on his system" soon after the disastrous

From: S. Goldstein, A. Bayés-de-Luna, J. Guindo-Soldevila: *Sudden Cardiac Death.* Armonk, NY: Futura Publishing Co., Inc., © 1994.

overthrow of his army by Manfred, and King Philip V is said to have dropped dead when he realized the Spaniards had been defeated. Chilon of Lacedaemon is alleged to have died from joy while embracing his son who had borne away the prize at the Olympic games. Benjamin Rush claimed that the doorkeeper of Congress, an aged man, died immediately upon hearing the capture of Lord Cornwallis's army. "His death was universally ascribed to a violent emotion of political joy." In more modern times the power of vengeful deities is no longer invoked, but the belief that intense emotional distress may induce sudden death persists unabated in average people. Novelists and playwrights have no compunction about arranging for their characters to succumb to a fatal heart attack or stroke in the midst of emotional crisis.

Greene et al.[2] examined the setting in which sudden death occurred, drawing from interviews with the patient's family and coworkers. This has provided a clearer description of the psychological and emotional setting of the patient prior to sudden death. With an even broader brush, Wolf[3] studied the closely knit community of Roseto, Pennsylvania, which, as long as it maintained its social and geographic isolation and integrity, was seemingly protected from death from coronary heart disease. Closely related to these emotional factors is the brain (particularly the hypothalamus) and the autonomic nervous system, both of which have a major influence on the cardiovascular system.

Neurophysiological Control of the Heart

The central nervous system is continually functioning as a cardiac regulator. This control is maintained through the limbic system, which functions as the area in the brain that handles input from the visceral and somatic sensory nerves as well as cortical areas and interprets realized or perceived experiences. This system establishes an interaction between the frontal lobes, the hypothalamus, and the autonomic effectors in the medulla. The medulla is the modulator of the rate and rhythm of the heart. The hypothalamus appears to be a highly integrated series of centers which function as servomechanisms and which integrate response patterns and functions not only as a mediator of autonomic responses but also as an effector of somatomotor and hormonal components of the central nervous system. However, it also generates responses free of cortically-controlled emotional involvement. The defense reaction is an example of the corticohypothalamic response pattern. The resultant elevation of arterial pressure and tachycardia are manifestations of the hypothalamic stimulation of the sympathetic cholinergic and adrenergic fibers which result in marked inotropic and chronotropic response. Within a few short minutes, a stress or anger response can place large loads on the heart, and, in the susceptible person with a narrow margin of safety, it can be fatal. Such was the case of John Hunter,[4] who predicted the manner of his own death when he said, "My life is at the mercy of any scoundrel who chooses to put me in a passion." Hunter, long plagued with angina pectoris, died suddenly, following a heated exchange with his medical associates.

Some animals, rather than developing a response characterized by fight or flight, respond in what has been termed "a conservation-withdrawal pattern," or as Folkow suggests, "playing dead."[5] The animal, when cornered, may play dead, fall in its tracks, become flaccid, apneic, hypotensive, and develop a profound bradycardia. This reaction may be so convincing that its predator may either miss its prey or turn away after sniffing the carcass. This reflex, originating in the hypothalamus, can be closely mimicked by the stimulation of the medullary depressor area. This "playing dead" reaction is probably present in all species to a greater or lesser extent, and is expressed in humans when, in the setting of severe emotional shock, he becomes weak, dizzy, and slumps into a chair. Some individuals, when confronted with certain types of stressful situations, are especially prone to respond by slumping into a faint, thereby gaining respite from the "slings and arrows of outrageous fortune," at least temporarily.

Wolf[6,7] suggested that sudden death may be a manifestation of the primitive medulla-controlled diving reflex.[8] In its purest form it is expressed as maximal vasoconstriction in order to minimize peripheral oxygen loss with a similar decrease in oxygen to other systems, including skeletal muscle. As a result, most of the blood essentially circulates between the heart and the brain. With the onset of diving, immediate bradycardia and vasoconstriction with a marked decrease in cardiac output occurs. At the same time arterial pressure is maintained by means of intense vasoconstriction. According to Folkow,[9] different species have varying degrees of adaptability. Ducks, for instance, may dive for 15 minutes, seals as long as 20 to 30 minutes, and whales as long as 2 hours. Bradycardia in humans, however, can lead to severe ischemia and provide the electrophysiological environment in which ventricular ectopy and fibrillation can occur.

In classic experiments by Richter,[10] sudden death resulted when dewhiskered rats were immersed in water, a stress that rats can withstand when their whiskers are intact. Richter hypothesized that the whiskers represent one of the animal's main contacts with the outside world. During immersion, electrocardiographic recording of the rat demonstrates severe bradycardia. The rat's situation at death was not characterized by a fight or flight reaction, but one of giving up. This hopelessness or giving up could be prevented by training the rats and allowing them to come to the surface. The rats will realize that their situation is not totally hopeless. Corley et al.[11] elicited in a monkey exposed to chronic and recurrent environmental stress, similar vagal-induced severe bradycardia that developed after periods of stress tachycardia. Other experiments by Schneider[12] found that, among patients who have had a past myocardial infarction, those with the greatest tendency to bradycardia in response to startle, had the poorest prognosis.

LeRiche et al.,[13] in 1931, and Ebert et al.[14] demonstrated that the electrical instability that develops following ligation of the left anterior descending coronary artery in dogs can be prevented by cardiac denervation. In contrast, Van Citters et al.[15] produced ventricular tachycardia in dogs with chronic heart block by stimulating the H_1 field of Forel. Using a Pavlovian model in which fear and trembling were induced in a group of dogs, Lown et al.[16] observed that the threshold for ventricular fibrillation was lowered in the test animals as compared to a control group. These studies all support the importance of the central nervous system in the physiological control and genesis of cardiac rate and rhythm.

The possibility that emotional stress can lead to large swings in cardiovascular physiology is supported by the work of Levi,[17] who examined the sympathoadrenal responses to stress and distress under various psychosocial stimuli. In these studies, increased catecholamine excretion was noted in various stressful situations. It is possible that catecholamines may be a predominant factor modifying the cardiovascular system, leading to increased hemodynamic stress in patients at high risk. Catecholamines appear to play an important role not only on blood pressure and pulse rate, but also upon the electrophysiological integrity of the heart, allowing for the emergence of ventricular ectopy and fibrillation, particularly in ischemic hearts.

The importance of acute psychological events as predictors of cardiac arrhythmias has been extensively explored. These studies indicate that in some instances, psychological stress can precipitate significant arrhythmias. Taggart and colleagues[18] demonstrated that ST segment electrocardiographic abnormalities associated with increased ectopic ventricular beats occurred during the stress of driving and public speaking. They suggested that these effects may be related to the sympathetic nervous system discharge. Increased fibrillation vulnerability has been described in animal models in which imbalance of the sympathetic nervous system has been demonstrated by interval stimulation. There is evidence to suggest that lateral asymmetry in the sympathetic nervous system control of the heart may also lead to increased ventricular arrhythmias.[19] Increased cognitive challenges also appear to be associated with increased ventricular arrhythmias that can be suppressed with the β-adrenergic blocking agent, oxyprenolol.[20]

In addition, vagal control of the heart rate has also been an important modulator of mortality. The lack of heart rate variability has been associated with increased arrhythmic death. Martin et al.[21] demonstrated that low heart rate variability was common before death in a group of sudden death victims. After acute myocardial infarction, Kleiger et al.[22] demonstrated that this lack of heart variability also was an important predictor of subsequent mortality. It was an independent risk factor even when such factors as low ejection fraction and ventricular premature beat frequency were included in the mortality analysis.

In the idiopathic prolonged QT syndrome, it is well known that stress can precipitate syncope in patients as a result of ventricular fibrillation (see Chapter XII). This phenomenon can be suppressed by β-adrenergic blocking agents or ablation of the stellate ganglion (see Chapter XVIII). In addition, mental stress has been demonstrated to be a triggering event in the development of silent ischemia. Deanfield et al.[23] provided evidence to indicate that there is a decrease in myocardial blood flow during arithmetic tasks. Other investigators suggest that stress-induced silent ischemia may be much more frequent than is detectable by clinical electrophysiological criteria. Ischemia due to mental stress appears to occur at a lower level of myocardial work requirement than that associated with physical exercise. This suggests that increased vasomotor tone is a factor in the supply and demand balance of the myocardium. Rebecca et al.[24] found significant reduction in a cross-sectional area of coronary artery disease during mental arithmetic tasks in 10 coronary patients with exertional chest pain. Coupled with increased myocardial oxygen demand-associated stress, these abnormalities can lead to ischemia. Cold-pressor tests have also been shown to produce a decrease in coronary artery diameter and an increase in coronary vascular resistance. This effect can be modified with the use of α-adrenergic blockers such as phentolamine. Angiographic studies of patients with coronary artery disease indicate that the endothelial changes associated with atherosclerosis can result in vasoconstriction during mental stress. This decrease in coronary blood flow is independent of heart rate, blood pressure, or plasma norepinephrine.[25] It is suggested from this study that atherosclerosis prevents the normal endothelium-dependent dilatation to occur during stress.

Lester et al.,[26] studying the effect of sleep on ventricular arrhythmias, noted that in patients with coronary heart disease, the greatest number of arrhythmias occurred in the transition from waking to stage I, from stage I to stage II, and during the period of rapid eye movements (REM). They also observed that there were more arrhythmias recorded when the patient was in the coronary care unit compared to the sleep laboratory. Nocturnal angina occurs more frequently during the REM phase of sleep.[27] Other investigators failed to corroborate an increase in frequency of arrhythmias occurring during sleep.[28] In fact, a 50% decrease in frequency of ventricular premature beats and a decrease in the Lown grade of ventricular premature beats from 2.75 to 1.78 occurred in sleep. DeSilva[29] used psychological stress tests in order to identify patients who were at risk of life-threatening arrhythmias (Fig. 1). The electrocardiographic recording in one such patient demonstrated a run of ventricular tachycardia during mental stress. A remarkable example of ventricular fibrillation is reported by Wellens et al.,[30] triggered by awakening to an alarm clock (Fig. 2). Similarly, Figure 3 shows the development of bidirectional ventricular tachycardia during the recollection and description of a previous stressful experience with a close friend.[31]

The cardiovascular response to acute psychological stress has a variety of hemodynamic and physiological expressions. DeSilva proposed that there were three types of responses[32] (Table 1). Both types I and II appear to be fairly self-limited and with little danger of morbidity and mortality. Vasovagal syncope can occur in type II and can result in some significant slowing of the heart rate and fainting. Type III responses may lead to significant ventricular arrhythmias, including ventricular tachycardia and ventricular fibrillation as a result of acute psychological stress and represent the greatest hazard to individuals.

Control

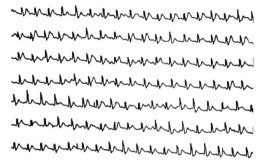

Psychologic Stress Testing

Figure 1. Psychologic stress testing in a man with previous myocardial infarction and recurrent cardiac arrest. The control tracing (upper panel) shows normal sinus rhythem at 65 beats per minute. During a discussion of his illness and possible death, he wept, basal heart rate increased, and recurrent runs of supraventricular and ventricular tachycardia were recorded (lower panel) (from Lown and DeSilva. *Am J Cardiol* 1978;41:979).

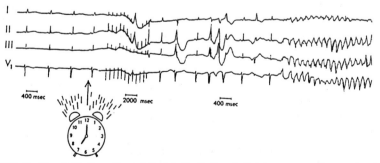

Figure 2. The initiation of ventricular fibrillation following an auditory stimulus (alarm clock). QT segment changes are followed by ventricular premature beats and ventricular fibrillation. The middle of the record is taken at a slower speed than the beginning and end (from Wellens et al.[30]).

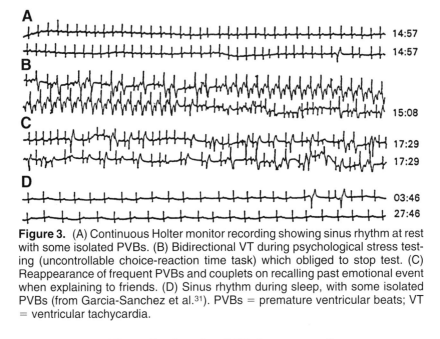

Figure 3. (A) Continuous Holter monitor recording showing sinus rhythm at rest with some isolated PVBs. (B) Bidirectional VT during psychological stress testing (uncontrollable choice-reaction time task) which obliged to stop test. (C) Reappearance of frequent PVBs and couplets on recalling past emotional event when explaining to friends. (D) Sinus rhythm during sleep, with some isolated PVBs (from Garcia-Sanchez et al.[31]). PVBs = premature ventricular beats; VT = ventricular tachycardia.

Psychological Triggers of Sudden Death

Engel,[1] in his remarkably entertaining and stimulating article entitled "Sudden and Rapid Death during Psychological Stress: Folklore or Folk Wisdom," suggests that perhaps the lethality of the emotional stress may not be in the exaggeration of either the fight or flight mechanism or the conservation-withdrawal reaction. Rather, he suggests that it may be due to an instability or a tendency for major swings from sympathetically stimulated tachycardia and hypertension to parasympathetic bradycardia and hypotension. Gellhorn[33] observed that with continued reapplication of stressful stimuli, the parasympathetic response may dominate. This type of reaction is seen in vasodepressor syncope, when tachycardia is replaced by bradycardia and when the impulse to flee is inhibited. With this background, Engel reviewed accounts of sudden death that came to his attention by verbal or written communication of interested colleagues and from newspaper accounts. He could characterize sudden death as occurring in eight different settings:

Table 1

Cardiovascular Responses to Acute Psychological Stress

Type of Response	ECG Rhythm	Somatic Correlates	Clinical Outcome
Type I (usual response)	Sinus tachycardia (hypertension)	Flushing, anxiety, tremor, sweating, rapid pulse	Self-limited recovery
Type II (unusual response)	(A) Bradycardia (hypertension)	Pallor, sweating, fainting, syncope	Spontaneous recovery, may need medical intervention
	(B) Atrial arrhythmias	Palpitations, dizziness, fatigue, chest pain, syncope	Spontaneous recovery, may need medical intervention
	(C) Isolated PVB	Palpitations, chest discomfort, syncope	Self-limited or may require medical treatment
Type III (extreme response)	Arrhythmias of sudden death (VF, asystole, electromechanical dissociation)	Cardiac arrest	Death if untreated

VF = ventricular fibrillation; PVB = premature ventricular beats.
(DeSilva PA. Electrocardiographic responses to behavioral stimuli. In: Herd JA, Gotto AM, Weiss SM, eds. Cardiovascular Instrumentation: Proceedings of the Working Conference on Applicability of New Technology to Behavioral Research. Washington, DC: 1984, US Dept of Health and Human Services, NIH Publication No. 84–1654; 121.[29] Reprinted with permission.)

1. on the impact, collapse, or death of a close person
2. during acute grief
3. on the threat of loss of a close person
4. during mourning or on an anniversary of death
5. on the loss of status or self-esteem
6. after danger is over
7. reunion
8. triumph or happy ending.

Common to these situations is intense stimulation or excitement or giving up or both, when confronted with a situation that is impossible to ignore. His hypothesis suggested that these wide swings of emotional content had representation in similar instability in the autonomic nervous system, which in patients with preexisting heart disease led to sudden death. Most of the patients and individuals died suddenly with preexisting coronary or other forms of heart disease. An experience that includes a number of these settings is recounted by Greene:[2]

> John was having a mastectomy . . . He decided to enter the hospital in August. The operation went smoothly, but in spite of the fact that he had no prior history of heart disease, John had a heart attack the evening following surgery while recovering from anesthesia. He survived and eventually was discharged. On returning home, however, he became increasingly depressed. According to his wife, he was particularly disturbed that he could not return to work.
>
> That Halloween, a group of local children exploded fireworks in his mailbox, damaging it severely. When John surveyed the damage to his property, to which he was deeply attached, his wife said he became 'not angry' but overwhelmed and utterly filled with despair. After all, he was recuperating from a heart attack, which prevented him from taking any action. John kept these feelings of despair inside, his typical way of coping.
>
> Several days later his wife persuaded him to take the first stroll of his convalescence in their garden, hoping to cheer him up. As they ventured outside they noticed that an arbor, which John had built earlier that summer and of which he was very proud, had been sprayed with black tar paint by the Halloween pranksters. John was again overwhelmed and stared helplessly at his beloved construction while his wife fumed and expressed her anger. Then he remarked that he did not feel well and wished to return to the house. He turned, walked twenty yards, and collapsed. As he did so, his wife asked if he was experiencing pain, and he said no. Within five minutes he was dead.
>
> Later on, John's physicians interviewed his wife. They wondered if his mastectomy had any special meaning for him. 'It's strange you should ask that question,' she replied. She revealed that John's sister had died one year earlier on November 3 following mastectomy. As if this were not momentous enough, John's older and favorite brother had dropped dead of a heart attack one year earlier on November 12. John's death occurred on November 6.
>
> The wife added that she was glad John had not gone further into the garden. Had he done so, he would have discovered that their new trailer had also been spray-painted in black.

Extensive literature suggests that many precipitating causes of death, yet only a few reports support the observations that death actually can be postponed in relation to a symbolically meaningful occasion. Phillips and King[34] examined cultural phenomena that had important symbolic meaning. They demonstrated that Jewish mortality fell sharply below the expected level just before Passover holidays and rose by an equal amount immediately afterward. In contrast, non-Jewish controls showed no significant fluctuation of mortality. To replicate this phenomenon in another culture, a similar study was carried out in Chinese women and the Harvest Moon Festival.[35] This festival is considered "an old woman's festival," one of great importance. The mortality rate in Chinese females in the week before and after the Harvest Moon Festival was examined using the previous Jewish population as the control. They observed a decrease by 35% in the week before the festival and a similar increase in the week following the event. These studies suggest that individuals could postpone death until after an important occasion such as a golden wedding anniversary or other important family functions. Phillips suggests that family structure is a specific physiological phenomenon that allows for this type of delay. In contrast, a stressful environment may increase the incidence of infarction. A significant increase in myocardial infarction was observed in Israel during the "SCUD" attacks that occurred during the Kuwait-Iraq war.[36] This may have been, in part, due to the necessity of wearing gas masks during the attack, some of which were said to be defective, resulting in transitory hypoxia.

Dying of fright, particularly if it was felt to be preordained, has been described by many researchers. As described by Walter Cannon,[37] voodoo deaths fit into this category when, for various reasons, the witch doctor decided certain actions are a "crime." Australian aboriginal witch doctors would point a bone at the offending individual, the sign for the individual's capitulation, and imminent death occurred within 24 hours. Basedow, in his book *The Australian Aborigine*,[38] in 1925, described the effect of being "boned":

> The man who discovers that he is being boned by an enemy is, indeed, a pitiable sight. He stands aghast with his eyes staring at the treacherous pointer, and with his hands lifted to ward off the lethal medium, which he imagines is pouring into his body. His cheeks blanch, and his eyes become glassy, and the expression of his face becomes horribly distorted. He attempts to shriek but usually the sound chokes in his throat, and all that one might see is froth at his mouth. His body begins to tremble

and his muscles twitch involuntarily. He sways backward and falls to the ground, and after a short time appears to be in a swoon. He finally composes himself, goes to his hut and there frets to death.

Greene et al.,[39] in studying the psychological background of sudden death by retrospective interviews with the family of the deceased and coworkers, describes the setting of the individual who dies suddenly as one who "has been running sad or disappointed." They are in a state of chronic depression with disappointments both in the family and at home. When aroused or pushed into activity, they suddenly die. These characteristics are in addition to the type A personality disorder with its predisposition to coronary heart disease as described by Friedman and Rosenman.[40,41] Those individuals would rather die than face the dependence and helplessness attending a myocardial infarction. Greene suggests that this helplessness and the reluctance to face illness occurring in the setting of the hard-driving and self-demanding individual, represents one of the characteristic behavior patterns seen in those dying suddenly of acute coronary heart disease. It is possible that the ingredient of survival in the type A personality (those with sustained drive, intensity, and competitiveness) is the ability of that individual to psychologically accept the dependence required of his illness.

Friedman and Rosenman[40] studied the occurrence of behavioral characteristics of patients with coronary heart disease and correlated their behavior patterns with cholesterol, diet, and activity. They observed that in the type A personality, the serum cholesterol, frequency of arcus senilis, and incidence of coronary artery disease was greater than in the type B personality who did not have this behavior pattern. They propose that elevation of various metabolic phenomena set the stage for the development of coronary heart disease that was ultimately expressed by the behavior pattern of the type A male. A study by Brackett and Powell[42] examined the role of the type A personality and sudden cardiac death and observed that an interview measure of type A behavior was a predictor of sudden death but not of nonsudden death in nonheart disease patients.

The concept that the stress in an individual's life may play a role in precipitating cardiovascular events has been under investigation for some time. Life change was measured retrospectively in both survivors of myocardial infarction and sudden death victims by Rahe et al.[43] They observed that there was a marked elevation in life change during the six months prior to infarction or death compared to the same interval one year earlier. This elevation was particularly apparent in sudden death victims. In a similar study, Cottington et al.[44] interviewed family members of female sudden cardiac death victims and observed that many events such as the loss of close friends and family occurred in the six months preceding their deaths. A prospective study by Ruberman et al.[45] in the β-Blocker Heart Attack Trial, using psychosocial interviews several months after recovery from a myocardial infarction, indicated that among the significant predictors of sudden cardiac death were increased scales of life stress and social isolation in those with increased mortality. They also observed that a lower education status was an important predictor of sudden cardiac death mortality in heart attack survivors.

The effect of bereavement and loss of a close person was studied by Rees and Lutkins.[46] In bereaved relatives, the mortality rate in the year following the event was higher for males than females. In the first year following the death of a close person, 12.2% of the widowed died, as compared to 0.56% in a control comparison group. The risk of a close relative dying during the first year of bereavement was doubled when the primary death causing bereavement occurred in a hospital compared with at home.

Over a seven-year period, Wolf[47] followed a series of 65 individuals who had experienced an acute myocardial infarction and noted a high degree of dejection and dissatisfaction in the study group. He also noted a marked increase in this postinfarct group of physiological lability in daily blood pressure, serum cholesterol, coronary blood flow, and variation in blood clotting factors when compared to a control population. When evaluating these patients, Wolf attempted to predict which of the control and study group would succumb first. Based primarily on expressed and observed depression in the patients, he was able to prospectively predict the first 10 individuals to die. Two of these died by suicide and the remaining eight died suddenly. All of these patients were judged to be alienated from their cultural and social setting and had the highest depression scores by emotional test scores.

The emotional reactions of patients in a coronary care unit to cardiac catastrophes involving other patients were investigated by Bruhn et al.[48] Of the 17 patients studied, 13 developed severe anxiety, depression, and premonition of death in association with hypertension, increased numbers of ventricular premature contractions, ventricular tachycardia, hyperventilation, and angina. Cardiac arrest and death occurred in one of these patients. In 4 patients who did not develop any anxiety reaction, there were no observed physiological events.

The effect of community support on the mortality of coronary artery disease has enfolded in the study of Roseto, Pennsylvania.[3,49,50] This highly structured and supportive Italian-American community of 1700 persons was noted to have a remarkably low coronary heart disease mortality rate, in spite of a relatively increased prevalence of the risk factors usually considered to predispose to myocardial infarction. The social structure was striking in its supportive nature to all its individual members and to the high degree of social cohesiveness. The male members particularly were inviolate and the unchallenged head of the family. The few deaths that did occur were found in individuals who somehow or other were outside the society. Although intriguing in concept, Keys[51] suggests that there is little to suggest a lower incidence of coronary disease in Roseto. A follow-up study by the original investigator suggests that the incidence of coronary disease in Roseto increased in the community due to development of societal dislocation occurring over time in this formerly isolated town.[52]

Yet death may come, as Wolf[53] has suggested, "as adaptation." In the setting of an intolerable situation, death may be the only way out and is particularly welcomed by the individual with heart disease. Shelley wrote, "How wonderful is Death, Death and his brother Sleep," and Shakespeare in (*Othello*, Act I, Scene iii) has Rodrigo say, "It is silliness to live when to live is torment, and then we have a prescription to die when death is our physician." Wolf quotes an Israeli physician who was remonstrated by a patient whom he had just resuscitated from a cardiac arrest: "For two years I have been trying to summon up courage to kill myself, and now when I die legitimately, you have to bring me back to life."

Jenkins,[54] in a review of current research of emotional and social factors relating to coronary heart disease, suggested that of the factors in the development of coronary heart disease, social mobility was of questionable importance whereas anxiety and neuroses appeared more frequently in patients with coronary disease. Life dissatisfaction and environmental stress were common. Social isolation and economic deprivation are predictors of poor prognosis after a myocardial infarction.[55,56] In addition, the coronary prone behavior pattern had a certain degree of validity. Individuals with this coronary-prone behavior pattern or the type A personality as described by Friedman and Rosenman,[40] not only have a greater incidence of angina and myocardial infarction, but also a greater incidence of sudden death.

The difficulties in modeling emotional variables should not deter us from continuing our investigations into the relationship between the social and psychological factors with sudden death. It is also possible that pharmacologic agents may make it possible to dampen the stress-induced physiological swings of high-risk patients and thereby improve their outlook. Investigation may demonstrate if emotional variables can be manipulated and if this type of personality modeling can be effective in changing the risks of subsequent coronary events. The importance of these investigations indicates that social and psychological factors cannot be ignored in epidemiologic studies of coronary disease and must be considered important when related to the more traditional biological risk factors. As Jenkins[54] points out, these social and psychological variables cannot be controlled any more than the variable of a family history of coronary disease or diabetes.

The complexity of the interrelationship between psychological stress and ischemic phenomenon has led to the suggestion by investigators that psychological stress tests should be a component of stress assessment in patients with coronary heart disease. The ability of certain drugs such as β-adrenergic blocking agents to modify this process further suggests an intimate relationship between the central nervous system and physiological phenomena occurring in ischemic heart disease. It has been suggested that β-adrenergic blocking agents with lipophilic properties, such as metoprolol, are able more readily to enter the brain tissue, thereby modulating cerebral control of heart rhythm and ventricular fibrillation threshold. In addition, the use of biofeedback or relaxation training has been demonstrated to decrease the frequency of ventricular ectopic beats. Although exercise rehabilitation may present an important strategy for physical conditioning, psychological reassurance and the integration of psychological rehabilitation into cardiac management of patients with coronary heart disease may be an important additional, unplanned, and uncontrolled therapeutic measure. These observations all suggest the importance of the central nervous system as a modulator of ischemic phenomena and sudden death.

References

1. Engel GL. Sudden and rapid death during psychological stress: Folklore or folk wisdom? *Ann Intern Med* 1971;74:771.
2. Greene WA, Moss AJ, Goldstein S. Delay, denial and death in coronary heart disease. In: *Stress and the Heart*. Eliot RS, ed. New York: Futura Publishing Company; 1974;143.

3. Wolf S. Mortality from myocardial infarction in Roseto. *JAMA* 1966;195:142.
4. Hunter J. *A Treatise on the Blood, Inflammation and Gunshot to which is Prefixed a Short Account of the Author's Life, by his Brother-in-law, Everard Home.* London: Richardson; 1794.
5. Folkow B, Neil E. *Circulation.* New York: Oxford University Press; 1971;349.
6. Wolf S. The end of the rope: The role of the brain in cardiac death. *Can Med Assoc J* 1967;97:1022.
7. Wolf S. Sudden death and the oxygen-conserving reflex. *Am Heart J* 1966;71:840.
8. Anderson HT. Physiological adaptions in diving vertebrates. *Physiol Rev* 1966;46:121.
9. Folkow B, Neil E. *Circulation.* New York: Oxford University Press; 1971;354.
10. Richter CP. On the phenomenon of sudden death in animals and man. *Psychosom Med* 1951;19:191.
11. Corley KC, Greenhoot J, Mauck HP, et al. Abnormalities of cardiac rhythm associated with environmental stress. *Fed Proc* 1970;29:517. Abstract.
12. Schneider RA. Patterns of autonomic response to startle in subjects with and without coronary artery disease. *Clin Res* 1957;15:59. Abstract.
13. LeRiche R, Herrmann L, Fontaine R. Ligature de la coronaire gauche et fonction cardiaque chez l'animal intact. *Comptes Rendus Soc Biol* 1931;107:545.
14. Ebert PA, Allgood RJ, Sabiston DC Jr. Effect of cardiac denervation on arrhythmia following coronary artery occlusion. *Surg Forum* 1967;18:114.
15. Van Citters RL, Smith OA Jr, Ruttenberg HD. Subthalamically induced paroxysmal ventricular tachycardia after complete heart block. *Am J Physiol* 1966;211:293.
16. Lown B, Verrier R, Corbalan R. Psychologic stress and threshold for repetitive ventricular response. *Science* 1973;182:834.
17. Levi L. Stress and distress in response to psychosocial stimuli. *Acta Med Scand* 1972;528(suppl):1.
18. Taggart P, Gibbons D, Somerville W. Some effects of motor car driving on the normal and abnormal heart. *Br Med J* 1969;4:130.
19. Randall, WC, ed. *Neural Regulation of the Heart.* New York: Oxford University Press; 1977.
20. Taggart P, Carruthers M, Somerville W. Electrocardiogram, plasma catecholamines, and lipids, and their modification by oxyprenolol when speaking before an audience. *Lancet* 1973;2:341.
21. Martin GJ, Magid NM, Myers G, et al. Heart rate variability and sudden death secondary to coronary artery disease during ambulatory electrocardiographic monitoring. *Am J Cardiol* 1987;60:86.
22. Kleiger RE, Miller P, Bigger JT, Moss AJ, and the Multicenter Post-Infarction Research Group. Decreased heart rate variability and its association with increased mortality after acute myocardial infarction. *Am J Cardiol* 1987;59:256.

23. Deanfield JE, Shea M, Kensett M, et al. Silent myocardial ischaemia due to mental stress. *Lancet* 1984;2:1001.

24. Rebecca G, Wayne R, Zebede J, et al. Pathogenic mechanisms causing transient myocardial ischemia with mental arousal in patients with coronary artery disease. *Clin Res* 1986;34:338A. Abstract.

25. Yeung AC, Vekshtein VI, Krantz DS, et al. The effect of atherosclerosis on the vasomotor response of coronary arteries to mental stress. *N Engl J Med* 1991;325:1551.

26. Lester BK, Block R, Gunn CG. Relation of cardiac arrhythmias to phases of sleep. *Clin Res* 1969;17:456. Abstract.

27. Nowlin JB, Troyer WG Jr, Collins WS, et al. The association of nocturnal angina pectoris with dreaming. *Ann Intern Med* 1965;63:1040.

28. Lown B, Tykocinski M, Garfein A, et al. Sleep and ventricular premature beats. *Circulation* 1973;48:691.

29. DeSilva RA. Electrocardiographic responses to behavioral stimuli. In: Herd JA, Gotto AM, Weiss SM, eds. *Cardiovascular Instrumentation: Proceedings of the Working Conference on Applicability of New Technology to Biobehavioral Research*. Washington, DC: 1984; US Dept of Health and Human Services NIH publication 84–1654;121.

30. Wellens HJJ, Vermeulen A, Durrer D. Ventricular fibrillation on arousal from sleep by auditory stimuli. *Circulation* 1972;46:665.

31. Garcia-Sanchez S, Guindo J, Bayés de Luna A. Psychological stress and sudden cardiac death. In: Bayés de Luna A, Brugada P, Cosin J, Navarro Lopez F, eds. *Sudden Cardiac Death*. Dordrecht, The Netherlands: Kluwer Academic Publishers; 1991;71.

32. DeSilva RA, Dimsdale JE. Biobehavioral issues in the assessment, continuing care and rehabilitation of patients at risk for life-threatening arrhythmias. In: *Biobehavioral Factors in Sudden Cardiac Death*. Inst Medicine Interim Rpt No 3. Washington, DC: National Academy of Sciences Press; 1982;97.

33. Gellhorn E. *Principles of Autonomic-Somatic Integrations*. Minneapolis: University of Minnesota Press; 1967.

34. Phillips DP, King EW. Death takes a holiday: Mortality surrounding major social occasions. *Lancet* 1988;2:728.

35. Phillips DP, Smith DG. Postponement of death until symbolically meaningful occasions. *JAMA* 1990:263:1947.

36. Meisel SR, Kutz I, Dayan K, et al. Effect of Iraqi missile war on incidence of acute myocardial infarction and sudden death in Israeli citizens. *Lancet* 1991;338:660.

37. Cannon WB. "Voodoo" death. *Psychosom Med* 1957;19:182.

38. Basedow H. *The Australian Aborigine*. Adelaide; Preece; 1925;178.

39. Greene WA, Goldstein S, Moss AJ. Psychosocial aspects of sudden death. A preliminary report. *Arch Int Med* 1972;1;29:725.

40. Friedman M, Rosenman RH. Association of specific overt behavior pattern with blood and cardiovascular findings. Blood cholesterol level, blood clotting time, incidence of arcus senilis, and clinical coronary artery disease. *JAMA* 1959;169:1286.

41. Rosenman RH, Friedman M, Jenkins CD, et al. Recurring and fatal myocardial infarction in the Western Collaborative Group Study. *Am J Cardiol* 1967;19:771.

42. Brackett CD, Powell LH. Psychosocial and physiological predictors of sudden cardiac death after healing of acute myocardial infarction. *Am J Cardiol* 1988;61:979.
43. Rahe RH, Romo M, Bennett L, et al. Recent life changes, myocardial infarction, and abrupt coronary death. *Arch Int Med* 1974;133:221.
44. Cottington EM, Matthews KA, Talbott E, et al. Environmental events preceding sudden death in women. *Psychosom Med* 1980;42:567.
45. Ruberman W, Weinblatt E, Goldberg JD, et al. Psychosocial influences on mortality after myocardial infarction. *N Engl J Med* 1984;311:552.
46. Rees WD, Lutkins SG. Mortality of bereavement. *Br Med J* 1967;4:13.
47. Wolf S. Psychosocial forces in myocardial infarction and sudden death. In: Levi L, ed. *Society, Stress, and Disease.* New York: Oxford University Press; 1974;I:324.
48. Bruhn JG, Thurman AE, Chandler BC, et al. Pateints' reactions to death in a coronary care unit. *J Psychosom Res* 1970;14:65.
49. Stout C, Morrow J, Brandt EN, et al. Unusually low incidence of death from myocardial infarction: Study of an Italian-American community in Pennsylvania. *JAMA* 1964;18:353.
50. Bruhn JG. An epidemiological study of myocardial infarctions in an Italian-American community. *J Chron Dis* 1965;18:353.
51. Keys A. Arteriosclerotic heart disease in Roseto, Pennsylvania. *JAMA* 1966:195:93.
52. Wolf S, Grace KL, Bruhn J, et al. Further data on death from myocardial infarction in Roseto, Pennsylvania and neighboring communities. *Internat Res Comm Sys;* 1973.
53. Wolf S. Psychosocial forces in myocardial infarction and sudden death. *Circulation* 1969;40(IV):74.
54. Jenkins CD. Psychologic and social precursors of coronary disease. *N Engl J Med* 1971;284:244,307.
55. Case R, Moss AJ. Living alone after myocardial infarction. *JAMA* 1992;267:515.
56. Williams RB. Prognostic importance of social and economic resources among medically treated patients with angiographic documented coronary artery disease. *JAMA* 1992;267:520.

Chapter VII

Evaluation of High-Risk Patients:
Electrocardiographic Techniques

The development of the electrocardiogram at the end of the 19th Century provided an important insight into cardiac physiology. In the last three decades, the technological advances have expanded its application to clinical decision-making and therapy. These technologies have particular applications to issues of sudden death, its mechanism and prevention. The specific technologies of electrocardiography, ambulatory recording, programmed electrophysiological stimulation, and signal-averaged electrocardiograms reviewed in this chapter provide an expanded dimension to our understanding of the electropathophysiology of sudden death.

Electrocardiogram

Epidemiologic studies have examined the value of the electrocardiogram for the detection of patients at risk of sudden death in different expressions of heart disease. The surface electrocardiogram as a technique for the identification of individuals at risk for sudden death[1] has been demonstrated to be related to the underlying disease.

The Framingham study[2] observed that a number of electrocardiographic abnormalities were shown to be associated with sudden death. Using multiple regression analysis, including nonelectrocar-

From: S. Goldstein, A. Bayés-de-Luna, J. Guindo-Soldevila: *Sudden Cardiac Death*. Armonk, NY: Futura Publishing Co., Inc., © 1994.

diographic variables, premature ventricular complexes failed to demonstrate an independent influence. However, the presence of a prior myocardial infarction, intraventricular conduction disturbances in patients with ischemic heart disease, left ventricular hypertrophy and tachycardia in males and females without ischemic heart disease, and nonspecific ST-T wave changes in males only were independent electrocardiographic predictors of sudden death. The presence of electrocardiographic criteria of left ventricular hypertrophy in individuals with one or more risk factors increased the probability that the patient has significant coronary lesions and is associated with a fivefold greater risk of sudden death than do those patients without electrocardiographic abnormalities.[3]

The prognostic importance of the surface electrocardiogram was also examined in the Coronary Drug Project.[4,5] Survivors of a myocardial infarction who demonstrate one or more premature ventricular contractions on their resting electrocardiogram have a three-year mortality, about twice that of those without premature ventricular contractions (21.7% versus 11.4%).[5] Excess long-term risk, including sudden death, was associated with the frequency and complexity of premature ventricular contractions. This excess risk was independent of other risks associated with electrocardiographic and clinical characteristics.[5] In the Tecumseh study,[6] patients with known ischemic heart disease, signs of left ventricular hypertrophy, intraventricular conduction disturbances, and anterior infarction also had an increased incidence of sudden death. Pedoe[7] reported that sudden death was more frequent in patients with electrocardiograms in which Q waves and ST-T abnormalities were present. The Canadian Air Force Study[8] was designed to investigate the predictive value of electrocardiograms for sudden death in an apparently normal population. Over a 30-year followup, 70% of those who died suddenly showed electrocardiographic abnormalities including ST-T, left ventricular hypertrophy, left bundle branch block, or premature ventricular contractions.

The extent and location of the infarction is also an important prognostic implication.[9–15] In patients with anterior myocardial infarction the prognosis is worse than that in patients with inferior myocardial infarction. Infarct site influences prognosis, independent of its size.[9] Patients with anterior myocardial infarction had an increased one-year mortality. Multivariate analysis with proportional hazards regression indicates that the prognostic significance of location of infarction is independent of its size based on peak CK levels.[9]

Patients with non-Q wave myocardial infarctions have a natural history that differs from that of patients with Q wave infarction.[12-15] The acute mortality in patients with non-Q wave infarcts is approximately half that of patients with Q wave infarcts, but patients with non-Q wave infarcts have an increased risk of reinfarction and late mortality (Fig. 1). The total cardiac mortality during the two-year follow-up was only slightly greater in patients with anterior non-Q infarction compared to inferoposterior infarction.[15] The extension of the infarction in the acute phase, defined as recurrent pain, new electrocardiographic changes, and a new peak of CPK, was not a predictor of poor prognosis in patients with Q wave infarcts but was the

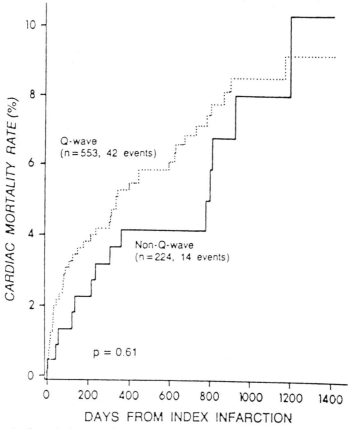

Figure 1. Cumulative cardiac mortality rate by the type of first infarction (Q wave versus non-Q wave)(from Benhorin et al.[15]).

strongest univariate predictor of one-year mortality in those with non-Q wave infarction.[12]

The presence of an intraventricular or bifasicular block as an independent marker of sudden death is controversial and depends on the clinical setting in which it occurs. Chronic right bundle branch block without apparent heart disease has no importance in sudden death, although this opinion is not without contrary views.[16,17] Bundle branch block occurring in the course of an acute infarction, particularly right bundle branch block, has a poor prognosis and is frequently associated with malignant ventricular arrhythmias in the first weeks after infarction.[18]

Other electrocardiographic parameters associated with increased cardiac mortality are the persistence of ST segment depression and Q waves in multiple leads, atrial arrhythmias, and voltage criteria for left ventricular hypertrophy.[19] Abnormalities of the P wave in coronary patients have also been associated with poor prognosis.[20] Several QRS point scores appear to identify patients with an ejection fraction of less than 50%.[21,22] In addition, some studies indicate that patients with prolongation of the QT interval have increased risk of sudden death (Table 1).[23]

In summary, the electrocardiogram provides important markers of sudden death. Nevertheless, the electrocardiogram may be normal or show only minor alterations in many coronary patients: 50% of patients with stable angina without myocardial infarction, 10% to 20% of patients with previous infarction, and 25% of patients with three-vessel disease, and in as many as 10% the electrocardiogram is normal during angina. Nevertheless, in most sudden cardiac death victims, the electrocardiogram is abnormal, independent of the associated heart disease.

Exercise Test

The exercise test provides data regarding:

1. myocardial ischemia including the development of angina, dyspnea, and ST alterations;
2. functional capacity including peak heart rate, blood pressure, work load; and
3. electrical instability, including atrial and ventricular arrhythmias and intraventricular blocks.

Table 1

Summary of Studies Relating QT Duration to Prognosis

Author	Study Size	Time since MI	Result
Schwartz and Wolf, 1978	55 pts, 55 controls	2 months–6 years	+
Haynes et al., 1978	125 SCD, 98 MI-No VT	14 months. SCD; 20 months, MI-No VT	+
Moller, 1981	91 MI	Prospective	+
Ahnve et al., 1984	865 MI	Prospective	+
Whelan et al., 1986	533 MI	Prospective	+
Boudelas et al., 1982	100 MI	14 months	–
Pohjola-Sintonen, 1986	457 MI	28 days	–
Juul-Muller, 1986	101 MI	Prospective	+
Peters, 1984	686 MI	Prospective	+
Case, 1984	686 MI	Prospective	+
Gupta, 1984	100 MI, 25 normals	Prospective	+

From (Cripps T.[23]) MI = myocardial infarction; SCD = sudden cardiac death; VT = ventricular tachycardia.

A number of procedures including the exercise test may be used to study exercise performance.[24] Although in itself the exercise test lacks sensitivity or specificity to detect patients at high risk of sudden death in the general population, it may be of value in some subgroups of patients, particularly if correlated with other techniques.[25]

In postmyocardial infarction patients, the exercise test, when carried out in the second to third week following myocardial infarction, is considered one of the most useful procedures to stratify risk. In patients without heart failure, ST segment depression is an important predictor of total and sudden cardiac death,[26-30] while in patients with heart failure,[31-37] parameters such as exercise duration and blood pressure response have a greater predictive value than ST segment depression.

Theroux et al.[26] performed exercise tests in 210 postmyocardial infarction patients without heart failure. During a follow-up of one year, only 1 of 146 patients with a normal ST response to exercise died suddenly (0.7%), compared to 10 of 64 patients with an abnormal response (15.7%). ST segment depression without angina did not correlate with the appearance of nonfatal myocardial infarction, stable or unstable angina, during one year of follow-up.[26,27] In similar studies, Sami,[28] Davidson,[29] and De Busk[30] reached similar conclusions.

Williams et al.[31] found that in postmyocardial infarction patients with moderate heart failure, the only alteration in the exercise test which defined a poor prognosis was a duration of exercise of less than three minutes. In patients with severe ventricular dysfunction,[32] ST depression was less predictive of mortality than variables which reflected the ventricular performance. Podrid et al.[33] observed that survival was related to exercise tolerance rather than the degree of ST depression. Degenais et al.[34] reported that in patients with ST depression, survival was again correlated to the duration of exercise. Waters et al.[35] found that an abnormal response of the ST segment was the strongest predictor of mortality in the first year after myocardial infarction since it was a marker of residual ischemia. Late mortality was related to markers of poor ventricular function rather than to arrhythmias induced by exercise. Studies that include patients with moderate heart failure[24,31-36] explain why the parameters which examine functional capacity are more important in the long-term follow-up than those which examine ischemia, such as ST depression. In reality, postinfarction patients at increased risk are those who have limited exercise performance for whatever the cause.[37]

The importance of ventricular arrhythmias occurring during the exercise test as a marker of sudden death in postmyocardial infarction patients remains controversial.[25,26] Theroux et al.[25] observed that the risk of sudden death was 22.4 times greater in patients with an abnormal ST response and only 2.9 times greater in those with ventricular arrhythmias induced by exercise. Waters et al.[35] observed that ventricular arrhythmias during the predischarge exercise test were predictive of increased mortality in the first year of follow-up. In contrast, the abnormal ST segment response was a predictor of mortality during the first year after myocardial infarction, but not thereafter.[35] Weld et al.[32] reported that the duration of exercise and ventricular arrhythmias, but not ST segment depression, were predictors of increased cardiac mortality. However, more than 50% of the patients had congestive heart failure. Thus, it seems that the relationship of exercise-induced ventricular arrhythmias to left ventricular dysfunction is the most important predictor.

In patients with chronic stable coronary heart disease, regardless of previous myocardial infarction, ST depression and exercise duration have a unique predictive value as a marker of poor prognosis.[25] In the pioneering work of McNeer,[38] duration of exercise, the maximum heart rate and, to a lesser extent, the ST segment depression, differentiated high- and low-risk groups independent of the extent of the coronary artery disease. Survival of patients who reached phase IV of the Bruce protocol or a heart rate above 169 beats per minute was greater than 90% during four years of follow-up. In contrast, fewer than 60% of patients who failed to reach stage 1 and whose heart rate did not exceed 120 per minute, were living at four years. In patients with an abnormal ST segment at onset of exercise, 77% were living at four years. Survival decreased to 63% if they could not complete phase II of the Bruce protocol. The Coronary Artery Surgical Study (CASS)[39] confirmed this result. At five years, total survival varied from 72% in patients with ST depression of greater than 1 mm during the first stage of exercise, to 95% in which the ST segment was normal at stage 3.

In patients with chronic stable coronary heart disease, the prognostic value of exercise-induced ventricular arrhythmias depends on the clinical characteristics of the patients studied. In the presence of ST segment depression, ventricular arrhythmias provoked by exercise are associated with more extensive coronary artery disease and left ventricular dysfunction, but do not constitute an independent risk factor of cardiac mortality.[40,41]

In summary, in patients with ischemic heart disease with a well-preserved ventricular function, ST segment depression is an important predictor of prognosis. In patients with depressed ventricular function, hemodynamic performance is of greater value. It is also evident that although sudden death is generally caused by ventricular arrhythmias,[42,43] ventricular arrhythmias during exercise testing are not an independent risk marker of sudden cardiac death.

In patients without overt coronary artery disease but with coronary risk factors, the Myocardial Risk Factor Intervention Trial (MRFIT) reported that the ST segment depression is an important predictor of poor prognosis.[44] In that study, an abnormal response to exercise, defined as an ST depression integral of 16 microvolts or more, was observed in 12.2% of the males. A fourfold increase in the seven-year coronary mortality (2/1000 versus 7.61/1000) was observed in males with an abnormal response to exercise, compared to males with a normal ST segment response during exercise (risk ratio 3.8% and 95% confidence limits 2.5 to 5.5).

The value of the exercise test for the detection of sudden death in the general population is very poor, in part due to the low incidence of sudden death. Some studies[45] observed that a positive exercise test in apparently healthy individuals is a predictor of future angina but not of myocardial infarction or sudden death. The appearance of ventricular arrhythmias during exercise in healthy individuals is frequent and has no prognostic significance.[46]

The prognostic value of the exercise test in relation to the appearance of cardiac morbidity, including sudden death, in patients with other forms of heart disease has also been examined. Following surgery for Fallot's tetralogy, the occurrence of complex ventricular arrhythmias induced during exercise is associated with hemodynamic alterations of the right ventricle and increased risk of sudden death.[47,48] The exercise test may also be useful to evaluate antiarrhythmic efficacy in patients with history of malignant ventricular arrhythmias.[49,50] The measurement of the QT interval during the exercise test is also useful in patients taking some antiarrhythmic drugs in order to identify risks of proarrhythmia. Kadish et al.[51] observed a paradoxical increase in the QT_c interval in patients who experienced a proarrhythmic effect due to class IA antiarrhythmic drugs. The exercise test may also determine which patients with Wolff-Parkinson-White syndrome are at risk of sudden death. The disappearance of preexcitation with effort is considered to be an indicator of a better prognosis[52,53] (See Chapter XIII).

Ambulatory Electrocardiographic Recording

Ventricular Premature Beats

Ambulatory electrocardiographic recordings have been used to stratify sudden death risk in postinfarction patients. The presence of premature ventricular contractions recorded on ambulatory electrocardiograms after an acute myocardial infarction adversely affects the prognosis of patients after discharge.[54] Clinical studies clearly demonstrate that ventricular ectopic activity has prognostic value independent of its relationship with left ventricular dysfunction.[55-60]

Ruberman[55] was one of the first investigators to call attention to the importance of ventricular premature beats recorded in patients after an acute myocardial infarction. Complex premature ventricular contractions and heart failure were independent and cumulative risk factors of sudden death during follow-up (Fig. 2). In the Multicenter Postinfarction Program[56] (Fig. 3), frequent and/or repetitive premature ventricular contractions were predictors of sudden death. They were, however, of lesser importance than decreased left ventricular function and pulmonary rales. Frequent and repetitive premature ventricular contractions also predicted poor prognosis in the Myocardial Infarct Limitation study.[57] This was particularly evident in the presence of left ventricular dysfunction.[57,58] In the Blocker Heart Attack Trial,[59] premature ventricular contractions after acute myocardial infarction were an important and independent marker of both total and sudden mortality. The recently published results of the GISSI-2 Trial[60] have demonstrated that although the incidence of ventricular arrhythmias is lowered by thrombolysis, frequent ventricular premature beats remain an independent risk factor of total and sudden death.[60]

Heart Rate and QT Variability

The ambulatory electrocardiogram can also determine other markers and triggers of sudden death including RR variability,[61] variation in the QT interval,[62,63] and other parameters of the autonomic nervous system function.[64] Kleiger et al.[61] demonstrated that

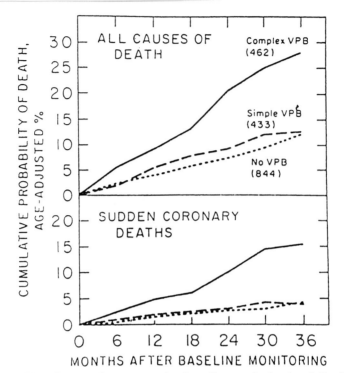

Figure 2. Mortality over three years after baseline monitoring in relation to ventricular premature beats (VPB) in the monitoring hour (from Ruberman et al.[55]).

postinfarction patients who lack variability of the RR interval (< 50 msec) are at increased risk of sudden death than those with RR variability of greater than 100 milliseconds. The sudden death risk can be predicted more precisely from this parameter than from premature ventricular contractions. Heart rate variability was used to predict death after resuscitation of out-of-hospital sudden death. Those survivors with the greatest variability had the best survival experience.[65]

The dynamic behavior of QT_c is also a predictor of malignant ventricular arrhythmias.[62,63] Our study of serial QT measurements on ambulatory recordings indicates that malignant ventricular arrhythmias were more frequent in patients with QT_c peaks of greater than 500 milliseconds (Fig. 4). These studies emphasize the importance of ambulatory electrocardiography as a measure of vagosympathetic variations of the autonomic nervous system.[64]

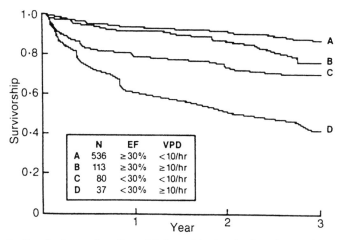

Figure 3. Survival as a function of left ventricular dysfunction and ventricular arrhythmias. The survival curves were calculated by the Kaplan-Meier method. EF = ejection fraction; VPD = ventricular premature depolarization (from Bigger et al.[58]).

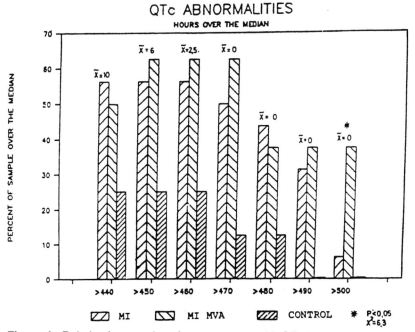

Figure 4. Relative frequencies of measurement with QT above several values. MI = myocardial infarction; MVA = malignant ventricular arrhythmias (from Marti et al. [62]).

Antiarrhythmic Drug Evaluation

The ambulatory electrocardiogram has also been useful to evaluate the efficacy of antiarrhythmic treatment in patients with a malignant ventricular arrhythmia. When evaluating the efficacy of antiarrhythmic treatment, it must be emphasized that premature ventricular contractions have a significant intraindividual variability. The ambulatory electrocardiogram may, however, be useful in deciding whether or not there is a proarrhythmic response. Morganroth[66] suggested that an increase in the number of premature ventricular contractions above a predetermined value can be considered as a proarrhythmic response.

Silent Ischemia

The ambulatory electrocardiogram is also an important tool for the detection of silent myocardial ischemia.[67–70] Recently Rocco et al.[70] demonstrated that the ambulatory ST segment depression in coronary patients defines a subgroup of patients at increased risk (Table 2). Its presence has been suggested as a marker of both cardiac events and death in patients with chronic coronary heart disease[69,70] and unstable angina[71,72] (Fig. 5) (see Chapter IX).

Other Situations

The presence of ambulatory rhythm abnormalities is also useful for the study of mortality predictors in resuscitated patients of out-of-hospital cardiac arrest.[73] Complex ventricular arrhythmias including bigeminy and trigeminy, repetitive forms or frequent multiforms, were observed in 56% of patients who developed subsequent cardiac arrest, compared with 18% of survivors. Temesy-Armos et al.[74] also examined the relationship of ventricular ectopy on survival and observed a progressive increase in mortality related to ventricular premature beat complexity (Fig. 6).

The ambulatory electrocardiogram is also useful in determining patients at risk of sudden death in other forms of heart disease. This is particularly true for dilated and hypertrophic cardiomyopathy,[75,76] in which the presence of frequent or repetitive premature ventricu-

Table 2

Prognostic Importance of Myocardial Ischemia Detected by Ambulatory Monitoring in Patients with Stable Coronary Artery Disease

	ST Depression	*No ST Depression*
Death	2	0
Myocardial infarction	4	0
Unstable angina	3	1
Revascularization for progressive symptoms	11	0
Total	20	0

Coronary events during follow-up of 12.5 ± 7.5 months.
(From Rocco et al.[70])

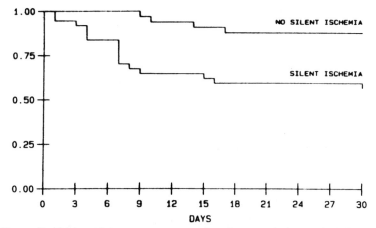

Figure 5. Kaplan-Meier curves comparing the cumulative probabilities of not experiencing myocardial infarction or revascularization for recurrent angina during a period of 30 days for the 37 patients with silent ischemia (group 1) and the 33 patients without it (group 2), as detected by continuous electrocardiographic monitoring ($P < 0.002$) (from Gottlieb et al.[71]).

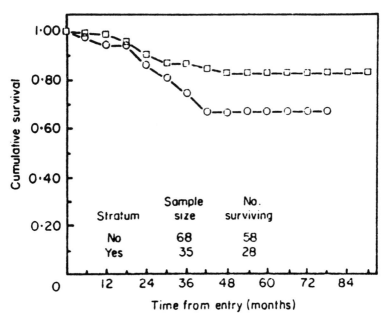

Figure 6. Comparison in incidence of recurrent sudden death for patients grouped by the presence (○) or absence (□) of the combinations of frequent and repetitive VPCs. VPC = ventricular premature contractions (from Temesy-Armos et al.[74]).

lar contractions may be a marker of sudden death. In mitral valve prolapse, complex ventricular arrhythmias are common but may not uniformly predict sudden death.[77,78] The presence of premature ventricular contractions also identifies patients after correction of Fallot's tetralogy, as well as other congenital heart disease at increased risk of sudden death.[79]

Programmed Electrical Stimulation

Programmed electrical stimulation has been used to guide antiarrhythmic treatment in patients with sustained and nonsustained ventricular tachycardia[80,81] and symptomatic arrhythmias. Induction of a sustained ventricular tachycardia of similar characteristics as that present spontaneously is presumed to be a demonstration of the anatomical substrate of arrhythmias.[82] Suppression by medication of that arrhythmia indicates that this drug may be effective in preventing the arrhythmia.[80] Nevertheless, the lack of suppression of induced sustained ventricular tachycardia with some antiarrhythmic drugs such as amiodarone or propafenone does not imply that these drugs are not efficient. The induction of ventricular fibrillation, polymorphic ventricular tachycardia, or salvos of nonsustained ventricular tachycardia is of less predictive value and is considered a nonspecific finding.[81]

There are few studies, the results of which are contradictory, comparing the prevention of malignant ventricular arrhythmias using treatment guided by electrophysiological studies or with ambulatory electrocardiographic guidance.[83-85] (see Chapter XVII).

The role of programmed electrical stimulation after acute myocardial infarction to stratify risk has been controversial. Some studies[86,87] suggest that programmed electrical stimulation predicts postinfarction patients who are at risk of sudden death. However, other studies[88,89] do not support this thesis. Induction of ventricular tachyarrhythmias did not identify patients at risk of sudden death, while a low ejection fraction and presence of a ventricular aneurysm did identify high-risk patients. Current opinion indicates that electrophysiological studies should not be performed routinely in postmyocardial infarction patients. Randomized treatment trials have not been carried out to test the suppression hypothesis. There is sufficient data available to suggest that, just as in the Cardiac Arrhythmia Suppression Trial (CAST)[90] using ambulatory electrocardiographically guided therapy, electrophysiologically guided suppression identifies only those patients at low risk of recurrent events.

Electrophysiological studies may also assist in determining those patients requiring a pacemaker.[91,92] They may also be important in patients without ischemic heart disease. In patients with Wolff-Parkinson-White syndrome, electrophysiological studies can identify those at risk of sudden death.[52,53] In Wolff-Parkinson-White syndrome, predictors of increased risk are the presence of more than one anomalous pathway and rapid atrioventricular conduction during atrial fibrillation (RR < 240 msec) (Chapter XIII).[52,53]

Electrophysiological studies are not useful in identifying the risk of sudden death in patients with long QT syndrome[93] or in patients after surgical correction of tetralogy of Fallot.[94] In patients with hypertrophic cardiomyopathy, the prognostic value of programmed electrical stimulation is not well understood.[95] Electrophysiological studies, however, are necessary as part of the implantation of an automatic implantable defibrillator and must precede its implantation to test efficacy after implantation.

Signal-Averaged Electrocardiogram

Ventricular late potentials in postmyocardial infarction patients have been proposed as markers of malignant ventricular arrhythmias and sudden death.[96–99] The presence of late potentials suggests that an arrhythmogenic substrate for sustained ventricular tachycardia is present. Although the sensitivity is high, specificity is marginal and the positive predictive value for the development of malignant ventricular arrhythmias or sudden cardiac death is only 20%. It is probably unjustified to expect that any one method can identify the individual patient at risk of sustained ventricular tachycardia or sudden death. According to Breithardt and Borggrefe,[97] ambulatory electrocardiography and signal averaging may be useful as screening methods, whereas programmed ventricular stimulation may be useful for patients at increased risk. Abnormal signal-averaged electrocardiography, combined with other testing after acute myocardial infarction, improves the positive predictive value.[100–102] The clinical value of ventricular late potentials as a marker of sustained ventricular tachyarrhythmias or sudden death in cardiomyopathies has also been suggested.[103] Mancini et al.[104] examined the prognostic value of signal-averaged electrocardiograms in patients with nonischemic congestive cardiomyopathy. Patients with abnormal signal-averaged electrocardiograms had an increased occurrence of sustained ventricular arrhythmia and death compared to those in whom abnormalities were absent and had an excellent prognosis.

It is important to emphasize that since sudden cardiac death is a multifactorial problem, multiple approaches to risk stratification are mandatory. In many previous studies of postinfarction patients, the statistical approach has allowed us to focus the risk factors of sudden death on ischemic events in a multifactorial way. Recent studies[100–102] demonstrate that the combined use of different parameters shows greater sensitivity, specificity, and positive predictive

Table 3

Relation Among the Signal-Averaged ECG, Ejection Fraction, Ambulatory Electrocardiographic Monitoring and Arrhythmic Events

	Normal (%)	Abnormal (%)	P Value	Odds Ratio
SA-ECG	2/57 (3/5)	13/45 (29)	0.003	11
EF	3/47 (6)	12/50 (24)	0.01	4.6
Holter	3/32 (9)	12/52 (23)	0.09	2.9
SA-ECG + EF	0/26 (0)	10/28 (36)	0.0007	30.1
SA-ECG + Holter	0/14 (0)	9/26 (35)	0.001	15.7
EF + Holter	1/16 (6)	11/30 (37)	0.025	8.68
SA-ECG + EF + Holter	0/9 (0)	8/16) (50)	0.01	19

ECG = electrocardiogram; EF = ejection fraction; SA-ECG = signal-averaged electrocardiogram.
(Gomes et al.[100])

accuracy in detecting patients at risk of a new arrhythmic event. Gomes et al.[100] observed that in patients with an abnormal signal-averaged electrocardiogram and an ejection fraction below 40%, complex ventricular arrhythmias during ambulatory recording occurred at an increased frequency. No arrhythmic events occurred in patients in whom all three variables were absent (Table 3). Kuchar et al.[101] demonstrated that an abnormal signal-averaged electrocardiogram in the presence of an ejection fraction of less than 40% identified patients with a 35% probability of the occurrence of an arrhythmic event, including sudden death or sustained symptomatic ventricular tachycardia during a follow-up of 14 months (Fig. 7). In contrast, the risk of arrhythmic events was 4% in patients with left ventricular dysfunction with normal signal-averaged tracing.

In summary, since sudden cardiac death is a multifactorial problem, risk stratification requires a multifactorial approach. This obviously also implies different and often multidimensional diagnostic procedures. Although electrocardiographic factors are important, the state of left ventricular function remains the most significant predictor of sudden death. The many electrocardio-

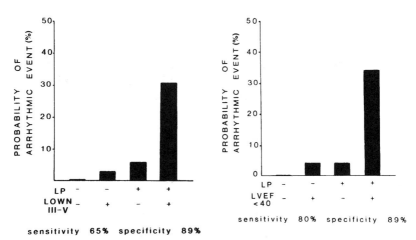

Figure 7. Predictive value of abnormal signal-averaged electrocardiogram (LP) and left ventricular ejection fraction (LVEF) < 40% and Lown 3–5 category of ventricular premature beats (from Kuchar et al.[101]).

graphic approaches reviewed in this chapter develop indices that contribute to a more accurate identification of patients at risk of sudden death.

References

1. Fisch C. Role of the electrocardiogram in identifying the patient at increased risk for sudden death. *J Am Coll Cardiol* 1985;5:6B.
2. Kreger BE, Cupples LA, Kannel WB. The electrocardiogram in prediction of sudden death: Framingham study experience. *Am Heart J* 1987; 113:377.
3. Kannel WB, Doyle JT, McNamara PM, et al. Precursors of sudden coronary death: Factors related to the incidence of sudden death. *Circulation* 1975;51:606.
4. The Coronary Drug Project Research Group. The prognostic importance of the electrocardiogram after myocardial infarction. *Ann Intern Med* 1972;77:677.
5. The Coronary Drug Project Research Group. Prognostic importance of premature beats following myocardial infarction: Experience in the Coronary Drug Project. *JAMA* 1973;223:1116.
6. Chiang BN, Perlman LV, Fulton M, et al. Predisposing factors in sudden cardiac death in Tecumseh, Michigan: A prospective study. *Circulation* 1970;41:31.

7. Pedoe HDT. Predictability of sudden death from resting electrocardiogram: Effect of previous manifestation of previous heart disease. *Br Heart J* 1978;40:630.

8. Rose G, Baxter PJ, Reid DD, et al. The Canadian Air Force study. Prevalence and prognosis of electrocardiographic findings in middle-aged men. *Br Heart J* 1978;40:636.

9. Hands ME, Lloyd BL, Robinson JS, et al. Prognostic significance of electrocardiographic site of infarction after correction for enzymatic size of infarction. *Circulation* 1986;73:885.

10. Thanavaro S, Kleiger RE, Province MA, et al. Effect of infarct localization on the in-hospital prognosis of patients with first transmural myocardial infarction. *Circulation* 1982;66:742.

11. Maisel AS, Gilpin E, Holt B, et al. Survival after hospital discharge in matched populations with inferior or anterior myocardial infarction. *J Am Coll Cardiol* 1985;6:731.

12. Maisel AS, Ahnve S, Gilpun E, et al. Prognosis after extension of myocardial infarct: The role of Q-wave and non-Q-wave infarction. *Circulation* 1985;71:211.

13. Hutter AM, DeSanctis RW, Flynn T, et al. Non-transmural myocardial infarction: A comparison of hospital and late clinical course of patients with that of matched patients with transmural anterior or transmural inferior myocardial infarction. *Am J Cardiol* 1981;48:595.

14. Nicholson MR, Roubin GS, Bernstein L, et al. Prognosis after an initial non-Q-wave myocardial infarction related to coronary artery anatomy. *Am J Cardiol* 1983;52:462.

15. Benhorin J, Moss A, Oakes D, et al. The prognostic significance of first myocardial infarction type (Q wave versus non-Q wave) and Q wave location. *J Am Coll Cardiol* 1990;15:1201.

16. Rotman N, Frietchwaser J. A clinical and follow-up study of right and left bundle branch block. *Circulation* 1975;51:477.

17. Schroeider JF. Newly acquired right bundle branch block. *Ann Intern Med* 1980;91:37.

18. Lie KI, Liem KL, Schrlenburgh RM, et al. Early identification of patients developing late in-hospital ventricular fibrillation after discharge from the coronary unit: A 5.5 year retrospective and prospective study of 1987 patients. *Am J Cardiol* 1978;41:674.

19. Pasternak RC, Braunwald E, Sobel BE. Acute myocardial infarction. In: Braunwald E, ed. *Heart Disease: Textbook of Cardiovascular Medicine.* Philadelphia: WB Saunders; 1992;1200.

20. Rios JC. *Clinical Electrocardiographic Correlations.* Philadelphia: FA Davis Company; 1977.

21. Askenazi P, Parisi AF, Cohen PF, et al. Value of the QRS complex in assessing left ventricular ejection fraction. *Am J Cardiol* 1978; 41:494.

22. Hamby RI, Murphy D, Hoffman I. Clinical predictability of left ventricular function post-myocardial infarction from the electrocardiogram. *Am Heart J* 1985;109:338.

23. Cripps T. The QT interval and its relationship to heart rate in patients after acute myocardial infarction. In: Butrous GS, Schwartz PJ, eds.

Clinical Aspects of Ventricular Repolarization. London: Farrand Press; 1989;369.

24. DeBusk RF. Specialized testing after recent acute myocardial infarction. *Ann Intern Med* 1989;110:470.

25. McHenry PL. Role of exercise testing in predicting sudden death. *J Am Coll Cardiol* 1985;5(suppl B):9.

26. Theroux P, Waters D, Halphen C, et al. Prognostic value of exercise testing soon after myocardial infarction. *N Engl J Med* 1979;301:341.

27. Waters DD, Theroux P, Halphen E, et al. Clinical predictors of angina following myocardial infarction. *Am J Med* 1979;66:991.

28. Sami M, Kraemer H, DeBusk RF. The prognostic significance of serial exercise testing after myocardial infarction. *Circulation* 1979;60:1238.

29. Davidson DM, DeBusk RF. Prognostic significance of a single exercise test 3 weeks after acute myocardial infarction. *Circulation* 1980; 61:236.

30. DeBusk RF, Blomqvist CG, Kouchoukos NT, et al. Identification and treatment of low risk patients after acute myocardial infarction and coronary artery bypass graft surgery. *N Engl J Med* 1986;314:16.

31. Williams WL, Nair RC, Higginson LAJ, et al. Comparison of clinical and treadmill variables for prediction of outcome after myocardial infarction. *J Am Coll Cardiol* 1984;4:477.

32. Weld FM, Chu KL, Bigger JT, et al. Risk stratification with low-level exercise testing 2 weeks after acute myocardial infarction. *Circulation* 1981;64:306.

33. Podrid JP, Graboys TB, Lown B. Prognosis of medically treated patients with coronary artery disease with profound ST segment depression during exercise testing. *N Engl J Med* 1981;305:1111.

34. Degenais GR, Rouleau JR, Christen A, et al. Survival of patients with strongly positive exercise electrocardiogram. *Circulation* 1982;65:452.

35. Waters DD, Bosch X, Bouchard A, et al. Comparison of clinical variables derived from a limited predischarge exercise testing as predictors of early and late mortality after myocardial infarction. *J Am Coll Cardiol* 1985;5:1.

36. Bruce RA, DeRoyden TA, Peterson DR, et al. Non-invasive predictors of sudden cardiac death in men with coronary heart disease: Predictive value of maximal stress testing. *Am J Cardiol* 1977;39:833.

37. Fioretti P, Brower RW, Somoons ML, et al. Relative value of clinical variables, bicycle ergometry, rest radionuclide ventriculography, and 24-hour ambulatory electrocardiographic monitoring at discharge to predict 1 year survival after acute myocardial infarction. *J Am Coll Cardiol* 1986;8:40.

38. McNeer JF, Margilis JR, Lee KL, et al. The role of the exercise test in the evaluation of patients for ischemic heart disease. *Circulation* 1978;57:64.

39. Weiner DA, Ryan TJ, McCabe CH, et al. Prognostic importance of the clinical profile and exercise test in medically treated patients with coronary artery disease. *J Am Coll Cardiol* 1984;3:772.

40. Nair CK, Aronow WS, Sketch NH, et al. Diagnostic and prognostic significance of exercise-induced premature ventricular complexes in men and women: A 4-year follow-up. *J Am Coll Cardiol* 1983;1:1201.

41. Califf RM, McKinnes RA, McNeer F, et al. Prognostic value of ventricular arrhythmias associated with treadmill exercise testing in patients studied with ventricular catheterization for suspected ischemic heart disease. *J Am Coll Cardiol* 1983;2:1060.

42. Bayés de Luna A, Coumel PH, Leclercq JF. Ambulatory sudden death: Mechanisms of production of fatal arrhythmia on the basis of data from 157 cases. *Am Heart J* 1989;117:151.

43. Bayés de Luna A, Guindo J, Rivera J. Ambulatory sudden death in patients wearing Holter devices. *J Ambulat Monitoring* 1989;2:3.

44. Rautaharju PM, Prineas RJ, Eifler WJ, et al. Prognostic value of exercise electrocardiogram in men at high risk of future coronary heart disease: Multiple Risk Factor Intervention Trial experience. *J Am Coll Cardiol* 1986;8:1.

45. McHenry PL, O'Donnell J, Morris SN, et al. The abnormal exercise electrocardiogram in apparently healthy men: A predictor of angina pectoris as an initial event during long-term follow-up. *Circulation* 1984;70:547.

46. Froelicher VF, Thomas MM, Pillow C, et al. Epidemiologic study of asymptomatic men screened by maximal treadmill testing for latent coronary artery disease. *Am J Cardiol* 1974;34:770.

47. James FW, Kaplan S, Schwartz DC, et al. Response to exercise in patients after total correction of tetralogy of Fallot. *Circulation* 1976;54:671.

48. Garson A, Gillette PC, Gutgesell HP, et al. Stress-induced ventricular arrhythmias after repair of tetralogy of Fallot. *Am J Cardiol* 1980;46:1006.

49. Graboys TB, Lown B, Podrid P, et al. Long-term survival of patients with malignant ventricular arrhythmias treated with antiarrhythmic drugs. *Am J Cardiol* 1982;50:437.

50. Bayés de Luna A, Guindo-Soldevila J, Torner P, et al. Value of effort test and acute drug testing in the evaluation of antiarrhythmic treatment. *Eur Heart J* 1987;8(suppl A):77.

51. Kadish AH, Weisman HF, Veltri EP, et al. Paradoxical effects of exercise on the QT interval in patients with polymorphic ventricular tachycardia receiving type Ia antiarrhythmic agents. *Circulation* 1990;81:14.

52. Torner P, Brugada P, Smeets J, et al. Ventricular fibrillation in the Wolff-Parkinson-White syndrome. *Eur Heart J* 1991;12:144.

53. Klein GJ, Bashore TM, Sellers TD, et al. Ventricular fibrillation in Wolff-Parkinson-White syndrome. *N Engl J Med* 1979;301:1080.

54. Armstrong WF, McHenry PL. Ambulatory electrocardiographic monitoring: Can we predict sudden death? *J Am Coll Cardiol* 1985;5(suppl B):13.

55. Ruberman W, Wienblatt E, Golberg J, et al. Ventricular premature beats and mortality after myocardial infarction. *N Engl J Med* 1977;297:750.

56. Moss AJ, Bigger JT, Case RB. Risk stratification and survival after myocardial infarction. *N Engl J Med* 1983;309:331.

57. Mukharji J, Rude RE, Poole WK, et al. The MILIS Study Group. Risk factors of sudden death after acute myocardial infarction: Two year follow-up. *Am J Cardiol* 1984;54:31.

58. Bigger JT, Fleiss JL, Kleiger R, et al. The relationships among ventricular arrhythmias, left ventricular dysfunction, and mortality in the 2 years after myocardial infarction. *Circulation* 1984;69:250.
59. Kostis JB, Byington R, Friedman LM, et al. and the BHAT study group. Prognostic significance of ventricular ectopic activity in survivors of acute myocardial infarction. *J Am Coll Cardiol* 1987;10:231.
60. Maggioni AP, Zuanetti G, Franzosi MG, et al, on behalf of GISSI-2 Investigators. Prevalence and prognostic significance of ventricular arrhythmias after acute myocardial infarction in the fibrinolytic era: GISSI-2 results. *Circulation* 1993;87:312.
61. Kleiger RE, Miller J Ph, Bigger JT, et al. Decreased heart rate variability and its association with increased mortality after acute myocardial infarction. *Am J Cardiol* 1987;59:256.
62. Martí V, Guindo-Soldevila J, Homs E, et al. Peaks of QT_c lengthening measures in Holter recordings as a marker of life-threatening arrhythmias in postmyocardial infarction patients. *Am Heart J* 1992;124:234.
63. Homs E, Viñolas X, Guindo J, et al. Automatic QT_c lengthening measurement in Holter ECG as a marker of life-threatening arrhythmias in postmyocardial infarction. *J Am Coll Cardiol* 1993;21;274A.
64. Leclerq JF, Maison-Blanche P, Cuchemezand B, et al. Respective role of sympathetic tone and of cardiac pauses in the genesis of 62 cases of ventricular fibrillation recorded during Holter monitoring. *Eur Heart J* 1988;9:1276.
65. Dougherty CM, Burr RL. Comparison of heart rate variability in survivors and nonsurvivors of sudden cardiac arrest. *Am J Cardiol* 1992;70:441.
66. Morganroth J, Borland M, Chao G. Application of a frequency definition of ventricular proarrhythmia. *Am J Cardiol* 1987;59:97.
67. Stern S, Tzivoni D. Early detection of silent ischemic heart disease by 24-hour electrocardiographic monitoring of active subjects. *Br Heart J* 1974:36:481.
68. Deanfield J, Shea M, Ribiero P, et al. Transient ST-segment depression as a marker of myocardial ischemia during daily life. *Am J Cardiol* 1984:54:1195.
69. Tzivoni D, Gavish A, Gottlieb S, et al. Prognostic significance of ischemic episodes in patients. *Am J Cardiol* 1988;62:661.
70. Rocco MB, Nabel EG, Campbell S, et al. Prognostic importance of myocardial ischemia detected by ambulatory monitoring in patients with stable coronary artery disease. *Circulation* 1988;78:877.
71. Gottlieb LS, Weisfeldt M, Ouyang P, et al. Silent ischemia as a marker for early unfavorable outcomes in patients with unstable angina. *N Engl J Med* 1986;314:1214.
72. Nademanee K, Intrarachot V, Singh PN, et al. Prognostic significance of silent myocardial ischemia in patients with unstable angina. *J Am Coll Cardiol* 1987;10:1.
73. Weaver WD, Cobb LA, Hallstrom AP. Ambulatory arrhythmias in resuscitated victims of cardiac arrest. *Circulation* 1982;66:212.
74. Temesy-Armos PN, Medendorp SV, Goldstein S, et al. Predictive value of ventricular arrhythmias in resuscitated out-of-hospital cardiac arrest victims. *Eur Heart J* 1988;9:625.

75. Meinertz T, Hofmann T, Kasper W, et al. Significance of ventricular arrhythmias in idiopathic dilated cardiomyopathy. *Am J Cardiol* 1984;53:902.
76. McKenna WJ, England D, Doi YL, et al. Arrhythmia in hypertrophic cardiomyopathy, I: Influence on prognosis. *Br Heart J* 1981;46:168.
77. Winkle RA, Lopes MG, Fitzgerland JW, et al. Arrhythmias in patients with mitral valve prolapse. *Circulation* 1975;52:73.
78. DeMaria AN, Amsterdam EA, Vismara LA, et al. Arrhythmias in mitral valve prolapse syndrome. *Ann Intern Med* 1976;84:656.
79. Kavey RW, Blackman MS, Sondheimer HM. Incidence and severity of chronic ventricular arrhythmias after repair of tetralogy of Fallot. *Am Heart J* 1982;103:342.
80. Horowitz LN, Josephson ME, Farshidi A, et al. Recurrent sustained ventricular tachycardiam, III: Role of the electrophysiologic study in selection of antiarrhythmic regimens. *Circulation* 1978;58:986.
81. Wellens HJJ, Brugada P, Stevenson WG. Programmed electrical stimulation of the heart: What is the significance of induced arrhythmias and what is the correct stimulation protocol? *Circulation* 1985;72:1.
82. Iesaka Y, Nogami A, Aonuma K, et al. Prognostic significance of sustained monomorphic ventricular tachycardia induced by programmed ventricular stimulation using up to triple extrastimuli in survivors of acute myocardial infarction. *Am J Cardiol* 1990;65:1057.
83. Mitchell LB, Duff HJ, Manyari DE, et al. A randomized clinical trial of the noninvasive approaches to drug therapy of ventricular tachycardia. *N Engl J Med* 1987;317:1681.
84. Mason JW, for the ESVEM investigators. A comparison of electrophysiologic testing with Holter monitoring to predict antiarrhythmic drug efficacy for ventricular tachyarrhythmias. *N Engl J Med* 1993;329;445.
85. Moro C, Almendral J, Fiol M, et al. Randomized trial comparing empiric amiodarone versus guided pharmacologic therapy for malignant ventricular arrhythmias (Spanish Trial on Sudden Death). *Circulation* 1991;84(II):126.
86. Hamer A, Vohra J, Hunt D, et al. Prediction of sudden death by electrophysiological studies in high risk patients surviving acute myocardial infarction. *Am J Cardiol* 1982;50:223.
87. Richards DA, Byth K, Ross DL, et al. What is the best predictor of spontaneous ventricular tachycardia and sudden death after myocardial infarction. *Circulation* 1991;83:756.
88. Marchlinski RE, Buxton AE, Waxman HL, et al. Identifying patients at risk of sudden death after myocardial infarction: Value of the response to programmed stimulation, degree of ventricular ectopic activity, and severity of left ventricular dysfunction. *Am J Cardiol* 1983;52:1190.
89. Roy D, Marchand E, Theroux P, et al. Programmed ventricular stimulation in predicting one-year mortality after acute myocardial infarction. *Circulation* 1985;72:487.
90. Echt DS, Liebson PR, Mitchell LB, et al, and the CAST Investigators. Mortality and morbidity in patients receiving encainide and flecainide, or placebo. *N Engl J Med* 1991;324:781.
91. Frye RJ. Report of the joint ACC/AHA. Guidelines for permanent cardiac pacemaker implantation. *Circulation* 1989;70:331A.

92. Zipes DP, Akhtar M, Denes P, et al. Guidelines for clinical intracardiac electrophysiologic studies. *Circulation* 1989;80:1925.
93. Schwartz PJ, Locati E, Priori SG, et al. The long Q-T syndrome. In: Zipes DP, Jalife J, eds. *Cardiac Electrophysiology.* Philadelphia: WB Saunders; 1990:589.
94. Chandar GS, Wolff GS, Garson A Jr, et al. Ventricular arrhythmias in postoperative tetralogy of Fallot. *Am J Cardiol* 1990;65:655.
95. Fananapazir L, Tracy CM, Leon MB, et al. Electrophysiologic abnormalities in patients with hypertrophic cardiomyopathy. A consecutive analysis in 155 patients. *Circulation* 1989;80:1259.
96. Simson MB. Identification of patients with ventricular tachycardia after myocardial infarction from signals in the terminal QRS complex. *Circulation* 1981;64:235.
97. Breithardt G, Borggrefe M. Pathophysiological mechanisms and clinical significance of ventricular late potentials. *Eur Heart J* 1986;7:364.
98. El-Sherif N, Samet P, eds. *Cardiac Pacing and Electrophysiology.* Philadelphia: WB Saunders; 1991.
99. Breithardt G, Cain ME, El-Sherif N, et al. Standards for analysis of ventricular late potentials using high resolution or signal-averaged electrocardiography. A statement by a Task Force Committee between the European Society of Cardiology, the American Heart Association and the American College of Cardiology. *Eur Heart J* 1991;12:473.
100. Gomes JA, Winters SL, Stewart D, et al. A new noninvasive index to predict sustained ventricular tachycardia and sudden death in the first year after myocardial infarction: Based on signal-averaged electrocardiogram, radionuclide ejection fraction and Holter monitoring. *J Am Coll Cardiol* 1987;10:349.
101. Kuchar DL, Thorburn CW, Sammel NL. Prediction of serious arrhythmic events after myocardial infarction: Signal-averaged electrocardiogram, Holter monitoring, and radionuclide ventriculography. *J Am Coll Cardiol* 1987;9:531.
102. Cripps T, Bennet D, Camm J, et al. Prospective evaluation of clinical assessment, exercise testing and signal-averaged electrocardiogram in predicting outcome after acute myocardial infarction. *Am J Cardiol* 1988;62:995.
103. Cripps TR, Couninhan PJ, Frenneaux MP, et al. Signal-averaged electrocardiography in hypertrophic cardiomyopathy. *J Am Coll Cardiol* 1990;15:956.
104. Mancini DM, Wong KL, Simson MB. Prognostic value of an abnormal signal-averaged electrocardiogram in patients with nonischemic congestive cardiomyopathy. *Circulation* 1993;87:1083.

Chapter VIII

Evaluation of High-Risk Patients:
Imaging Techniques

Recent advances in cardiac imaging techniques including coronary angiography have improved not only the diagnostic accuracy, but also the prognostic evaluation of patients with heart disease. The role of the most recent techniques such as magnetic resonance imaging (MRI), monoclonal antibody imaging, etc., are yet to be evaluated.[1,2] In this chapter we review those procedures with a known prognostic value.

Chest Roentgenogram

Although modern diagnostic techniques offer greater prognostic information than the chest x-ray, we should not lose sight of its importance. In patients with acute myocardial infarction, the presence of cardiomegaly and signs of pulmonary congestion are markers of poor prognosis, not only during the acute phase of the infarction but also in long-term follow-up. Battler et al.[3] analyzed the prognostic value of the initial chest x-ray taken during the first 24 hours after the acute myocardial infarction. Patients with increased cardiothoracic ratio (≥ 0.50) or increased left heart dimension had respectively 2.7 and 4 times greater one-year mortality rates than patients with normal heart size. Similarly, the degree of pulmonary congestion was associated with a significant increase in early and late mortal-

From: S. Goldstein, A. Bayés-de-Luna, J. Guindo-Soldevila: *Sudden Cardiac Death*. Armonk, NY: Futura Publishing Co., Inc., © 1994.

127

ity. Patients with interstitial pulmonary edema or localized alveolar edema in the initial chest x-ray had a one-year mortality rate of approximately 50%. Patients with diffuse pulmonary edema had a 30-day survival of only 18% and after one year there were no survivors. In contrast, patients without pulmonary edema and normal left heart dimensions at the initial chest x-ray had a one-year probability of survival, including hospital mortality, of 94%. The prognostic significance of increased cardiac size on x-ray film as a risk marker of sudden death has also been demonstrated in the Aspirin Myocardial Infarction Study.[4] Cardiomegaly was present in 23.8% of patients who died suddenly, but only in 7.4% of survivors ($P < 0.01$). Cardiomegaly has also been a common denominator for reduced survival in other heart disease, including dilated cardiomyopathy,[5] valvular heart disease,[6] hypertensive heart disease,[7] or chronic stable coronary heart disease.[8,9]

Echocardiography

Bidimensional echocardiography and Doppler are key techniques in the diagnosis of heart disease. Nevertheless, they have been used occasionally for prognostic purposes only and their importance as a marker for sudden death is therefore not well known. Two-dimensional echocardiography provides important information to evaluate systolic and diastolic ventricular function, segmental contractility, wall thickening, presence of ventricular aneurysms, and the presence of intracavitary thrombus. Depressed left ventricular ejection fraction is a major risk marker in patients with heart disease. Preliminary studies suggest good overall agreement between abnormal left ventricular wall-motion score index assessed by two-dimensional echocardiography and depressed left ventricular ejection fraction determined angiographically (Fig. 1).[10] Both methods had a high predictive value in a prospective three-year follow-up of 50 post-myocardial infarction patients (Fig. 2).

Wall-motion score using bidimensional echocardiography during the acute phase can predict short-term complications.[11-14] The prognostic value of echocardiography has been determined in several trials.[15-17] Bhatnager et al.[15] demonstrated that alterations in ventricular contractility determined by bidimensional echocardiography prior to hospital discharge are useful in detecting cardiac events in the first and second year of follow-up. In 47 consecutive survivors of

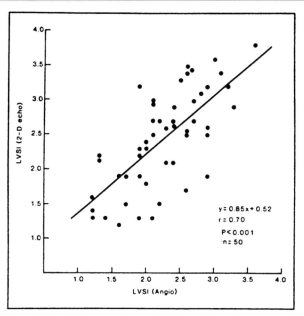

Figure 1. Correlation between left ventricular wall-motion score index (LVSI) determined with use of two-dimensional echocardiography and angiography (from Shiina et al.[10]).

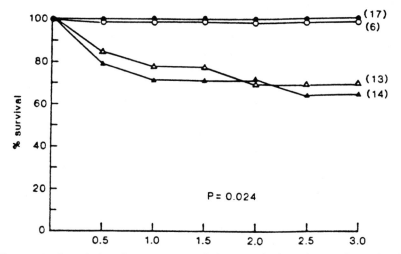

Figure 2. Correlation between cumulative survival and two-dimensional echocardiographic measurements of left ventricular wall-motion score index (LVSI). Closed circles = LVSI less than 2.0; open circles = LVSI 2.0 to 2.4; open triangles = LVSI 2.5 to 2.9; closed trianges = LVSI 3.0 or greater (from Shiina et al.[10]).

acute myocardial infarction followed during a mean of 47 months, 17 major cardiac events occurred, including sudden death. A left ventricular wall-motion score of ≥ 8.0 was present in 82% of patients with complications compared with 7% of those who remained asymptomatic. Patients who died had significantly higher wall-motion scores compared to those who survived (11.3 ± 0.9 versus 4.7 ± 0.5) ($P < 0.005$). Kan et al.[16] studied 345 patients with acute myocardial infarction, 61 who died within one year, 31 in-hospital and 38 after discharge, most of which were sudden deaths. A left ventricular segmental wall-motion score ≥ 10 predicted death within one year (88 sensitivity, 86% specificity, 61% positive predictive value and 97% negative predictive value). Other researchers[17] have reported that the prognostic value of segmental contractility is greater in anterior than in inferior myocardial infarctions.

The role of exercise echocardiography for risk stratification of postmyocardial infarction patients has been studied by various researchers.[18–20] It has been suggested that a decrease in ejection fraction or new worsening wall-motion abnormalities with exercise correlates with an increased risk of cardiac death and other cardiac events. Applegate et al.[18] studied 67 postmyocardial infarction patients. After a mean follow-up of 11 months, 16 patients had new cardiac events. A decrease in ejection fraction of more than 10% was seen in 7 of these 16 patients compared with only 4 of 51 without events ($P < 0.002$). Moreover, a new or worsening wall-motion abnormality during the recovery period of exercise had a 63% sensitivity and 80% specificity for cardiac events during the follow-up. Ryan et al.[19] studied 40 postmyocardial infarction patients and found that the exercise echocardiogram was negative in 19 of 20 patients with a good clinical outcome (95% specificity) and was positive in 16 of 20 patients with poor clinical outcome (80% sensitivity). The predictive value of positive exercise echocardiogram was 94% (Fig. 3). Jaarsma et al.[20] studied 113 patients with acute myocardial infarction and found that asynergy in a region remote from the infarct was associated with presence of three-vessel coronary artery disease in 75% of patients. The absence of compensatory regional hyperkinesis in patients with anterior myocardial infarction was associated with a particularly high mortality of 68%.[20]

In addition, preliminary studies indicate that intravascular high-frequency ultrasound provides an accurate image of coronary lumen and can identify and measure the severity of atherosclerotic plaque.[21] The prognostic value of this new technique remains unknown.

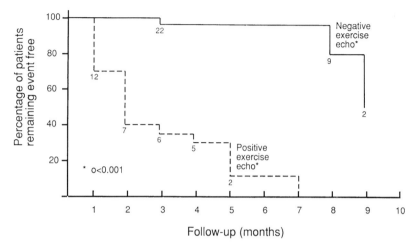

Figure 3. Cumulative survival curves as function of exercise echocardiographic results. Curves represent the proportion of patients remaining event free. Broken line indicates patients with negative exercise echocardiogram. Solid line represents patients with positive exercise echocardiogram. Follow-up is shown on abscissa. The two curves are statistically different at *P* < 0.001. Numbers under the curve represent total number of patients remaining at risk (from Ryan et al.[19]).

Nuclear Imaging Techniques

Radioisotopic studies for risk stratification have been helpful particularly in patients with coronary heart disease. They improve the value of the exercise ECG test alone for detecting ischemia and provide a description of left ventricular function at rest and during exercise.[22]

Resting Thallium Scintigraphy

The extent of myocardial damage after acute myocardial infarction may be accurately estimated by resting thallium scintigraphy. Silverman et al.[23] demonstrated the prognostic value of early resting thallium scintigraphy in 42 postmyocardial infarction patients. Fourteen patients died, 7 during hospitalization and 7 after discharge. A large thallium defect identified those patients who were likely to die (Fig. 4). Nonsurvivors had significantly larger defects and a mean defect score of 14.3 versus 2.3 in survivors (*P* < 0.001).

Only one of 28 patients alive at last follow-up had a total defect score of more than 7.0, while 12 of 14 patients who died had a score over 7.0. Mortality for patients at high risk (scintigraphic score ≥ 7.0) was significantly higher at two weeks ($P < .0001$), six months ($P < 0.001$) and at the end of follow-up ($P < 0.001$) than for patients at low risk (score < 7.0) (Fig. 5).

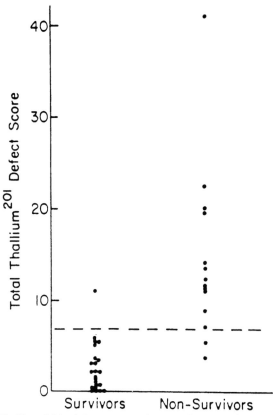

Figure 4. Thallium-201 defect score for survivors and nonsurvivors. The dashed line is drawn at a score of 7.0. All but one of the survivors had a score less than 7.0, while all but two of the nonsurvivors had a score greater than 7.0 (from Silverman et al.[23]).

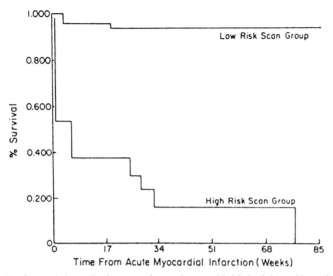

Figure 5. Actuarial survival curves for patients with high-risk and low-risk scintigrams (from Silverman et al.[23]).

Exercise Thallium Scintigraphy

Exercise thallium scintigraphy is more sensitive than exercise electrocardiography alone to detect the presence, localization, and extension of myocardial ischemia. This is especially true in patients with low functional capacity such as chronic pulmonary disease, peripheral vascular disease, and orthopedic problems, or in the presence of resting ECG abnormalities such as bundle branch block, digitalis therapy, or other causes of ST-T abnormalities.[2,24,25] As demonstrated by Gibson et al.,[24] in postmyocardial infarction patients, exercise thallium scintigraphy was better than submaximal exercise ECG and coronary angiography in predicting cardiac death and other cardiac events including reinfarctions, unstable angina, or necessity for bypass surgery. Predictors of adverse prognosis included delayed tracer redistribution, increased lung uptake, and perfusion defects in more than one vascular territory. They prospectively evaluated 140 consecutive patients with uncomplicated acute myocardial infarction. After a mean follow-up of 15 months, 50 patients experienced cardiac events, 5 of whom died suddenly. Scintigraphy identified 47 of the 50 high-risk patients (94% sensitivity). The overall sensitivity of angiography (71%) and exercise ECG testing (56%) was significantly lower than that of scintigraphy ($P < 0.01$ and $P < 0.001$, respectively). Surprisingly, in this study, resting ejection fraction did not predict adverse outcome. Hung et al.[25] observed that although thallium scintigraphy was useful to predict poor prognosis, its value was equal to that obtained with the ECG exercise test and inferior to the results of exercise radionuclide ventriculography.

In patients without prior myocardial infarction, exercise thallium scintigraphy has also been a powerful noninvasive prognostic tool. Brown et al.[26] found that the number of myocardial segments with transient thallium defects during exercise was the most important predictor of subsequent cardiac death or myocardial infarction in a study of 100 patients presenting for chest pain evaluation. Of the 78 patients with zero or one transient thallium defect, only two had cardiac events in a mean follow-up of 3.7 years. In contrast, in 22 patients with at least two transient thallium defects, 4 patients had cardiac events during the follow-up. These early results were subsequently confirmed in larger series,[27,28] demonstrating that the event rate was more than tenfold greater in patients with reversible thallium defects.[27]

Abnormal pulmonary uptake of thallium, a recognized marker of left ventricular dysfunction during exercise, is also a risk marker in coronary patients without prior myocardial infarction. Gill et al.[29] conducted a long-term follow-up of 525 consecutive patients who underwent exercise thallium scintigraphy. Increased pulmonary uptake was the single best predictor of cardiac death and other cardiac events during the follow-up. Cardiac events occurred in 5% with normal thallium scan; 25% with an abnormal thallium scan but normal lung activity; and 67% with increased thallium lung uptake ($P < 0.0001$). This latter parameter had 51% sensitivity, 92% specificity, 67% positive predictive value, 86% negative predictive value, and 82% diagnostic accuracy. More than 50% of cardiac deaths occurred in patients with abnormal pulmonary uptake.[29]

Resting Radionuclide Angiography

The left ventricular ejection fraction measured at rest after acute myocardial infarction is probably the most important noninvasive single predictor of risk in postmyocardial infarction patients.[2,30–33]

The Multicenter Post-Infarction Research Group[31] provided the most compelling evidence of the importance of the resting ejection fraction as a risk marker for subsequent cardiac death and sudden death after discharge from the hospital. They evaluated 866 patients with both 24-hour Holter monitoring and radionuclide ventriculography. After a mean follow-up of 22 months, 101 patients died; 82% of deaths were of cardiac origin and 37% of these were classified as sudden. Although both ejection fractions below 40% and the frequency of premature complexes were independent risk markers, ejection fraction was the main determinant of survival. Cardiac mortality was inversely related to the resting ejection fraction (Fig. 6). The MILIS study confirmed these results.[32] In a mean follow-up of 18 months, the incidence of sudden death was 11.6% in patients with an ejection fraction below 40% (21/181) and 2.3% in patients with an ejection fraction greater than 40% (8/352). Ahnve et al.[33] demonstrated that when used alone, left ventricular ejection fraction better defined the risk for total cardiac mortality and sudden cardiac death than ventricular arrhythmias. Ejection fraction below 45% had 62% sensitivity and 64% specificity for total cardiac death, and 77% sensitivity and 66% specificity for sudden cardiac death (Fig. 7).

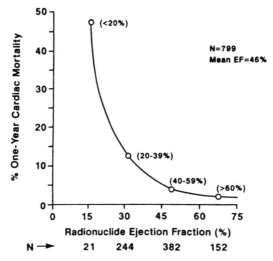

Figure 6. One-year cardiac mortality rate in four categories of radionuclide ejection fraction (EF), determined before discharge. N denotes the total number of patients in the population and in each category (from The Multicenter Postinfarction Research Group[31]).

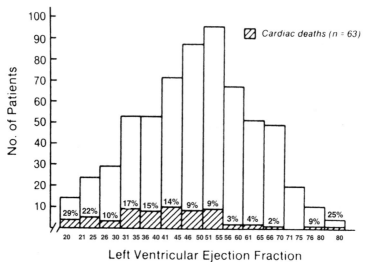

Figure 7. Distribution of discharge left ventricular ejection fraction (LVEF) among patients followed for one year (n = 632). The height of the bars represents the number of patients with LVEF in the interval indicated. The cross-notched portion indicates numbers of patients within the specific interval who suffered a cardiac death during the one-year follow-up. The percentage this represents of the total number of patients within the interval is indicated above the cross-notched portion of the bar (from Ahnve et al.[33]).

Exercise Radionuclide Angiography

The value of exercise and left ventricular ejection fraction has also been demonstrated to affect prognostic value in postmyocardial infarction patients. Corbet et al.[34] analyzed the results of exercise radionuclide ventriculography in 117 patients with uncomplicated myocardial infarction and observed that the change in ejection fraction with submaximal exercise was the most useful parameter for predicting subsequent events. Seventy of 74 patients who failed to increase their ejection fraction with exercise suffered events within six months. In contrast, only 4 of 43 patients who increased their ejection fraction with exercise had events. Dewhurst and Muir,[35] however, demonstrated that a resting ejection fraction of less than 35% identified a high-risk subgroup of patients with poor prognosis. Exercise assessment added little additional prognostic value in these patients. In patients with resting ejection fraction above 35%, a decline in ejection fraction of at least 5% during exercise significantly increased the risk for future events. Other researchers[36,37] suggest that the absolute value of ejection fraction during maximal exercise may be more predictive for prognosis than the change in left ventricular ejection fraction from rest to exercise. Morris et al.[37] observed an expected two-year mortality of 11% in patients with an exercise ejection fraction of 0.50, 25% when ejection fraction was 0.30, and 56% with an ejection fraction of 0.15. The change in ejection fraction with exercise predicted the time to bypass grafting for refractory angina, but not death or nonfatal myocardial infarction. In patients with chronic stable coronary artery disease, the exercise ejection fraction is the most important variable for predicting cardiac death or nonfatal myocardial infarction.[26,27]

Coronary Angiography

In patients with ischemic heart disease, cardiac angiography provides two important prognostic variables: the state of ventricular function and the severity and extent of coronary artery disease. Both the number of major coronary arteries severely obstructed and the degree of left ventricular dysfunction are independent risk markers, the latter exerting the dominant influence.[38,39]

Coronary angiography provides important prognostic implications related to:

A. Number of diseased coronary arteries (> 50% obstruction): Multiple studies demonstrate that survival is determined by the number of severely narrowed vessels. Patients with single-vessel disease experience a low cardiac mortality (< 2%/year) while patients with left main or three-vessel coronary artery disease have a high risk of death (> 10%/year) (Fig. 8). In the CASS registry, the four-year survival of medically treated patients was 92%, 84%, and 68% in patients with one-, two- and three-vessel disease, respectively.[39] Lesions of the main coronary artery are particularly life threatening.[40] Mortality of medically treated patients has been reported as 29% at 18 months,[41] 39% at two years,[42] and 43% at five years.[43]

B. Localization of the obstruction: As Proudfit et al.[44] demonstrated, survival rates were better in patients

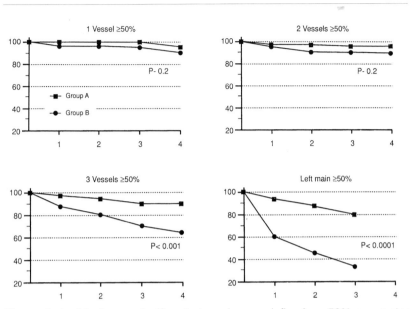

Figure 8. In this figure, significant stenosis was defined as 50% or greater narrowing. Within the one-, two- and three-vessel and left main coronary artery disease categories, the cumulative survival rates of patients in whom all diseased vessels were 75% or greater stenosed (group A) are compared with those in whom one or more of the diseased vessels were only 50% stenosed (group B). Patients with two- and three-vessel disease who were in group B had a mixture of 50% stenosed vessels and 75% or greater stenosed vessels (from Harris et al.[49]).

with right coronary artery disease than those with left anterior descending coronary artery involvement (Table 1).[44] In patients with anterior descending artery disease, proximal obstructions had a worse prognosis.[45–47] Califf et al.[48] reported a survival rate of 98% in patients with lesions after the first septal perforator and 90% in patients with lesions before the first septal perforator. After controlling for the effect of left ventricular ejection fraction on survival, the presence of proximal lesions remained significant ($P = 0.01$).[48]

C. Degree of the obstruction: In addition to the number of narrowed vessels, the severity of obstruction is also an

Table 1

Percent Survival According to the Coronary Artery Involved

Coronary Artery	5 Yr	10 Yr	15 Yr
Right	90	73	66
Circumflex	80	70	64
Left descending	81	56	46

$P < 0.05$ between right and circumflex coronary arteries compared to left anterior descending at 10 and 15 years.

important risk marker. Prognosis in patients with 50% to 75% narrowing is better than in those with more than 75% narrowing,[49] especially in patients with left main or three-vessel coronary artery disease.

Cardiac morbidity following acute myocardial infarction may also be influenced by the patency of the infarct-related artery,[50,51] and the presence of luminal irregularities or ulcerations.[52]

The degree of left ventricular dysfunction is a more important determinant of prognosis than the extent and severity of the lesions.[38,39] Sanz et al.[38] studied 259 consecutive men (< 60 years old) who survived an acute myocardial infarction and were studied within one month after hospital admission. In a mean follow-up of 34 months, 19 patients died, 17 suddenly and 2 of intractable heart failure. Ejection fraction was the best predictor of death. The probability of four years' survival was the best in patients with normal ejection fraction ($> 50\%$) and the worst in those with an ejection fraction below 20% (30% to 75%). The prognosis of patients with an ejection fraction between 21% and 49% was significantly worse (78%) than in those with normal ejection fraction only in the subgroup with three-vessel disease ($P < 0.01$). Similar results were reported in the CASS study[39] of 20,088 medically treated patients with chronic coronary artery disease, 48% of whom had a previous myocardial infarction. Although survival was related to the number of vessels affected, ejection fraction was the best risk factor (Fig. 9).

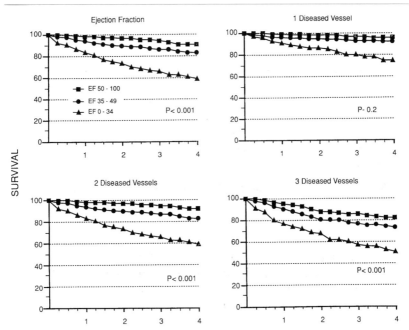

Figure 9. Four-year survival data for patients with at least one-vessel disease, less than 50% left main coronary artery obstruction, and a measured ejection fraction (EF)(from Mock et al.[39]).

Other markers of ventricular dysfunction also play an important role in prognosis. White et al.[53] studied 605 males after recovery from myocardial infarction. During a mean follow-up of 78 months, there were 101 cardiac deaths, 71 of which were sudden. Multivariate analysis demonstrated that left ventricular end-systolic volume was the primary predictor of survival. It was superior to both ejection fraction and severity and extension of the coronary artery lesions.

Finally, many studies have shown that the presence of ventricular aneurysm is a risk marker of malignant ventricular arrhythmias and sudden cardiac death.[54–56] A recent study revealed that decreased left ventricular ejection fraction was the best predictor for total cardiac death and nonsudden cardiac death, whereas sudden cardiac death was better predicted by the presence of left ventricular aneurysm[56] (Fig. 10).

The imaging techniques developed in the last three decades have added immensely to our ability to identify individuals at risk of sudden death. They have, however, not provided the mechanism by which death occurs. Their predictive occurrence also must be

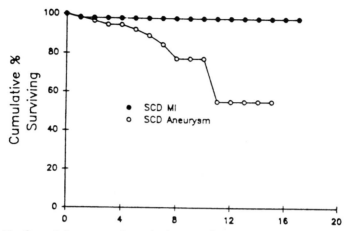

Figure 10. Cumulative percent survival comparing aneurysm and myocardial infarction (MI) groups for sudden cardiac death (SCD) (from Hassapoyannes et al.[56]).

balanced against the risks of individualized medical and surgical therapy.

References

1. Marcus ML, Schelbert HR, Skorton DJ, Wolf GL, eds. *Cardiac Imaging.* Philadelphia: WB Saunders; 1991.
2. DeBusk RF. Specialized testing after recent acute myocardial infarction. *Ann Intern Med* 1989;110:470.
3. Battler A, Karliner JS, Higgins CB, et al. The initial chest x-ray in acute myocardial infarction. Prediction of early and late mortality and survival. *Circulation* 1980;61:1004.
4. Goldstein S, Friedman L, Hutchinson R, et al., and the Aspirin Myocardial Infarction Study Research Group. Timing mechanism and clinical setting of witnessed death in postmyocardial infarction patients. *J Am Coll Cardiol* 1984;3:1111.
5. Fuster V, Gersh BJ, Giuliani ER, et al. The natural history of idiopathic dilated cardiomyopathy. *Am J Cardiol* 1981;47:525.
6. Hammermeister KE, Chikos PM, Fisher L, et al. Relationship of cardiothoracic ratio and plain film heart volume to late survival. *Circulation* 1979;59:89.
7. Sokolow M, Perloff D. The prognosis of essential hypertension treated conservatively. *Circulation* 1961;23:697.
8. Proudfit WL, Bruschke AVG, Sones FM. Natural history of obstructive coronary artery disease: ten-year study of 601 nonsurgical cases. *Prog Cardiovasc Dis* 1978;21:53.

9. Harlan WR, Oberman A, Grimm R, et al. Chronic congestive heart failure in coronary artery disease: Clinical criteria. *Ann Intern Med* 1977;86:133.

10. Shiina A, Tajik AJ, Smith HC, et al. Prognostic significance of regional motion abnormality in patients with prior myocardial infarction: A prospective correlative study of two-dimensional echocardiography and angiography. *Mayo Clin Proc* 1986;61:254.

11. Nishimura RA, Tajik AJ, Shub C, et al. Role of two-dimensional echocardiography in the prediction of in-hospital complications after acute myocardial infarction. *J Am Coll Cardiol* 1984;4:1080.

12. Heger JJ, Weyman AE, Wann LS, et al. Cross-sectional echocardiographic analysis of the extent of left ventricular asynergy in acute myocardial infarction. *Circulation* 1980;61:1113.

13. Gibson RS, Bishop HL, Stamm RB, et al. Value of early two dimensional echocardiography in patients with acute myocardial infarction. *Am J Cardiol* 1982;49:1110.

14. Bhatnagar SK, Al-Yusuf AR. Significance of early two-dimensional echocardiography after acute myocardial infarction. *Int J Cardiol* 1984;5:575.

15. Bhatnager SK, Moussa MAA, Al-Ysuf AR. The role of prehospital discharge two-dimensional echocardiography in determining the prognosis of survivors of first myocardial infarction. *Am Heart J* 1985;109:472.

16. Kan G, Visser CA, Koolen JJ, et al. Short- and long-term predictive value of admission wall-motion score in acute myocardial infarction: A cross-sectional echocardiographic study of 345 patients. *Br Heart J* 1986;56:422.

17. Domingo E, Alvarez A, Garcia del Castillo H, et al. Prognostic value of segmental contractility assessed by cross-sectional echocardiography in first acute myocardial infarction. *Eur Heart J* 1989;10:532.

18. Applegate RJ, Dell'Italia LJ, Crawford MH. Usefulness of two-dimensional echocardiography during low-level exercise testing early after uncomplicated acute myocardial infarction. *Am J Cardiol* 1987;60:10.

19. Ryan T, Amstrong WF, O'Donnell JA, et al. Risk stratification after acute myocardial infarction by means of exercise two-dimensional echocardiography. *Am Heart J* 1989;114:1305.

20. Jaarsma W, Visser CA, Kupper AJ, et al. Usefulness of two-dimensional exercise echocardiography shortly after myocardial infarction. *Am J Cardiol* 1986;57:86.

21. Potkin BN, Bartorelli AL, Gessert JM, et al. Coronary artery imaging with intravascular high-frequence ultrasound. *Circulation* 1990;81:1575.

22. Gibbons RJ. The use of radionuclide techniques for identification of severe coronary disease. *Curr Prob Cardiol* 1989;15:303.

23. Silverman KJ, Becker LC, Bulkley BH, et al. Value of early thallium-201 scintigraphy for predicting mortality in patients with acute myocardial infarction. *Circulation* 1980;61:996.

24. Gibson RS, Watson DD, Craddock GB, et al. Prediction of cardiac events after uncomplicated myocardial infarction: A propective study comparing predischarge exercise thallium-201 scintigraphy and coronary angiography. *Circulation* 1983;68:321.

25. Hung J, Goris ML, Nah E, et al. Comparative value of maximal treadmill testing exercise thallium myocardial perfusion scintigraphy and exercise radionuclide ventriculography for distinguishing high- and low-risk patients soon after myocardial infarction. *Am J Cardiol* 1984; 53:1221.

26. Brown KA, Boucher CA, Okada RD, et al. Prognostic value of exercise thallium-201 imaging in patients presenting for evaluation of chest pain. *J Am Coll Cardiol* 1983;1:994.

27. Staniloff HM, Forrester JS, Berman DS, et al. Prediction of death, myocardial infarction and worsening chest pain using thallium scintigraphy and exercise electrocardiography. *J Nuc Med* 1986;27:1842.

28. Ladenheim ML, Kotler TS, Pollock BH, et al. Incremental prognostic power of clinical history, exercise electrocardiography and myocardial perfusion scintigraphy in suspected coronary artery disease. *Am J Cardiol* 1987;59:270.

29. Gill JB, Ruddy TD, Newell JB, et al. Prognostic importance of thallium uptake by the lungs during exercise in coronary artery disease. *N Engl J Med* 1987;317:1485.

30. Schulze RA Jr, Rouleau J, Rigo P, et al. Ventricular arrhythmias in the late hospital phase of acute myocardial infarction: Relation to left ventricular function detected by gated cardiac blood pool scanning. *Circulation* 1975;52:1006.

31. The Multicenter Postinfarction Research Group. Risk stratification and survival after myocardial infarction. *N Engl J Med* 1983;309:331.

32. Mukharki J, Rude RE, Poole WK, et al, and the MILIS Study Group. Risk factors for sudden death after acute myocardial infarction: Two-year follow-up. *Am J Cardiol* 1984;54:31.

33. Ahnve S, Gilpin E, Henning H, et al. Limitations and advantages of the ejection fraction for defining high risk after acute myocardial infarction. *Am J Cardiol* 1986; 58: 872.

34. Corbett JR, Nicod PH, Huxley RL, et al. Left ventricular function alterations at rest and during submaximal exercise in patients with recent myocardial infarction. *Am J Med* 1983;74:577.

35. Dewhurst NG, Muir AL. Comparative prognostic value of radionuclide ventriculography at rest and during exercise in 100 patients after first myocardial infarction. *Br Heart J* 1983;49:111.

36. Abraham RD, Harris PJ, Roubin GS, et al. Usefulness of ejection fraction response to exercise one month after acute myocardial infarction in predicting coronary anatomy and prognosis. *Am J Cardiol* 1987;60:225.

37. Morris KG, Palmeri ST, Califf RM, et al. Value of radionuclide angiography for predicting specific cardiac events after acute myocardial infarction. *Am J Cardiol* 1985;55:318.

38. Sanz G, Castañer A, Betriu A, et al. Determinants of prognosis in survivors of myocardial infarction: A prospective clinical angiographic study. *N Eng J Med* 1982;306:1065.

39. Mock MB, Ringqvist I, Fisher LD, et al. Survival of medically treated patients in the Coronary Artery Surgery Study. *Circulation* 1982;66:562.

40. Conley MR, Ely R, Kisslo J, et al. The prognostic spectrum of left main stenosis. *Circulation* 1978;57:947.

41. Conti CR, Selvi JH, Christie LG. Left main coronary artery stenosis: Clinical spectrum, pathophysiology and management. *Prog Cardiovasc Dis* 1979;22:73.
42. Talano J, Scanlon P, Meadows W, et al. Influence of surgery on survival in 145 patients with left main coronary artery disease. *Circulation* 1975;51(suppl I):105.
43. Taylor HA, Deumile NJ, Chaitman BR, et al. Asymptomatic left main coronary artery disease in the Coronary Artery Surgery Study (CASS) registry. *Circulation* 1989;79:1171.
44. Proudfit WJ, Bruschke AVG, MacMillan JP, et al. Fifteen-year survival study of patients with coronary artery disease. *Circulation* 1983;68:986.
45. Schulman SP, Achuff SC, Griffit LSC, et al. Prognostic cardiac catheterization variables in survivors of acute myocardial infarction: A five-year prospective study. *J Am Coll Cardiol* 1988;11:1164.
46. DeFeyter PJ, Van Eenice MJ, Dighton DH, et al. Prognostic value of exercise testing, coronary angiography and left ventriculography six to eight weeks after acute myocardial infarction. *Circulation* 1982;66:527.
47. Rahimtoola SH. Left main equivalence is still unproved hypothesis but proximal left anterior descending coronary artery disease is a high risk lesion. *Am J Cardiol* 1984;53:1719.
48. Califf RM, Tomabechi Y, Lee KL, et al. Outcome in one-vessel coronary artery disease. *Circulation* 1983;67:287.
49. Harris PJ, Behar VS, Conley MJ, et al. The prognostic significance of 50% coronary stenosis in medically treated patients with coronary artery disease. *Circulation* 1980;62:240.
50. Cigarroa RG, Lange RA, Hillis LD. Prognosis after acute myocardial infarction in patients with and without residual antegrade coronary blood flow. *Am J Cardiol* 1989;64:155.
51. Dalen JE, Gore JM, Braunwald E, et al, and the TIMI Investigators. Six- and twelve-month follow-up of the phase I thrombolysis in myocardial infarction (TIMI) trial. *Am J Cardiol* 1988;62:179.
52. Ellis S, Alderman EL, Cain K, and the participants of the Coronary Artery Surgery Study (CASS). Morphology of left anterior descending coronary territory lesions as a predictor of anterior myocardial infarction. A CASS registry study. *J Am Coll Cardiol* 1989;13:1481.
53. White HD, Norris RM, Brown MA, et al. Left ventricular end-systolic volume as the major determinant of survival after recovery from myocardial infarction. *Circulation* 1987;76:44.
54. Cohen M, Wiener I, Prichard A, et al. Determinants of ventricular tachycardia in patients with coronary artery disease and ventricular aneurysm: Clinical, hemodynamic and angiographic factors. *Am J Cardiol* 1983;51:61.
55. Kanowky MS, Falcone RA, Dresden CA, et al. Identification of patients with ventricular tachycardia after myocardial infarction: Signal-averaged elctrocardiogram, Holter monitoring, and cardiac catheterization. *Circulation* 1984;70:264.
56. Hassapoyannes CA, Stuck LM, Hornung CA, et al. Effects of left ventricular aneurysm on risk of sudden and nonsudden cardiac death. *Am J Cardiol* 1991;67:454.

Chapter IX

Sudden Death in Ischemic Heart Disease

In this chapter we will review the relationship between sudden cardiac death and the different forms of ischemic heart disease: stable and unstable angina pectoris, silent myocardial ischemia, and myocardial infarction.

Stable Angina Pectoris

Unfortunately, there are few studies examining the incidence of sudden death in patients with stable angina pectoris. Studies published to date only mention total mortality, occasionally noting that "many of the deaths were sudden."

The Framingham study[1] observed an annual mortality of patients with stable effort angina pectoris, with or without previous infarction, of approximately 4%. In other studies the figures are slightly different.[2,3] Graham et al.[3] collected information on the long- term follow-up of 586 patients who survived an initial ischemic event, either unstable angina or myocardial infarction, and observed survival rates at 5, 10, and 15 years of 80%, 61%, and 43%, respectively. The differences between series may be attributed to variations in the study populations. The prognosis varies greatly in relationship to clinical, angiographic, and ergometric parameters, and with the treatment. According to the Veterans Administration Cooperative Study Group,[4] the main clinical factors affecting the prognosis of patients with stable angina pectoris are the severity of

From: S. Goldstein, A. Bayés-de-Luna, J. Guindo-Soldevila: *Sudden Cardiac Death.* Armonk, NY: Futura Publishing Co., Inc., © 1994.

symptoms, presence or absence of electrocardiographic changes, particularly depression of the ST segment, history of previous myocardial infarction, presence of associated arterial hypertension and NYHA functional classification III or IV.

Angiographic Factors

The angiographic extent of coronary arterial disease, as well as the severity of ventricular dysfunction, are major predictors of survival[5] (see Chapter VIII). Angiographic studies have shown that patients with coronary narrowing of over 70% of the left main coronary artery have a high mortality rate.[6–8] In patients who received medical treatment alone, mortality is 29% at 18 months,[6] 39% at 24 months,[7] and 50% at 36 months.[8] In subjects with 50% to 70% obstruction, survival is 91% at 12 months and 66% at 36 months.[8] In contrast to patients with left main coronary artery narrowing, patients with single-vessel disease experience an annual mortality as low as 2%.[5] It is slightly higher in patients with involvement of the left anterior descending or circumflex coronaries than in those with involvement of the right coronary artery.[2] Obstruction of the first portion of the left anterior descending artery, before the first septal artery, presents a worse prognosis (see Chapter VIII).

Exercise Testing

Physical stress is useful in the stratification of patients with stable angina pectoris, with or without previous infarction[9,10] (see Chapter VII). Individuals who reach stage IV of the Bruce protocol or attain heart rates of 160 beats per minute, with or without changes in the ST segment of more than 0.1 mV have a mortality rate in the first year of approximately 2%. However, when effort tests must be interrupted at level I or II of the Bruce protocol, the annual mortality increases to as high as 15% to 20%.[9,10] Exercise thallium scintigraphy which demonstrates a delay in tracer distribution, multiple perfusion defects, and abnormal pulmonary uptake are all markers of poor prognosis[11] (chapter VIII). Patients with chronic ischemic heart disease confirmed by angiography with a normal exercise thallium scintigraphy have an excellent prognosis, despite the existence of chest pain.[12,13] Finally, exercise left ventricular ejection fraction measured by means of radionuclide angiography is also an excellent marker of poor prognosis.[14] Patients with an ejection fraction of greater than 30% that declines during exercise often have critical lesions of the left main coronary artery or three-vessel disease, and present elevated mortality over the next two years.[14]

Unstable Angina Pectoris

Although patients who develop acute myocardial infarction often have clinical antecedents of angina, the outcome of unstable angina is very unpredictable.[15–17] Cardiac mortality rates vary widely in the different studies. As in acute myocardial infarction, mortality rate has decreased in the last years due to more aggressive treatment. Several studies performed in the 1970s and early 1980s demonstrated that the in-hospital mortality of patients with unstable angina is 1%, at 3 months it is 2% to 10%, and after 12 months it is 8% to 18%.[15,16] In contrast, in a recent study including 468 patients, mortality was 4% during the first year, and greater than 20% at five years.[18] Patients who continue to experience repeated episodes of angina after 48 hours of intensive pharmacologic treatment have an increased mortality rate.[17–19] Recent studies by Gottlieb et al.[20,21] and Nademanee et al.[22] demonstrate that frequent episodes of silent myocardial ischemia during unstable angina detected in Holter monitoring are a marker of unfavorable outcome.

Coronary Spasm

The role of coronary arterial spasm in stable and unstable angina and its relationship to intra-arterial platelet thrombi is unclear. The occurrence of coronary spasm can produce severe myocardial ischemia, which can result in alterations in ventricular function and myocardial excitability (Fig. 1) and can sometimes lead to myo-cardial infarction or sudden death.[23–25] This increased incidence of mortality due to coronary artery spasm occurs in patients with unstable angina during the first six months of follow-up, and particularly during the first month.[26,27] Satisfactory stabilization of spasm can be achieved with calcium antagonists or nitroglycerin preparations.

We studied 20 apparently stable ambulatory patients with episodes of coronary spasm manifested by ST elevation (Fig. 1). In a

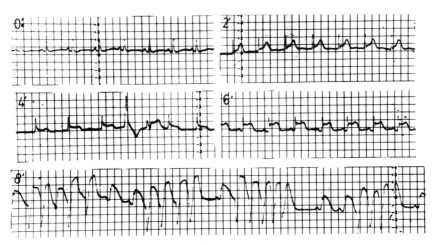

Figure 1. Sequence of an attack of Prinzmetal angina with the appearance of ventricular tachycardia runs at the moment of maximum ST segment elevation (from Bayes-de-Lana, et al [23]).

mean follow-up of 7.3 ± 2.5 years, one patient experienced sudden death that occurred at six months after the initial onset of symptoms.[23] This low incidence of sudden death may be explained by the fact that most of these patients were seen as outpatients in a stable condition and calcium antagonist treatment was begun immediately.

Acute Myocardial Infarction

Most patients who die suddenly exhibit evidence of a previous myocardial infarction. In contrast, evidence of new myocardial necrosis is observed in only 20% of those who experience sudden death.

The natural history of acute myocardial infarction has changed with the development of new techniques and the introduction of thrombolytic therapy. In studies published during the early 1980s, the in-hospital mortality in acute myocardial infarction approximated 20%.[28,29] About 10% of patients discharged from the hospital die in the first year of follow-up.[30–33] Of these, death is sudden in approximately 50% of cases.[30–33] In contrast, reports in the last four years[34–37] report in-hospital mortality rates of approximately 15%, with an additional 3% during the first year after discharge (Table 1).

Observations made by the Minnesota Heart Survey[38] suggest that improvement of survival for both males and females has oc-

Table 1

Cardiac Mortality of Postmyocardial Infarction Patients after Hospital Discharge

Trial	Cardiac Mortality	Sudden Death	Follow-Up
GISSI II[34]	2.6%	1.1%	6 months
TIMI II[35]	1.2%	—	42 days
CAST[36]	2.3%	1.2%	300 days
STSD[37]	7.7%	4%	28 months

curred between 1970 and 1985. The three-year mortality for both males and females decreased in 1970 to 1985 (Figs. 2 and 3). The incidence of sudden death is lower than 2%, although it varies greatly according to different subgroups. In patients with a very low ejection fraction and frequent or complex ventricular arrhythmias which represent less than 5% of all patients, the risk of sudden death during the first year is between 10% and 15%.

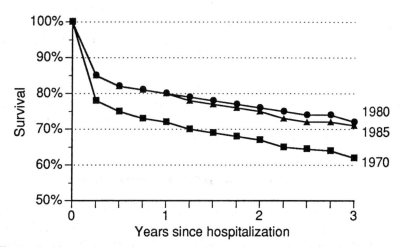

Figure 2. Years since hospitalization. Three-year survival among twin cities (Minneapolis and St. Paul, MN) males hospitalized with definite myocardial infarction in 1970, 1980, and 1985: The Minnesota Heart Survey (McGovern et al.[38]).

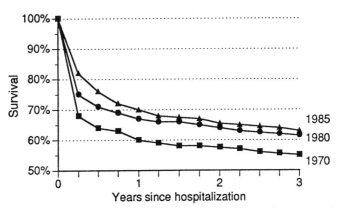

Figure 3. Years since hospitalization. Three-year survival among twin cities (Minneapolis and St. Paul, MN) females hospitalized with definite myocardial infarction in 1970, 1980, and 1985: The Minnesota Heart Survey (McGovern et al.[38]).

Patients who exhibit ventricular conduction disorders, particularly right bundle branch block in the acute phase of infarction,[39] together with sustained ventricular tachycardia or ventricular fibrillation after the acute phase of myocardial infarction, have a much higher total and sudden death mortality (see Chapter VII).

We can use a number of different techniques to identify the post-myocardial infarction patients at risk of malignant ventricular arrhythmias and sudden cardiac death. The existence and severity of left ventricular dysfunction, residual ischemia, and electrical instability are all important factors. Since sudden cardiac death is a multifactorial problem, the detection of different triggers or markers determines those patients at risk. The combined use of different parameters greatly improves the sensitivity and specificity of the prediction of sudden death[40–42] (see Chapters II and VII).

Silent Myocardial Ischemia

In the last few years, numerous studies have investigated the prognostic value of silent myocardial ischemia in the general population and in different clinical forms of ischemic heart disease[43] (Fig. 4). Studies have demonstrated a link between the frequency and duration of episodes of silent myocardial ischemia and sudden death.[44,45] Nevertheless, the role of silent myocardial ischemia in

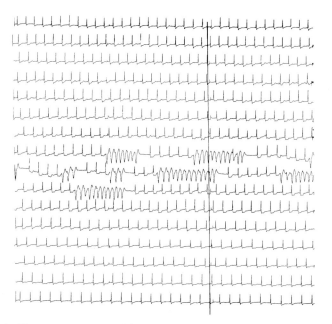

Figure 4. The occurrence of ST segment elevation preceding nonsustained ventricular tachycardia recorded during ambulatory electrocardiogram.

sudden cardiac death remains unclear. That silent myocardial is-chemia can trigger sudden death, as in the case of malignant ventricular arrhythmia preceded by ST segment depression, is a clear possibility. An indirect association can occur in which sudden death occurs in the presence of silent ischemia. A direct relationship, however, requires a cause and effect mechanism. While the indirect relationship suggests that silent myocardial ischemia can lead to sudden death, this may be an associated phenomenon only.

It is undoubtedly important to determine the relationship between silent myocardial ischemia and sudden cardiac death since treatment directed at suppressing silent ischemia may influence sudden ischemic episodes and death, particularly if the relationship is direct.

Reports of silent ischemia and sudden death have been published as isolated cases[44,45] and represent a relatively small percentage of cases in both Gomes et al.[46] and our own series of ambulatory sudden death recorded with Holter devices.[47,48] Sharma et al.[49] and Warnes and Roberts[50] observed sudden cardiac death in patients with silent myocardial ischemia. The Framingham study[51,52] suggests that silent myocardial ischemia can be the triggering mechanism in cases of sudden death appearing as painless myocardial infarction. Nevertheless, the importance of silent myocardial ischemia as a mechanism of sudden death remains uncertain.

The prognostic significance of silent myocardial ischemia depends upon its clinical setting. In the general population Erikssen and Thaulow[53] studied 2014 males between 45 and 59 years old, and detected 50 patients with silent myocardial ischemia occurring during exercise testing. Three of these individuals died suddenly during a follow-up of 8.5 years. Hickman et al.[54] observed 78 males with silent myocardial ischemia, three of whom died in a three-year follow-up, again showing an annual mortality rate close to 1%. In patients with stable angina pectoris, Mody et al.[55] demonstrated that subjects with over 60 minutes of silent ischemia per day had more severe angiographic abnormalities and thus, an unfavorable prognosis. More recently, Rocco et al.[56] demonstrated that silent myocardial ischemia is associated with a higher mortality rate and cardiac events in patients with stable coronary artery disease. Gottlieb et al.[20,21] and Nademanee et al.[22] observed that in unstable angina, the presence of silent myocardial ischemia is a marker of poor prognosis in spite of intensive medical treatment. This is particularly true when silent ischemia lasts for more than 60 minutes per day. Silent ischemia represented approximately 35% of all ischemic episodes in patients with vasospastic angina.[23] The presence of ventricular arrhythmias during attacks is related to the degree of ST segment elevation and the duration of the crisis. Arrhythmias were presumed to be due to reperfusion in about 30% of cases. Myerburg[57] observed episodes of silent ischemia and coronary spasm in 356 survivors of out-of-hospital cardiac arrest. In all five patients, arrhythmic events were observed to be associated with induced spasm and ischemia. Maseri et al.[58,59] observed that in 7000 episodes of ST segment elevations recorded in patients admitted to the coronary unit, 70% occurred without pain. The importance of silent myocardial ischemia occurring immediately after a myocardial infarction is not yet established. The occurrence of silent ischemia during an exercise stress test has a negative prognostic value. Theroux et al.[60] observed an incidence of sudden death in patients with depression of the ST segment during exercise testing of 16%. It was independent of the presence of anginal pain. Tzivoni et al.[61] reported that the presence of ST depression on Holter monitoring in postmyocardial infarction patients, with or without positive exercise testing, is a marker of poor prognosis. In a review of the relationship of arrhythmic sudden death and silent ischemia, Stern and Tzivoni were unable to establish a close relationship although the conceded the importance of ischemia as a mechanism of sudden death.[62] Moss[63] recently reported that angina, but not silent ischemia detected by exercise testing, Holter ECG, or other techniques, is a predictor of poor outcome in postmyocardial infarction patients. We must wait for the results of ongoing large scale trials to know the actual role of silent ischemia in risk assessment after myocardial infarction.

In summary, an indirect relationship between myocardial ischemia and sudden cardiac death clearly exists.[64] However, a direct relationship between silent ischemia is present in but a few instances when the cause of sudden cardiac death is ventricular fibrillation. Ambulatory sudden death occurring in coronary patients with silent ischemia often have other markers of a vulnerable myocardium. A new exacerbation of silent or symptomatic ischemia can explain some, but not all, cases of ambulatory sudden death. It is therefore necessary to search for other triggering mechanisms in order to explain all instances of ambulatory sudden death. Further studies are required to determine the interactions between triggers such as ventricular arrhythmias and the vulnerable myocardium.

References

1. Kannel WB, Feinlieb M. Natural history of angina pectoris in the Framingham study: Progress and survival. *Am J Cardiol* 1972;29:154.
2. Frank CW, Weinblatt W, Shapiro S. Angina pectoris in men: Prognostic significance of related medical factors. *Circulation* 1973;47:509.
3. Graham I, Mulcahy R, Hickey N, et al. Natural history of coronary heart disease: A study of 586 men surviving an initial acute attack. *Am Heart J* 1983;105:249.
4. Detre K, Peduzzi P, Murphy M, et al. Effect of bypass surgery on survival in patients with low- and high-risk groups delineated by the use of simple clinical variables. *Circulation* 1981;63:1329.
5. Reeves TJ. Relation and independence of angina pectoris and sudden death in persons with coronary atherosclerotic heart disease. *J Am Coll Cardiol* 1985;5:167B.
6. Conti CR, Selby JH, Christie LG. Left main coronary artery stenosis: Clinical spectrum pathophysiology and management. *Prog Cardiovasc Dis* 1979;22:73.

7. Talano J, Scanlon P, Meadows W, et al. Influence of surgery on survival in 145 patients with left main coronary artery disease. *Circulation* 1975;52(suppl I):105.

8. Conley MJ, Ely RL, Kisslo J, et al. The prognostic spectrum of left main stenosis. *Circulation* 1978;57:947.

9. Dagenais GR, Rouleau JR, Christen A, Fabia J. Survival of patients with a strongly positive exercise electrocardiogram. *Circulation* 1982; 65:452.

10. McNeer JF, Margolis JR, Lee KL, et al. The role of the exercise test in the evaluation of patients with ischemic heart disease. *Circulation* 1978;57:64.

11. Rutherford JD, Braunwald E. Chronic ischemic heart disease. In: Braunwald E, ed. *Heart Disease: A Textbook of Cardiovascular Medicine.* Philadelphia: WB Saunders; 1992;1292.

12. Wahl J, Hakki AH, Iskadrian AS. Prognostic implications of normal exercise thalium-201 images. *Arch Intern Med* 1985;145:253.

13. Pamelia FX, Gibson RS, Watson DD, et al. Prognosis with chest pain and normal thallium-201 exercise scintigrams. *Am J Cardiol* 1985; 55:920.

14. Beller GA, Gibson RS, Watson DD. Radionuclide methods of identifying patients who may require coronary artery bypass surgery. *Circulation* 1985;72(suppl V):9.

15. Roberts KB, Califf RM, Harrell FE, et al. The prognosis for patients with new-onset angina who have undergone cardiac catheterization. *Circulation* 1983;68:970.

16. Gazes PC, Mobley EM, Faris HM, et al. Preinfarction (unstable) angina: A prospective study: Ten year follow-up. Prognostic significance of electrocardiographic changes. *Circulation* 1973;48:331.

17. Mulcahy R, Awadhi AHA, deBuitleor M, et al. Natural history and prognosis of unstable angina. *Am Heart J* 1985;109:753.

18. Parisi AF, Khuri S, Deupree RH, et al. Medical compared with surgical treatment of unstable angina: 5-year mortality and morbidity in the Veterans Administration study. *Circulation* 1989;80:1176.

19. Victor MF, Likoff MJ, Mintz GS, et al. Unstable angina pectoris of new onset: A prospective clinical and arteriographic study of 75 patients. *Am J Cardiol* 1981;47:228.

20. Gottlieb LS, Weisfeldt M, Ouyang P, et al. Silent ischemia as a marker for early unfavorable outcomes in patients with unstable angina. *N Engl J Med* 1986;314:1214.

21. Gottlieb SO, Weisfeldt ML, Ouyang P, et al. Silent ischemia predicts infarction and death during 2 years follow-up of unstable angina. *J Am Coll Cardiol* 1987;10:756.

22. Nademanee K, Intarachot V, Josephson M, et al. Prognostic significance of silent myocardial ischemia in patients with unstable angina. *J Am Coll Cardiol* 1987;10:1.

23. Bayés de Luna A, Carreras F, Cladellas M, et al. Holter ECG study of the electrocardiographic phenomena in Prinzmetal angina attacks with enphasis on the study of ventricular arrhythmias. *J Electrocardiol* 1985;18:267.

24. Puddu PE, Bourassa M, Waters DD, et al. Sudden death in two patients with variant angina and apparently minimal fixed coronary stenoses. *J Electrocardiol* 1983;16:213.
25. Miller DD, Waters DD, Szlachcic J, et al. Clinical characteristics associated with sudden death in patients with variant angina. *Circulation* 1982;66:588.
26. Waters DD, Szlachcic J, Miller DD, et al. Clinical characteristics of patients with variant angina complicated by myocardial infarction or death within one month. *Am J Cardiol* 1982;49:658.
27. Severi S, Davies G, Maseri A, et al. Long-term prognosis of variant angina with medical treatment. *Am J Cardiol* 1980;46:226.
28. Rosenthal ME, Oseran DS, Gang E, et al. Sudden cardiac death following acute myocardial infarction. *Am Heart J* 1985;109:865.
29. Moss AJ. Prognosis after myocardial infarction. *Am J Cardiol* 1982; 52:667.
30. Kannel WB, Sorlie P, McNamara PM. Prognosis after initial myocardial infarction: The Framingham study. *Am J Cardiol* 1979;44:53.
31. Mukharji J, Rude RE, Poole WK, et al. and the MILIS study group. Risk factors of sudden death after acute myocardial infarction: Two year follow-up. *Am J Cardiol* 1984;54:31.
32. Bigger JT, Fleiss JL, Kleiger R, et al. The Multicenter Postinfarction Research Group: The relationships among ventricular arrhythmias, left ventricular dysfunction, and mortality in the 2 years after myocardial infarction. *Circulation* 1984;69:250.
33. The Multicenter Postinfarction Research Group. Risk stratification and survival after myocardial infarction. *N Engl J Med* 1983;309:331.
34. Gruppo Italiano per lo Studio della Sopravvivenza nell' Infarto miocardico: GISSI-2. A factorial randomized trial of alteplase versus streptokinase and heparin versus no heparin among 12,490 patients with acute myocardial infarction. *Lancet* 1990;336:65.
35. The TIMI Study Group. Comparison of invasive and conservative strategies after treatment with intravenous tissue plasminogen activator in acute myocardial infarction. *N Engl J Med* 1989;320:618.
36. CAST Investigators. Preliminary Report: Effect of encainide and flecainide on mortality in a randomised trial of arrhythmia suppression after myocardial infarction. *N Eng J Med* 1989;321:406.
37. Navarro-Lopez F, Cosin J, Marrugat J, Guindo J, Bayés de Luna A, Navarro-Lopez F, et al. for Spanish Trial of Sudden Death (SSSD) Investigators. Comparison of the effects of amiodarone versus metoprolo on the frequency of ventricular arrhythmias and mortality after acute myocardial infarction. *Am J Cardiol* 1993;72:1243.
38. McGovern PG, Folsom AR, Sprafka M, et al. Trends in survival of hospitalized myocardial infarction patients between 1970 and 1985: The Minnesota Heart Survey. *Circulation* 1991;85:172.
39. Lie KL, Lien KL, Schullenberg RM, et al. Early identification of patients developing late in-hospital ventricular fibrillation after discharge from the coronary care unit. *Am J Cardiol* 1978;41:674.
40. Gomes JA, Winters SL, Stewart D, et al. A new noninvasive index to predict sustained ventricular tachycardia and sudden death in the first

year after myocardial infarction: Based on signal-averaged electrocardiogram, radionuclide ejection fraction, and Holter monitoring. *J Am Coll Cardiol* 1987;10:349.

41. Kuchar DL, Thorburn CW, Sammel NL. Prediction of serious arrhythmic events after myocardial infarction: Signal-averaged electrocardiogram, Holter monitoring and radionuclide ventriculography. *J Am Coll Cardiol* 1987;9:531.

42. Cripps T, Bennet D, Camm J, Ward D. Prospective evaluation of clinical assessment, exercise testing and signal-averaged electrocardiogram in predicting outcome after acute myocardial infarction. *Am J Cardiol* 1988;62:995.

43. Cohn PF, ed. *Silent Myocardial Ischemia and Infarction.* New York: Marcel Dekker, Inc; 1989.

44. Hong R, Bhandari A, McKay C, et al. Life-threatening ventricular tachycardial and fibrillation induced by painless myocardial ischemia during exercise test. *JAMA* 1987;257:1937.

45. Gradman AH, Bell PA, DeBusj RF. Sudden death during ambulatory monitoring: Clinical and electrocardiographic correlations. Report of a case. *Circulation* 1977;55:210.

46. Gomes JA, Alexopoulos D, Winters SL, et al. The role of silent ischemia, the arrhythmic substrate and the short-long sequence in the genesis of sudden cardiac death. *J Am Coll Cardiol* 1989;14:1618.

47. Bayés de Luna A, Guindo J, Rivera I. Ambulatory sudden death in patients wearing Holter devices. *J Amb Monitor* 1989;2:3.

48. Bayés de Luna A, Coumel Ph, Leclercq JF. Ambulatory sudden death: Mechanisms of production of fatal arrhythmia on the basis of data from 157 cases. *Am Heart J* 1989;117:151.

49. Sharma B, Asinger R, Francis G, et al. Demonstration of exercise-induced painless myocardial ischemia in survivors of out-of-hospital ventricular fibrillation. *Am J Cardiol* 1987;59:740.

50. Warnes C, Roberts W. Sudden coronary death: Relation of amount and distribution of coronary narrowing at necropsy to previous symptoms of myocardial ischemia, left ventricular scarring and heart weight. *Am J Cardiol* 1984;54:65.

51. Kannel WB, Abbot RD. Incidence and prognosis of unrecognized myocardial infarction: An update on the Framingham study. *N Eng J Med* 1984;311:1144.

52. Kannel WB. Silent myocardial ischemia and infarction: Insights from the Framingham study. *Cardiol Clin* 1986;4:583.

53. Erikssen J, Thaulow E. Follow-up of patients with asymptomatic myocardial ischemia. In: Rutishauser W, Roskman H, eds. *Silent Myocardial Ischemia.* Berlin: Springer Verlag; 1984;156.

54. Hickman JR, Uhl GS, Cook RL, et al. A natural history study of asymptomatic coronary disease. *Am J Cardiol* 1980;45:422.

55. Mody F, Nademanee K, Interachot V, et al. Prognostic significance of silent ischemia in chronic stable angina based on correlations with coronary angiography. *Circulation* 1987;76(suppl IV):78.

56. Rocco MB, Nabel EG, Campbell S, et al. Prognostic significance of myocardial ischemia detected by ambulatory monitoring in patients with stable coronary artery disease. *Circulation* 1988;78:877.

57. Myerburg RJ, Kessler KM, Mallon SM, et al. Life-threatening ventricular arrhythmias in patients with silent myocardial ischemia due to coronary artery spasm. *N Engl J Med* 1992;326:1451.
58. Maseri A. Role of coronary artery spasm in symptomatic and silent myocardial ischemia. *J Am Coll Cardiol* 1987;8:249.
59. Maseri A, Severi S, Marzullo P. Role of coronary arterial spasm in sudden coronary ischemic death. *Ann NY Acad Sci* 1982;382:204.
60. Théroux P, Waters DD, Halphen C, et al. Prognostic value of exercised testing soon after myocardial infarction. *N Engl J Med* 1979;301:341.
61. Tzivoni D, Gavish A, Gottlieb S, et al. Prognostic significance of ischemic episodes in patients with previous myocardial infarction. *Am J Cardiol* 1988;62:661.
62. Stern S, Tzivoni D. Ventricular arrhythmias, sudden death, and silent myocardial ischemia. *Prog Cardiovasc Dis* 1992;35:19.
63. Goldstein RE, Moss AJ, Greenberg H, et al. Prognosis in patients with silent myocardial ischemia after recovery from a myocardial infarction. *Circulation* 1992;86:I115.
64. Bayés de Luna A, Guindo J, Viñolas X. Do silent myocardial ischemia and ventricular arrhythmias interact to result in sudden death? *Cardiol Clin* 1992;10:449.

Chapter X

Sudden Death in Cardiomyopathies

Sudden death has been studied mainly in dilated and hypertrophic cardiomyopathy. The close relationship between impaired ventricular function and malignant ventricular ectopy provides a fertile pathophysiological environment in which sudden death can occur. It may also occur in the natural history of other less well-known myopathic syndromes such as arrhythmogenic right ventricular dysplasia and cardiomyopathies secondary to amyloidosis and chronic alcoholism.

Dilated Cardiomyopathy

Dilated cardiomyopathy is becoming increasingly more common. It is estimated that approximately 7.5 cases per 100,000 inhabitants occur each year[1-4] The one-year mortality rate varies between 10% to 50%, depending upon the New York Heart Association (NYHA) functional class.[5-8] The natural history of patients with dilated cardiomyopathy is uncertain. Some patients experience an accelerated course while others may experience a striking improvement and stabilization.[3] Fuster et al.[3] followed 104 patients with idiopathic dilated cardiomyopathy from 6 to 20 years. Eighty patients died (77%), with two-thirds of the deaths occurring within the first two years after diagnosis (Fig. 1). In contrast, the condition of most of the remaining patients subjectively improved and stabilized. Eighteen of 24 survivors had clinical improvement and a normal or

From: S. Goldstein, A. Bayés-de-Luna, J. Guindo-Soldevila: *Sudden Cardiac Death.* Armonk, NY: Futura Publishing Co., Inc., © 1994.

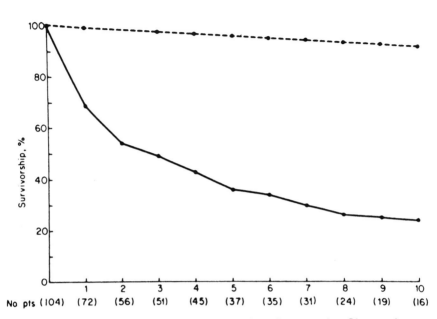

Figure 1. Natural history of idiopathic dilated cardiomyopathy. Observed survival plotted against time in years in 104 patients (pts) with the diagnosis of idiopathic dilated cardiomyopathy (solid line). The dashed line represents the control expected survival, on the basis of age and sex distribution, according to the death rates of the Minnesota 1970 White Population Life Table. The number of alive patients under observation at each follow-up interval is indicated in parentheses (from Fuster et al.[3]).

reduced heart size.[3] The natural history of dilated cardiomyopathy in children is similar to adults. Akagi et al.[4] investigated 25 children with a mean age of 9.6 years with dilated cardiomyopathy and symptoms of congestive heart failure. During an average follow-up of 15.6 months, 18 children (72%) died, 14 (78%) of whom died within the first year.[4]

In the United States about 10,000 people die annually as a result of dilated cardiomyopathy.[9] It has been estimated that approximately 50% of these deaths are sudden.[5,8–20] Table 1 shows the annual incidence of sudden cardiac death in 13 series of patients with dilated cardiomyopathy.[9–20] The mean frequency of sudden death is 44%. The occurrence of sudden death is particularly devastating in patients with mild symptoms[21,22] and in those patients with severe left ventricular dysfunction who are awaiting cardiac transplantation.[22] Stevenson et al.[22] investigated the outcome of 615 patients

Table 1

Sudden Death in Patients with Dilated Cardiomyopathy

Study	Patients (n)	Mortality Total	Sudden	Percentage of Sudden Death
Von Olshausen et al.[9]	60	7	3	43
Chakko & Gheorghiade[10]	43	16	10	63
Huang et al.[11]	35	4	2	50
Wilson et al.[12]	77	50	19	38
Holmes et al.[13]	31	14	12	86
Meinhertz et al.[14]	74	19	12	63
Francis.[15]	159	73	46	63
V-HEFT*	346	145	80	55
Maskin et al.[16]	35	25	1	4
Sukaurai & Kawai.[17]	190	87	19	22
Massie et al.[18]	56	29	10	34
Lee & Packer.[19]	203	155	58	37
Franciosa et al.[20]	182	88	40	45
Total	1491	712	312	44

*Results from Francis.[15]

with advanced heart failure referred for cardiac transplantation. Transplant was deemed appropriate in 53% of patients. While on the transplant list, with an average waiting time of 152 ± 133 days, sudden death occurred in 15% of patients and represented 75% of all deaths. In 288 patients who were not candidates for transplantation, the six-month survival was 80%. In these patients followed over one year, 15% died suddenly and accounted for 19% of all deaths (Fig. 2). Patients with a history of ventricular arrhythmias may require aggressive antiarrhythmic therapy, including automatic defibrillator, in order to avoid sudden death until symptoms become severe enough to indicate transplantation.[22]

Patients with dilated cardiomyopathy have an increased incidence of both spontaneous[9-20] and induced[23-25] ventricular arrhythmias. In a review of 701 patients by Francis et al.,[15] 87% of patients had multiform ventricular premature complexes and 54% had runs of ventricular tachycardia (Table 2). The possible mechanisms that

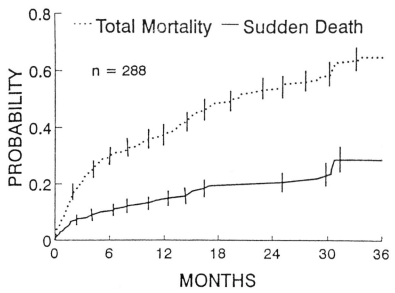

Figure 2. Actuarial risk for all causes of mortality (dotted line) and sudden death (solid line) in 288 patients with advanced heart failure who were not candidates for cardiac transplantation. All patients were stabilized on medical therapy and discharged to their homes. One standard error is indicated by the vertical bar (from Stevenson et al.[22]).

Table 2

Complex Ventricular Arrhythmias in Patients with Dilated Cardiomyopathy

Study	Patients (n)	Lown Classification 3 & 4A	4B
Von Olshausen et al.[9]	60	95	80
Chakko & Gheorghiade.[10]	43	88	51
Huang et al.[11]	35	93	60
Wilson et al.[12]	77	71	50
Holmes et al.[13]	31	87	49
Meinertz et al.[14]	74	87	49
Maskin et al.[16]	34	92	71
V-HEFT.*	346	81	28
Total	701	87%	54%

*Results from Francis.[5]

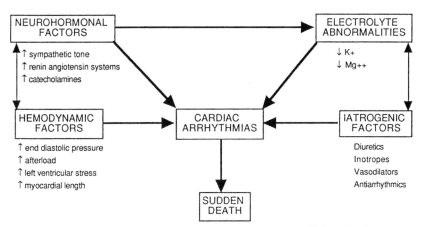

Figure 3. Pathogenesis of arrhythmias in patients with heart failure.

trigger malignant ventricular arrhythmias and sudden death in these patients were uncertain (Fig. 3). The most important hemodynamic predictor was an increase in the end-diastolic pressure. Neurohormonal activation can also increase cardiac arrhythmic automatism, produce electrolyte abnormalities, and facilitate the appearance of ventricular arrhythmias. Lastly, patients with heart failure are especially prone to develop proarrhythmia in response to many drugs used in the treatment of heart failure. Antiarrhythmics, inotropic agents, and diuretics may precipitate the appearance of ventricular arrhythmias (Fig. 3).

The predictive value of ventricular arrhythmias detected on ambulatory electrocardiographic recording for sudden death in patients with dilated cardiomyopathy is debatable. Its importance varies greatly from one series to another (Table 3). While some researchers consider the presence of arrhythmias a marker of risk of sudden death,[10,13,14] others have found no significant differences.[9,11,12] In a study of 74 patients with dilated cardiomyopathy followed for 11 months, Meinertz et al.[14] found that 75% of the patients who died suddenly presented more than 20 pairs or runs of ventricular tachycardia in a 24-hour ambulatory electrocardiographic recording, while patients who died from heart failure did not. In contrast, Olshausen et al.[9,26] studied 73 patients with dilated cardiomyopathy for over three years and found a mortality rate of 38%, half due to sudden death and half due to heart failure. The only marker of sudden death was a low ejection fraction (< 40%) and the presence of left bundle branch block. The presence of ventricular arrhythmias did not identify patients at increased risk. Two important reasons may

Table 3

Influence of Ventricular Arrhythmias On the Survival of Patients with Dilated Cardiomyopathy

Study	Patients (n)	Mean Follow-up (months)	Conclusions
Von Olshausen et al.[9]	60	12	No association
Chakko & Gheorghiada[10]	43	16	Association
Huang et al.[11]	35	34	No association
Wilson et al.[12]	77	12	No association
Holmes et al.[13]	43	14	Association
Meinertz et al.[14]	74	11	Association

explain the lack of relation between ambulatory ventricular arrhythmias and sudden death in patients with dilated cardiomyopathy.[27] First, complex ventricular arrhythmias may be a nonspecific manifestation of a dying left ventricle rather than an indication of a specific arrhythmogenic substrate. In the Captopril-Digoxin Multicenter Trial,[28] asymptomatic ventricular tachycardia in patients receiving placebo was a marker of hemodynamic and clinical instability and sudden death. In that study, asymptomatic runs of ventricular tachycardia reflected the severity of the underlying defect in cardiac function more accurately than ejection fraction or exercise tolerance. Secondly, in patients with dilated cardiomyopathy, sudden death may be related to events other than malignant ventricular tachyarrhythmias. The final event before sudden death in patients with advanced heart failure is different from that preceding sudden death in the general population. Bradyarrhythmia or electromechanical dissociation are more common in patients with advanced heart failure.[29] In a study of 21 unexpected cardiac arrests occurring in monitored heart failure patients who were stable, awaiting discharge after transplant evaluation, 38% of patients had ventricular tachycardia or fibrillation at the time of arrest. The remaining patients had severe sinus bradycardia, atrioventricular block, or electromechanical dissociation. In our study of ambulatory sudden death,[30] most patients who died of bradyarrhythmias had a history of advanced heart failure (Chapter III). Lethal bradyarrhythmias and electromechanical dissociation can be triggered by circulatory reflexes that are evoked by sudden increases in intraventricular pressure and volume, which are likely to occur during the terminal stages of contractile failure.[27,31]

Ventricular arrhythmia suppression with antiarrhythmic drugs does not reduce mortality in patients with heart failure.[32] Three main limitations of antiarrhythmic treatment explain the lack of efficacy in these patients. Several studies have shown the decreased efficacy of antiarrhythmic drugs in patients with dilated cardiomyopathy.[33–37] It has also been shown[37] that in spite of preventing tachyarrhythmia, sudden death was not prevented. It is well known that the lower the ejection fraction, the more difficult it is to suppress ventricular ectopy and the greater the number of therapeutic failures. There is also a greater risk of proarrhythmias.[38] Proarrhythmic events are more common in the setting of a severely depressed myocardium, electrolyte and neurohormonal alterations, and with treatments with inotropic drugs and diuretics. In addition, a number of antiarrhythmic drugs have a significant negative inotropic effect.[39–41]

Antiarrhythmic treatment is therefore justified only in patients with dilated cardiomyopathy and symptomatic ventricular arrhythmias such as syncope or previous resuscitated arrest. In those cases, a history of sustained ventricular tachycardia or ventricular fibrillation and, in some cases, with salvos of rapid and frequent ventricular tachycardia, amiodarone has proven to be an efficient drug, with a good hemodynamic tolerance[42,43] (Chapter XVII). In patients with overt heart failure, type I antiarrhythmic agents should not be used due to their negative inotropic effect and risk of proarrhythmia. In patients with ventricular fibrillation and depressed ejection fraction, nonpharmacological techniques[44–46] are required, particularly an implanted defibrillator[44,45] (Chapter XVIII).

Arrhythmogenic Right Ventricular Dysplasia

Right ventricular dysplasia is a special form of cardiomyopathy characterized by a decrease in right ventricular wall thickness, disappearance of contractile cells, and partial or total replacement of a portion of the right ventricular musculature with adipose and fibrous tissue.[47,48] In its extreme, Uhl's anomaly, there is apposition of endocardial and epicardial layers of the affected areas.[49,50] It is more common in men than in women, and in the young. Patients may present signs and symptoms of right ventricular failure and very often some type of ventricular arrhythmias, including sustained ventricular tachycardia of left bundle branch block morphology.

Sustained ventricular tachycardia or ventricular fibrillation, syncope, and sudden death are frequently associated with exercise.[51–54] Although arrhythmogenic right ventricular dysplasia is not classically considered a major cause of sudden death in young athletes,[55] it has been responsible for 20% of sudden deaths in one series.[56]

Although these patients often have premature ventricular complexes and even sustained ventricular tachycardia during electrocardiographic recording, there is a relatively low incidence of ventricular fibrillation and sudden death. Leclerq and Coumel[51] recently published their experience with 58 patients with arrhythmogenic right ventricular dysplasia and severe ventricular arrhythmias. Although sustained ventricular tachycardia was present in 50 patients, ventricular fibrillation occurred only in three, and nonsustained ventricular tachycardia in seven. After a mean follow-up of 8.8 years only four cardiac deaths occurred: three due to acute heart failure and only one due to recurrent ventricular fibrillation. Similar results were reported by Marcus et al.[52] However, Thiene at al.[53] suggest that arrhythmogenic right ventricular dysplasia represents 10% to 15% of total sudden deaths in postmortem studies performed in patients under 35 years. In many, sudden death was the first manifestation of the disease. Thus, it is possible that two different subgroups of patients exist: one composed of young people in whom sudden death may be the first manifestation of the disease, and another composed of young adults with symptomatic recurrent sustained ventricular tachycardias, but with a relatively low risk of sudden death.

There is no uniform opinion regarding treatment.[48,57–61] If the patient demonstrates frequent and symptomatic salvos of ventricular tachycardia without syncope or out-of-hospital cardiac arrest, flecainide, propafenone, sotalol, or amiodarone may be useful.[57] The best results probably are achieved with sotalol. If there is evidence of syncope or cardiac arrest, an electrophysiological study should be carried out with endomyocardial mapping to evaluate the possibility of electrode catheter ablation[58,59] or surgical therapy.[60,61] If it is not possible to carry out either of these techniques or if sustained ventricular tachycardia is still inducible, the implantation of an automatic defibrillator together with pharmacological treatment is justified (Chapters XVII and XVIII).

Hypertrophic Cardiomyopathy

Hypertrophic cardiomyopathy is a genetically autosomal dominant disorder characterized by unexplained left ventricular hypertrophy and myocyte disarray. It is often associated with ventricular arrhythmias and sudden cardiac death, especially in a young population[62-65] (Fig. 4). The annual incidence of sudden cardiac death is 2% to 4% in adults and 6% to 8% in children and adolescents.[65-70] Nevertheless, this high incidence comes from data generated in referral cardiac centers and may reflect a bias to patients with more severe disease. Kofflard et al.[71] observed, in a large, nonselected population with hypertrophic cardiomyopathy, that the risk of cardiac mortality and sudden death is relatively low (1% annual cardiac mortality).

The natural history of hypertrophic cardiomyopathy appearing in infants or children differs from the disease in adults. In infants, hypertrophic cardiomyopathy is thought to be responsible for a small proportion of crib deaths. The diagnosis is often missed. The first clinical manifestation is usually heart failure and cyanosis. In a study of 20 infants, the mortality rate over five years was 50%, and cardiac failure was the most common cause of death.[68] When hypertrophic cardiomyopathy is diagnosed in infancy, the prognosis is poor and is related to severely impaired left ventricular function. Sudden death appears to be uncommon in the first decade of life (Fig. 4A), although at present there are little data available on this subgroup of patients.

In adults the natural course of the disease, although not benign, is not as malignant. It is calculated that more than 60% of adult patients who die from hypertrophic cardiomyopathy do so suddenly,[62-66,69] The vast majority of young patients who die suddenly are asymptomatic or minimally symptomatic, and usually their disease has not been identified clinically (Fig. 4B). Most patients experience sudden death while sedentary or participating in mild exertional activities (Fig. 4C). However, in approximately 40% of

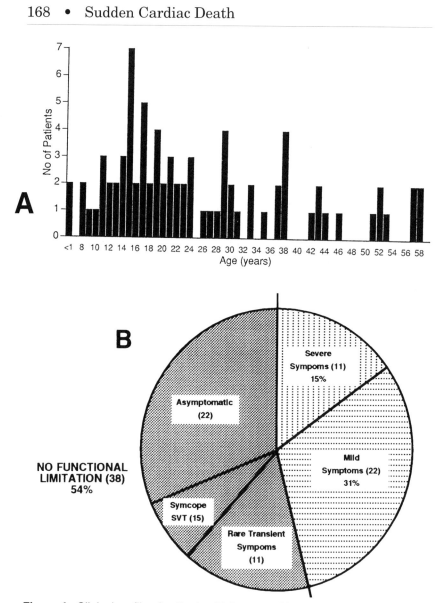

Figure 4. Clinical profile of patients with hypertrophic cardiomyopathy and sudden death. *Includes four patients who died during sleep (from Maron et al.[65]). (A) Bar graph showing age distribution for 78 patients who died suddenly or experienced cardiac arrest. (B) Circle graph showing functional state before sudden death or cardiac arrest. SVT = supraventricular tachycardia (Maron et al.[65])

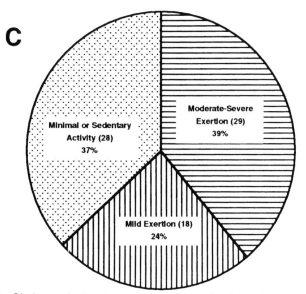

Figure 4C. Circle graph showing activity at time of sudden death or arrest.

cases, patients die during, or just after performing vigorous physical activities, including competitive athletics. Hypertrophic cardiomyopathy is often detected in postmortem studies of young athletes who die suddenly.[55]

Initial necropsy studies of patients who die suddenly showed a substantial increase in left ventricular wall thickness and mass.[71,72] Recent echocardiographic analyses of patients with hypertrophic cardiomyopathy demonstrated an association between marked and diffuse left ventricular hypertrophy and sudden cardiac death.[71] Spirito and Maron[73] observed that diffuse hypertrophy was eight times more common in patients with hypertrophic cardiomyopathy who died suddenly than in survivors. In addition, necropsy studies have shown that young patients who die suddenly had a more widespread distribution of disorganized cardiac muscle cells within the left ventricular wall than did patients with hypertrophic cardiomyopathy who died of congestive heart failure or other causes.[74] Sudden death has recently been reported in a patient with marked myocardial disarray and minor myocardial hypertrophy.[75]

The mechanism of sudden death in hypertrophic cardiomyopathy has not been established, although many potential mechanisms exist. Reports of complete heart block, asystole, myocardial infarc-

Table 4

Prediction of Sudden Death in Adults With Hypertrophic Cardiomyopathy

	Sensitivity	Specificity	Positive Predictive Accuracy	Negative Predictive Accuracy
Clinical-hemodynamic	70	68	24	94
Angiogram as diagnostic	82	72	32	96
Nonsustained ventricular tachycardia	69	80	22	97

(From McKenna and Camm.[83])

tion, and supraventricular tachycardia with atrioventricular node or accessory pathway have been published.[76–79] McKenna et al.[80] speculate that primary hemodynamic collapse is the most common initiating event, with the outcome determined by the electrical instability of the myocardium. They suggest that patients with widespread cellular disarray are more prone to develop ventricular fibrillation as a consequence of hemodynamic collapse. Tachycardia, whether physiological or secondary to an arrhythmia, may be thus indirectly associated with hypotension, impaired diastolic function, myocardial ischemia, angina, or syncope.[81] Frenneaux et al.[82] demonstrated an abnormality in the autonomic control of circulation in some patients with hypertrophic cardiomyopathy. In their study of 103 patients during exercise testing, 32 became hypotensive at a time when their cardiac output was rising. During exercise these patients either were unable to maintain stroke volume or systemic vascular resistance. To test this hypothesis, they performed invasive hemodynamic studies in 10 hypotensive responders and in 10 normal blood pressure responders.[82] Cardiac output increased appropriately and similarly in both groups, but there was an exaggerated fall in systemic vascular resistance in the hypotensive responders.

Retrospective analysis of clinical, hemodynamic, and angiographic parameters fails to identify patients who subsequently die suddenly.[83] In general, the most important risk factors for sudden death are a family history of hypertrophic cardiomyopathy and sudden death, early diagnosis of the disease in childhood or adolescence, frequent syncope, early appearance of atrial fibrillation, and the presence of nonsustained ventricular tachycardia during ambulatory electrocardiographic recording (Fig. 5). Primary electrical instability of the myocardium is an important determinant of sudden death in these patients. This is suggested by the fact that nonsustained ventricular tachycardia recorded in an ambulatory electrocardiographic recording is a major risk factor of sudden death in adult patients with hypertrophic cardiomyopathy.[84–87] Studies of McKenna et al.[85] and Maron et al.,[86] with a combined total of 170 patients, demonstrated that the incidence of sudden death after three years was nearly 7% (13/170). Most of these patients (9/13) had nonsustained ventricular tachycardia during ambulatory electrocardiographic recording ($P <$ 0.001). Although these data suggest that nonsustained ventricular tachycardia serves as a marker of increased risk for sudden cardiac death in patients with hypertrophic cardiomyopathy, it should be emphasized that it has a relatively low predictive accuracy. Paradoxically, the relation between nonsustained ventricular tachycardia and sudden death has proven to be weakest in young patients, the age when the risk of sudden death is perceived to be the greatest.[88] Spon-

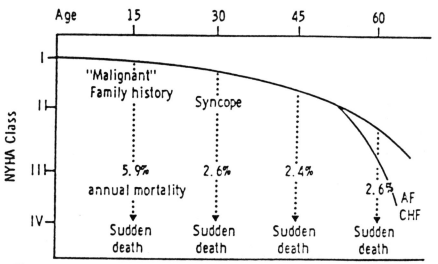

Figure 5. Natural history of hypertrophic cardiomyopathy (from McKenna et al.[91]). AF = atrial fibrillation; CHF - congestive heart failure.

taneous sustained ventricular tachycardia is rare[89] in patients with hypertrophic cardiomyopathy. The role of programmed ventricular stimulation in patients with hypertrophic cardiomyopathy is controversial. However, in 155 patients studied by Fananapazir et al.,[90] inducible sustained ventricular arrhythmias occurred in approximately 40% of cases. A strong association was observed between arrhythmia induction and prior cardiac arrest and syncope. In addition, supraventricular tachyarrhythmias were induced in approximately 25% of patients. Furthermore, the majority of patients also had abnormalities of sinoatrial, atrioventricular, or His-Purkinje conduction.[90]

Current treatment of these patients is also controversial. In asymptomatic patients, a 48-hour ECG should be obtained in order to detect the presence of salvos of nonsustained ventricular tachycardia. If present, treatment with low-dose amiodarone may be beneficial. McKenna et al.[91,92] suggested that treatment with amiodarone significantly reduces the risk for sudden death when compared to conventional antiarrhythmic treatment (Fig. 6). Twenty-one patients with hypertrophic cardiomyopathy and ventricular tachy-

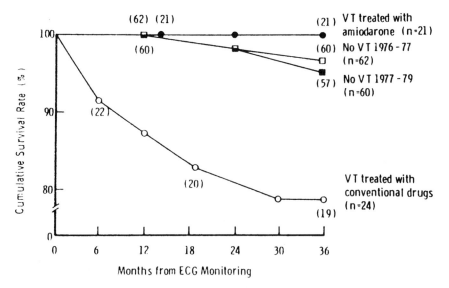

Figure 6. Cumulative survival in consecutive patients with hypertrophic cardiomyopathy. Patients with ventricular tachycardia (VT) detected between 1976 and 1977 received conventional antiarrhythmic drugs; those with VT between 1977 and 1979 received amiodarone (from McKenna et al.[91]).

cardia received an average of 300 mg/day of amiodarone. There were no deaths during the three-year follow-up. This contrasts with the 7% annual mortality of patients who received conventional treatment. Fananapazir[93] recently reported conflicting results in 49 patients with hypertrophic cardiomyopathy. He suggests that amiodarone has little effect on sudden death in patients with non-sustained ventricular tachycardia.[93] We must therefore wait for the results of large scale trials to be sure of the best approach for these patients. Moreover, it should be emphasized that although amiodarone is a potent antiarrhythmic, it is not beneficial for all patients.[94] It also has potential deleterious hemodynamic effects and may lead to clinical deterioration in patients with hypertrophic cardiomyopathy.

Other drugs such as β-blockers[95] or verapamil,[96] although useful in improving hemodynamics and symptomatology, have not proven to prolong life in patients with hypertrophic cardiomyopathy and may be deleterious in some patients.[97] Surgical treatment therapy using a myotomy-myectomy can improve symptoms and quality of life. Conclusive evidence to demonstrate its ability to prolong life is absent.[98]

Secondary Nonischemic Cardiomyopathies

Sudden death has also been described in other forms of cardiomyopathies including alcoholic cardiomyopathy, amyloidosis, sarcoidosis, hemochromatosis, neuromuscular disorders, connective tissue disorders, Chagas' disease, and toxic myocarditis.

Sudden cardiac death commonly occurs in the natural history of alcoholic cardiomyopathy.[99,100] Acute alcohol ingestion may induce malignant ventricular arrhythmias and sudden death.[101]

Cardiac amyloidosis is characterized by the presence of amyloid deposits, particularly within the cardiac conduction system. In the series of Wright and Calkins,[102] 30% of patients with primary amyloidosis died suddenly. In these patients sudden death may be due to either recurrent ventricular fibrillation[103] or advanced atrioventricular block.[104]

Sudden cardiac death frequently appears in the natural course of cardiac sarcoidosis.[105,106] Roberts et al.[105] reported that sudden arrhythmic death was the terminal event in 67% of patients with sarcoid heart disease. Sudden death was the initial manifestation of sarcoidosis in 11% of patients who died and its occurrence has been related to the extent of cardiac involvement.[106] In addition, there is evidence that sudden cardiac death also occurs in patients with hemochromatosis, neuromuscular disorders, and several connective disorders.[107–110]

Chagas' disease is one of the main public health problems in South and Central America. Between 20 to 30 million people worldwide are infected by *Trypanosoma cruzi,* and 90 million are at risk.[111] Although Chagas' heart disease is believed to be rare in the United States, its incidence is increasing.[112] The main manifestation of the disease is extensive myocarditis. Approximately 20% to 25% of infected patients present cardiac involvement including cardiac enlargement, congestive heart failure, thromboembolism, and arrhythmias. Conduction disorders and ventricular arrhythmias are a prominent feature of chronic Chagas' disease. Syncope and sudden death are a constant threat and may be the first manifestation of the disease.[113–116] Although the incidence of sudden death is not established, it is estimated that in Argentina alone, Chagas' heart disease is responsible for approximately 5000—6000 deaths per year, half of these being sudden.[117,118] Extensive acute myocarditis, malignant ventricular arrhythmias, and advanced heart block may be the cause of sudden death in these patients.

Cardiomyopathies represent a myocardial milieu in which arrhythmias are common. The relationship of the arrhythmia to the specific pathology is uncertain, yet it is clear that sudden death represents an important problem in the setting of progressive ventricular dysfunction regardless of the etiology of the myopathic process.

References

1. Gillum RF. Idiopathic cardiomyopathy in the United States, 1970—1982. *Am Heart J* 1986;111:752.
2. Franciosa JA, Wilen M, Ziesche S, et al. Survival in men with severe chronic left ventricular failure due to either coronary heart disease or idiopathic dilated cardiomyopathy. *Am J Cardiol* 1983;51:831.
3. Fuster V, Gersh BJ, Giuliani ER, et al. The natural history of idiopathic dilated cardiomyopathy. *Am J Cardiol* 1981;45:525.
4. Akagi T, Benson LN, Lightfoot NE, et al. Natural history of dilated cardiomyopathy in children. *Am Heart J* 1991;121:1502.
5. Likoff MJ, Chandler SL, Kay HR. Clinical determinants of mortality in chronic congestive heart failure secondary to idiopathic dilated or to ischemic cardiomyopathy. *Am J Cardiol* 1987:59:634.

6. Packer M. Sudden unexpected death in patients with congestive heart failure: A second frontier. *Circulation* 1985;72:681.

7. Bigger JT. Why patients with congestive heart failure die: Arrhythmias and sudden cardiac death. *Circulation* 1987;75:IV-28.

8. Anderson KP, Freedman RA, Mason JW. Sudden death in idiopathic dilated myocardiopathy. *Ann Intern Med* 1987;107:104.

9. Von Olshausen K, Schäfer A, Mehmel HC, et al. Ventricular arrhythmias in idiopathic dilated cardiomyopathy. *Br Heart J* 1984;51:195.

10. Chakko S, Georghiade M. Ventricular arrhythmias in severe heart failure: Incidence significance and effectiveness of antiarrhythmic therapy. *Am Heart J* 1985;109:497.

11. Huang SK, Messer JV, Denes P. Significance of ventricular tachycardia in idiopathic dilated cardiomyopathy: Observations in 35 patients. *Am J Cardiol* 1982;51:507.

12. Wilson JR, Schwartz JS, Sutton MSTJ, et al. Prognosis in severe heart failure: Relation to hemodynamic measurements and ventricular ectopic activity. *J Am Coll Cardiol* 1983;2:403.

13. Holmes J, Kubo SH, Codi RJ, et al. Arrhythmias in ischemic and nonischemic dilated cardiomyopathy: Prediction of mortality by ambulatory electrocardiography. *Am J Cardiol* 1985;55:146.

14. Meinertz T, Hofmann T, Kasper W, et al. Significance of ventricular arrhythmias in idiopathic dilated cardiomyopathy. *Am J Cardiol* 1984; 53:902.

15. Francis GS. Development of arrhythmias in the patient with congestive heart failure: Pathophysiology, prevalence, and prognosis. *Am J Cardiol* 1986;57:3B.

16. Maskin CS, Siskind SJ, LeJemtel TH. High prevalence of nonsustained ventricular tachycardia in severe congestive heart failure. *Am Heart J* 1984;107:896.

17. Sakurai T, Kawai C. Sudden death in idiopathic cardiomyopathy. *Jpn Circ J* 1983;47:581.

18. Massie B, Ports T, Chatterjee K, et al. Long-term vasodilator therapy for heart failure: Clinical response and its relationship to hemodynamic measurements. *Circulation* 1981;63:269.

19. Lee WH, Packer M. Prognostic importance of serum sodium concentration and its modification by converting-enzyme inhibition in patients with severe chronic heart failure. *Circulation* 1986;73:257.

20. Franciosa JA, Wilen M, Ziesche SM, et al. Survival in men with severe chronic left ventricular failure due to either coronary heart disease or idiopathic dilated cardiomyopathy. *Am J Cardiol* 1983;51:831.

21. Gradman A, Deedwania P, Cody R, et al. for the Captopril-Digoxin Study Group. Predictors of total mortality and sudden death in mild to moderate heart failure. *J Am Coll Cardiol* 1989;14:564.

22. Stevenson WG, Stevenson LW, Middlekauff HR, et al. Sudden death prevention in patients with advanced ventricular dysfunction. *Circulation* 1993;88:2953.

23. Stevenson WG, Stevenson LW, Weiss J, et al. Inducible ventricular arrhythmias and sudden death during vasodilator therapy of severe heart failure. *Am Heart J* 1988;116:1447.

24. Carlson MD, Schoenfeld MH, Garan H, et al. Programmed ventricular stimulation in patients with left ventricular dysfunction and ventricular tachycardia: Effects of acute hemodynamic improvement due to nitropusside. *J Am Coll Cardiol* 1989;14:1744.

25. Brachmann J, Dietz R, Kübler W, eds. *Heart Failure and Arrhythmias.* Berlin: Springer-Verlag, 1990.

26. Von Olshausen K, Stienen U, Math D, et al. Long-term prognostic significance of ventricular arrhythmias in idiopathic dilated cardiomyopathy. *Am J Cardiol* 1988;61:146.

27. Packer M. Lack of relation between ventricular arrhythmias and sudden death in patients with chronic heart failure. *Circulation* 1992; 85:I-50.

28. Packer M, for the Captopril-Digoxin Multicenter Research Group: Asymptomatic ventricular tachycardia identifies patients with heart failure at risk of clinical progression rather than sudden death. *Circulation* 1989;80:II-120.

29. Luu M, Stevenson WG, Stevenson LW, etc. Diverse mechanisms of unexpected cardiac arrest in advanced heart failure. *Circulation* 1989;80:1675.

30. Bayés de Luna A, Coumel P, Leclercq JF. Ambulatory sudden cardiac death: Mechanisms of production of fatal arrhythmia on the basis of data from 157 cases. *Am Heart J* 1989;117:151.

31. Greenberg HM. Bradycardia at onset of sudden death: Potential mechanisms. *Ann NY Acad Sci* 1984;427:241.

32. Guindo J, Bayés de Luna A, Torner P, et al. Treatment of heart failure: Impact on sudden death. In: Bayés de Luna A, Brugada P, Cosin J, Navarro Lopez F, eds. *Sudden Cardiac Death.* Dordrecht: Kluwer Academic Press; 1990.

33. Swan HJC, ed. Meeting of the minds: Treatment of arrhythmias in congestive heart failure. *Am Heart J* 1987;114:1265.

34. Bigger JT. Management of ventricular arrhythmias in patients with congestive heart failure. *Am J Cardiol* 1986;57:1B.

35. Gomes JAC, Hariman RI, Kang PS, et al. Programmed electrical stimulation in patients with high grade ventricular ectopy: Electrophysiological findings and prognosis for survival. *Circulation* 1984; 70:43.

36. Wilson JR. Use of antiarrhythmic drugs in patients with heart failure: Clinical efficacy, hemodynamic results and relation to survival. *Circulation* 1987;75:IV-64.

37. Poll DS, Marchlinski FE, Buxton AE, et al. Sustained ventricular tachycardia in patients with idiopathic dilated cardiomyopathy: Electrophysiologic testing and lack of response to antiarrhythmic drug therapy. *Circulation* 1984;70:451.

38. Slater W, Lampert S, Podrid PJ, et al. Clinical predictors of arrhythmia worsening by antiarrhythmic drugs. *Am J Cardiol* 1988;61:349.

39. Greene HL, Richardson DW, Hallstrom AP, et al. Congestive heart failure after acute myocardial infarction in patients receiving antiarrhythmic agents for ventricular premature complexes (Cardiac Arrhythmia Pilot Study). *Am J Cardiol* 1989;63:393.

40. Gottlieb SS. The use of antiarrhythmic agents in heart failure: Implications of CAST. *Am Heart J* 1989;118:1074.
41. Ravid S, Podrid PJ, Lambert S, et al. Congestive heart failure induced by six of the newer antiarrhythmic drugs. *J Am Coll Cardiol* 1989;14:1326.
42. Hamer AWF, Arkles LB, Johns JA. Beneficial effects of low dose amiodarone in patients with heart failure: A placebo controled trial. *J Am Coll Cardiol* 1989;14:1768.
43. Dominguez de Rozas JM, Garcia Picart J, Guindo J, et al. Amiodarone as a drug of first choice in the prevention of sustained ventricular tachycardia and/or fibrillation. In: Bayés de Luna A, Betriu A, Permanyer G. *Cardiovascular Therapy.* Dordrecht: Martinus Nijhoff; 1988.
44. Mirowski M, Reid PR, Mower MM, et al. Termination of malignant ventricular arrhythmias with an implanted automatic defibrillator in human beings. *N Engl J Med* 1980;303:322.
45. Tchou PJ, Kadri N, Anderson J, et al. Automatic implantable cardioverter defibrillators and survival of patients with left ventricular dysfunction and malignant ventricular arrhythmias. *Ann Intern Med* 1988;109:529.
46. Saksena S. Nonpharmacologic therapy for malignant ventricular arrhythmias in patients with congestive heart failure. In: Brachmann J, Dietz R, Kübler W, eds. *Heart Failure and Arrhythmias.* Berlin: Springer-Verlag; 1990.
47. Marcus FI, Fontaine GH, Guiraudon G, et al. Right ventricular dysplasia: A report of 24 adult cases. *Circulation* 1982;65:384.
48. Rizzon P, Breithardt G, Chiddo A, eds. Arrhythmogenic right ventricle. *Eur Heart J* 1989;10(suppl D):1.
49. Diggelmann U, Baur HR. Ramilial Uhl's anomaly in the adult. *Am J Cardiol* 1984;53:1402.
50. Bewick DJ, Chandler BM, Montague TJ. Dilated right ventricular cardiomyopathy: Uhl's disease. *Chest* 1986;90:300.
51. Leclercq JF, Coumel P. Characteristics, prognosis and treatment of the ventricular arrhythmias of right ventricular dysplasia. *Eur Heart J* 1989;10(suppl D):61.
52. Marcus FI, Fontaine GH, Frank R, et al. Long-term follow-up in patients with arrhythmogenic right ventricular disease. *Eur Heart J* 1989;10(suppl D):68.
53. Thiene G, Nava A, Corrado D, et al. Right ventricular cardiomyopathy and sudden death in young people. *N Engl J Med* 1988;318:129.
54. Maron BJ. Right ventricular cardiomypathy: another cause of sudden death in the young people. *N Engl J Med* 1988;318:178.
55. Maron BJ, Epstein SE, Roberts WC. Causes of sudden death in competitive athletes. *J Am Coll Cardiol* 1986;7:204.
56. Thiene G, Gambino A, Corrado D, et al. The pathological spectrum underlying sudden death in athletes. *New Trends Arrhyth* 1986;1:323.
57. Kunze KP, Hoffmann M, Kuck KH. A prospective study of intravenous and oral flecainide in right ventricular arrhythmia. *J Am Coll Cardiol* 1988;11:56A.

58. Leclercq JF, Chouty F, Cauchemez B, et al. Results of electrical fulguration in arrhythmogenic right ventricular disease. *Am J Cardiol* 1988;62:220.

59. Fontaine G, Frank R, Rougier I, et al. Electrode catheter ablation of resistant ventricular tachycardia in arrhythmogenic right ventricular dysplasia: Experience of 13 patients with a mean follow-up of 45 months. *Eur Heart J* 1989;10:74D.

60. Guiraudon GM, Klein GJ, Galamhusein SS, et al. Total disconnection of the right ventricular free wall: Surgical treatment of right ventricular tachycardia associated with ventricular dysplasia. *Circulation* 1983; 67;463.

61. Guiraudon GM, Klein GJ, Sharma AD, et al. Surgical therapy for arrhythmogenic right ventricular adiposis. *Eur Heart J* 1989;10:82D.

62. McKenna WJ, Krikler D. Arrhythmias in hypertrophic cardiomyopathy. In: Cosín J, Bayés de Luna A, García Civera R, Cabadés A, eds. *Cardiac Arrhythmias.* Oxford: Pergamon Press; 1988.

63. Maron BJ, Roberts WC, Epstein SE. Sudden death in hypertrophic cardiomyopathy: A profile of 78 patients. *Circulation* 1982;65:1388.

64. Nicod P, Polikar R, Peterson KL. Hypertrophic cardiomyopathy and sudden death. *N Engl J Med* 1988;318:1255.

65. Maron BJ, Fananapazir L. Sudden cardiac death in hypertrophic cardiomyopathy. *Circulation* 1992;85:I-57.

66. McKenna WJ, Deanfield J, Faruqui A, et al. Prognosis in hypertrophic cardiomyopathy: Role of age, and clinical, electrocardiographic and hemodynamic features. *Am J Cardiol* 1981;47:532.

67. Maron BJ, Tajik AJ, Ruttenberg HD, et al. Hypertrophic cardiomyopathy in infants: Clinical features and natural history. *Circulation* 1982;65:7.

68. McKenna WJ, Deanfield JE. Hypertrophic cardiomyopathy: An important cause of sudden death. *Arch Dis Child* 1984;59:971.

69. Fananapazir L, Chang AC, Epstein SE, et al. Prognostic determinants in hypertrophic cardiomyopathy. *Circulation* 1992;86:730.

70. Olsen EG. Anatomic and light microscopic characterization of hypertrophic obstructive and nonobstructive cardiomyopathy. *Eur Heart J* 1983;4:F-1.

71. Kofflard MJ, Waldstein DJ, Vos J, ten Cate FJ. Prognosis in hypertrophic cardiomyopathy observed in a large clinic population. *Am J Cardiol* 1993;72:939.

72. Roberts WC, Ferrans VJ. Pathologic anatomy of the cardiomyopathies: Idiopathic dilated and hypertrophic types, infiltrative types, and endomyocardial disease with and without eosinophilia. *Hum Pathol* 1975; 6:287.

73. Spirito P, Maron BJ. Relation between extent of left ventricular hypertrophy and occurrence of sudden cardiac death in hypertrophic cardiomyopathy. *J Am Coll Cardiol* 1990;15:1521.

74. Maron BJ, Roberts WC. Quantitative analysis of cardiac muscle cell disorganization in ventricular septum of patients with hypertrophic cardiomyopathy. *Circulation* 1979;59:689.

75. Maron BJ, Kragel AH, Roberts WC. Sudden death due to hypertrophic cardiomyopathy in the absence of increased myocardial mass. *Br Heart J* 1990;63:287.
76. Louie EK, Maron BJ. Familial spontaneous complete heart block in hypertrophic cardiomyopathy. *Br Heart J* 1986;55:469.
77. Chmielewski CA, Riley RS, Mahendran A, et al. Complete heart block as a cause of syncope in asymmetric septal hypertrophy. *Am Heart J* 1977;93:91.
78. Glancy DL, O'Brien KP, Gold HK, et al. Atrial fibrillation in patients with idiopathic hypertrophic subaortic stenosis. *Br Heart J* 1970; 32:652.
79. Krikler DM, Davies MJ, Rowland E, et al. Sudden death in hypertrophic cardiomyopathy: Associated accessory atrioventricular pathways. *Br Heart J* 1980;43:245.
80. McKenna WJ. The natural history of hypertrophic cardiomyopathy. *Cardiovasc Clin* 1988;19:135.
81. Stafford WJ, Trohman RG, Bilsker M, et al. Cardiac arrest in an adolescent with atrial fibrillation and hypertrophic cardiomyopathy. *J Am Coll Cardiol* 1986;7:701.
82. Frenneaux MP, Counihan PJ, Webb D, et al. Evidence for an abnormal vasodilator response in hypertrophic cardiomyopathy. *J Am Coll Cardiol* 1989;13:117A.
83. McKenna WJ, Camm AJ. Sudden death in hypertrophic cardiomyopathy: Assessment of patients at high risk. *Circulation* 1989;80:1489.
84. McKenna WJ, Chetty S, Oakley CM, et al. Arrhythmia in hypertrophic cardiomyopathy: exercise and 48 hour ambulatory electrocardiographic assessment with and without beta adrenergic blocking therapy. *Am J Cardiol* 1980;45:1.
85. McKenna WJ, England D, Doi YL, et al. Arrhythmia in hypertrophic cardiomyopathy. I. Influence on prognosis. *Br Heart J* 1981;46:168.
86. Maron BJ, Savage DD, Wolfson JK, et al. Prognostic significance of 24 hour ambulatory electrocardiographic monitoring in patients with hypertrophic cardiomyopathy: A prospective study. *Am J Cardiol* 1981; 48:252.
87. Fananapazir L, Epstein SE. Ventricular tachycardia and sudden death in hypertrophic cardiomyopathy patients. *Circulation* 1989;80:1923.
88. McKenna WJ, Franklin RCG, Nihoyannopoulos P, et al. Arrhythmia and prognosis in infants, children and adolescents with hypertrophic cardiomyopathy. *J Am Coll Cardiol* 1988;11:147.
89. Alfonso F, Frenneaux MP, McKenna WJ. Clinical sustained uniform ventricular tachycardia in hypertrophic cardiomyopathy: Association with left ventricular apical aneurysm. *Br Heart J* 1989,61:178.
90. Fananapazir L, Tracy CM, Leon MB, et al. Electrophysiologic abnormalities in patients with hypertrophic cardiomyopathy: A consecutive analysis in 155 patients. *Circulation* 1989;80:1259.
91. McKenna WJ, Harris L, Perez G, et al. Arrhythmias in hypertrophic cardiomyopathy: II. Comparison of amiodarone and verapamil in treatment. *Br Heart J* 1981;43:176.

92. McKenna WJ, Oakley CM, Krikler DM, et al. Improved survival with amiodarone in patients with hypertrophic cardiomyopathy and ventricular tachycardia. *Br Heart J* 1985;53:412.

93. Fananapazir L. Sudden cardiac death during amiodarone therapy in hypertrophic cardiomyopathy patients with ventricular tachycardia on Holter. *Circulation* 1990;83:III-333.

94. Paulus WJ, Nellens P, Heyndrickx GR, et al. Effects of long-term treatment with amiodarone on exercise hemodynamics and left ventricular relaxation in patients with hypertrophic cardiomyopathy. *Circulation* 1986;74:544.

95. Stenson RE, Flamm MD Jr, Harrison DC, et al. Hypertrophic subaortic stenosis: Clinical and hemodynamic effects of long-term propranolol therapy. *Am J Cardiol* 1973;31:763.

96. Rosing DR, Condit JR, Maron BJ, et al. Verapamil therapy: A new approach to the pharmacologic treatment of hypertrophic cardiomyopathy. III. Effects of long-term administration. *Am J Cardiol* 1981;48:545.

97. Epstein SE, Rosing DR. Verapamil: Its potential for causing serious complications in patients with hypertrophic cardiomyopathy. *Circulation* 1981;64:437.

98. Redwood DR, Goldstein RE, Hirshfeld J, et al. Exercise performance after septal myotomy and myectomy in patients with obstructive hypertrophic cardiomyopathy. *Am J Cardiol* 1979;44:215.

99. Vikhert AM, Tsiplenkova VG, Cherpachenko NM. Alcoholic cardiomyopathy and sudden cardiac death. *J Am Coll Cardiol* 1986;8:3A.

100. McCall D. Alcohol and the cardiovascular system. *Curr Probl Cardiol* 1987;12:351.

101. Panos RJ, Sutton FJ, Young-Hyman P, et al. Sudden death associated with alcohol consumption. *PACE* 1988;11:423.

102. Wright JR, Calkins E. Clinical-pathologic differentiation of common amyloid syndromes. *Medicine* (Baltimore) 1981;60:429.

103. Bharati S, Lev M, Denes P, et al. Infiltrative cardiomyopathy with conduction disease and ventricular arrhythmia: Electrophysiologic and pathologic correlations. *Am J Cardiol* 1980;45:163.

104. Lumb G, Shacklett RS. Human cardiac conduction tissue lesions. *Am J Pathol* 1960;36:411.

105. Roberts WC, McAllister HA, Ferrans VJ. Sarcoidosis of the heart. *Am J Cardiol* 1977;63:86.

106. Silverman KJ, Hutchins GM, Bulkley BH. Cardiac sarcoid: A clinicopathologic study of 84 unselected patients with systemic sarcoidosis. *Circulation* 1977;58:1204.

107. Lemery R, Brugada P, Havenith B, et al. Sudden death in hemochromatosis after closed-chest catheter ablation of the atrioventricular junction. *Am Heart J* 1988;61:941.

108. Cosh JA, Lever JV, eds. *Rheumatic Diseases and the Heart.* Berlin: Springer-Verlag, 1988.

109. Bulkley BH, Klacsman PG, Hutchins GM. Angina pectoris, myocardial infarction and sudden cardiac death with normal coronary arteries: A clinicopathological study of nine patients with progressive systemic sclerosis. *Am Heart J* 1978;95:563.

110. Vidosava R, Dubravka C, Slobodan A, et al. Myocarditis as a cause of sudden death in patients with myasthenia gravis. *Acta Cardiol* 1991;3:45.
111. Puigbo JJ, Acquatella H, Giordano H, et al. Chagas' disease: Overview and perspectives. In: Olsen EG, Sekiguchi M. *Restrictive Cardiomyopathy and Arrhythmias.* Tokyo: University of Tokyo Press; 1990; 347.
112. Hagar JM, Rahimtoola SH. Chagas' heart disease in the United States. *N Engl J Med* 1991;325:763.
113. Mendoza I, Camardo J, Moleiro F, et al. Sustained ventricular tachycardia in chronic chagasic myocarditis: Electrophysiologic and pharmacologic characteristics. *Am J Cardiol* 1986;57:423.
114. Pimenta J, Miranda M, Britto Pereira C. Electrophysiologic findings in long-term asymptomatic chagasic individuals. *Am Heart J* 1983; 106:374.
115. de Paola AA, Horowitz LN, Miyamoto MH, et al. Angiographic and electrophysiologic substrates of ventricular tachycardia in chronic Chagas' myocarditis. *Am J Cardiol* 1990;65:360.
116. Pinto Lima FX, Spiritus O, Tranchesi J. Arrhythmias and vector electrocardiographic analysis of complete bundle branch block in Chagas' disease: A study of 103 autopsied cases. *Am Heart J* 1958;56:501.
117. Monti E, Villa J, De Rosa M, et al. Cardiopatía chagásica crónica y su clasificación. *Rev Arg Cardiol* 1988;56:109.
118. Manzullo EC. Epidemiología de la Enfermedad de Chagas en la Argentina. *Rev Fed Arg Cardiol* 1988;17:141.

Chapter XI

Sudden Death in Valvular Heart Disease

Sudden death occurs frequently in the natural history of valvular heart diseases, especially in aortic valvular stenosis. In the last few years emphasis has also been placed on the relationship of mitral valve prolapse, ventricular arrhythmias, and sudden death.

Aortic Valve Stenosis

Before effective surgical treatment was available, aortic valvular stenosis was most frequently associated with noncoronary sudden death.[1] With early surgery, the incidence of sudden cardiac death has greatly declined.[2] Nevertheless, sudden death may be the first manifestation of the disease, particularly in young athletes (Chapter XVI). Patients with even severe aortic stenosis tend to be free of cardiovascular symptoms until late in the course of the disease.[3] Sudden cardiac death is the first manifestation of the disease in approximately 3% to 5% of cases in some series.[4,5]

Natural history studies of aortic stenosis[6] indicate that 52% of the symnptomatic patients treated medically die within five years and 90% within ten years of diagnosis. Other untreated series of patients with hemodynamically significant aortic stenosis report a five-year survival rate of 64%.[7] After the appearance of symptoms, the natural history of the disease is malignant and the mortality increases.[4,5] Thus, after appearance of angina or syncope, the average survival is two to three years; after appearance of congestive heart

From: S. Goldstein, A. Bayés-de-Luna, J. Guindo-Soldevila: *Sudden Cardiac Death.* Armonk, NY: Futura Publishing Co., Inc., © 1994.

failure it is 1.5 years[5,8](Fig. 1). Of those patients with aortic stenosis who died, death was sudden in most cases.[5,8,9]

The natural history of aortic stenosis is based primarily on retrospective clinical analysis with little hemodynamic information. Chizner et al.[8] published a series of 42 patients with hemodynamic documentation of isolated valvular aortic stenosis who did not undergo early valve replacement. Thirty-two were symptomatic and 10 asymptomatic at the time of cardiac catheterization. Of 32 symptomatic patients, 23 had moderate or severe stenosis and were followed until death or for an average of 64.4 months after catheterization. In this group of patients the mortality rate from onset of symptoms was 26% at one year, 57% at three years, and 64% at five years (Fig. 2). Fifty-six percent of the deaths were sudden; 25% were due to progressive heart failure; in 12.5% death occurred after acute myocardial infarction and cardiogenic shock; and in 6.5% of cases the mode of death was unknown. Four of 9 symptomatic patients with mild aortic stenosis died. All 4 had antecedent congestive heart failure and 3 had experienced angina. Asymptomatic patients had a good survival. Eight asymptomatic patients with moderate or severe aortic stenosis were followed for almost six

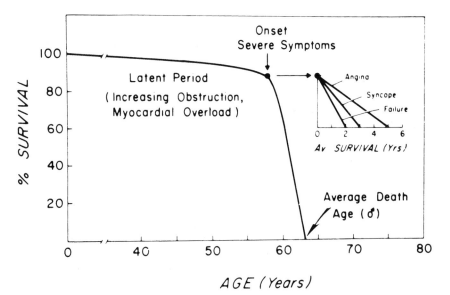

Figure 1. Natural history of aortic stenosis without surgical treatment. (Adapted with permission from Ross J, Braunwald E.[5])

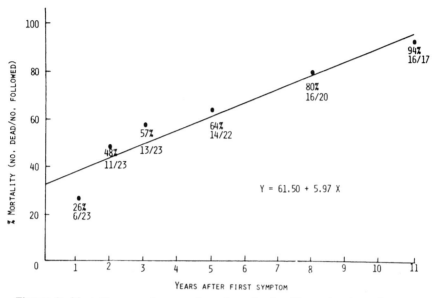

Figure 2. Mortality curve for symptomatic patients with moderate and severe aortic stenosis (from Chizner et al.[8]).

years and none died.[8] The mechanism of sudden death is unknown, although it is considered to be due to either malignant ventricular arrhythmia or bradyarrhythmia.[10–14]

In patients with aortic stenosis without symptoms the risk of sudden death is relatively low. Limitation of physical exercise to functional capacity is appropriate.[5,8,10] Patients at high risk are those who become symptomatic, particularly when syncope or heart failure appears.[11–13] In these patients, valve replacement is indicated.[15] Balloon valvuloplasty is a new technique used in the treatment of mitral and aortic stenosis.[16] In spite of the excellent results achieved in the treatment of mitral stenosis, in patients with aortic stenosis the results in general are unsatisfactory.

In totally asymptomatic patients we recommend clinical and echo-Doppler follow-up. When aortic stenosis becomes critical and the peak systolic pressure gradient is greater than 50 mm Hg or an effective calculated orifice is less than 0.75 cm^2/m^2 aortic valve replacement is indicated regardless of symptomatology. It should be kept in mind that sudden death can appear in totally asymptomatic patients and that at present, the surgical mortality in these patients is very low.

Mitral Valve Prolapse

The incidence (5%–7%) in the general population of mitral valve prolapse detected by echocardiography[17–19] is quite high, yet only 60 cases of sudden death have been reported worldwide.[20] It therefore appears that the risk of sudden death in these patients is low. For this reason, it is necessary to identify the subgroup of patients at increased risk (Table 1). Kligfield et al.[21] estimated that the incidence of sudden death varies according to the presence of symptoms and the severity of mitral regurgitation. In completely asymptomatic patients without hemodynamically significant mitral regurgitation, mortality is 1.9/10,000 patients per year. In symptomatic patients, mortality rises to 40/10,000 patients per year. If there is clinical evidence of mitral regurgitation, the annual mortality rate is 188/10,000 patients per year. An additional risk factor is the presence of frequent and complex ventricular arrhythmias.[22–25] Table 2 shows that prevalence of ventricular tachyarrhythmias is related to the presence of mitral regurgitation. Repolarization abnormalities and especially lengthening of the QT_c interval are also considered to be possible risk factors.[26–32] Puddu et al.[32] observed an increase in plasma catecholamine concentration in patients with mitral prolapse and long QT_c interval. It has been speculated that these patients have more arrhythmogenicity.[33] The detection by echocardiography of a redundant mitral valve[34] and a family history of sudden death[20,35] are also considered possible risk factors. Ventricular tachyarrhythmias are the main cause of sudden death in patients with mitral prolapse,[28,36–39] although

---

Table 1

Possible Factors of Risk of Sudden Death in Patients with Mitral Valve Prolapse

1. History of syncope, presyncope, palpitations
2. Hemodynamically significant mitral regurgitation
3. Complex ventricular arrhythmias
4. Long QT interval
5. Repolarization alterations on inferior leads
6. Redundant mitral leaflets
7. Family history of sudden cardiac death
8. Age and sex

Table 2

Prevalence of Ventricular Arrhythmias in Patients with Mitral Valve Prolapse with or without Regurgitation

| | *Mitral Valve Prolapse* | | |
	Without MR *N = 63* *(%)*	*With MR* *n = 17* *(%)*	*P*
VPC frequency:			
No VPC	37	0	< 0.01
Mean > 10/1000	3	41	< 0.005
VPC complexity:			
Multiform	43	88	< 0.005
Couplets	6	65	< 0.005
Runs of VT	5	35	< 0.005
Lown grade:			
0–2	56	6	< 0.001
3	33	24	NS
4[a]	3	35	< 0.005
4[b]	5	29	< 0.005
5	2	6	NS

(Adapted from Kligfield et al.[25]) VPC = ventricular premature complexes; VT = ventricular tachycardia; MR = mitral regurgitation.

some cases of death due to advanced atrioventricular block have been reported.[40]

Most patients with mitral valve prolapse do not require treatment since the incidence of sudden death is low. Preventive treatment of a patient with various risk factors should be individualized. Symptomatic patients with mitral valve prolapse and malignant arrhythmia should be advised of the possible risk of strenuous physical exercise,[20] since sudden death has been reported in competitive athletes (Chapter XVI). A maximal exercise test may be helpful in identifying patients at risk of exercise-induced arrhythmias and may provide a means by which antiarrhythmic therapy can be adjusted. At present there is little evidence that antiarrhythmic drugs prevent sudden death in these patients. In view of the evidence that these patients are more sensitive to catecholamines, β-blocking agents or sotalol have been proposed as the treatment of choice.

Sudden Death in Other Valvular Heart Disease

Sudden cardiac death may complicate any form of valvular heart disease.[41–44] With the advent of cardiac surgery, the natural history of valvular heart disease has improved significantly and the incidence of sudden death has been reduced.[2] Nevertheless, patients with prosthetic or heterograft valve replacements remain at some risk for sudden cardiac death due to ventricular arrhythmias, prosthetic valvular dysfunction, or coexistent coronary heart disease.[45–48] An increased incidence of ventricular arrhythmias has been observed during the follow-up of patients with valve replacement, especially in those who had aortic replacement, multiple valvular surgery, or cardiomegaly.[47] In one series, sudden cardiac death was reported as the second most important cause of death after valve replacement surgery, representing 21% of all deaths.[46] Sudden death occurred most frequently in the first three weeks after operation and then plateaued after eight months. Hoffmann and Burckhardt.[48] prospectively evaluated 100 patients after aortic valve replacement. Cardiac mortality rate was increased in patients with an ECG criteria of left ventricular hypertrophy and those with repetitive ventricular premature beats found during 24-hour ambulatory electrocardiographic recording.[48] All patients who died suddenly had ventricular ectopic activity or left ventricular hypertrophy ($P < 0.05$).

The importance of these characteristics as a mechanism of death or merely representing severity of left ventricular dysfunction is not clear. In general, sudden death remains a significant problem in patients with valvular heart disease and, in particular, aortic stenosis.

References

1. Rapaport E. Natural history of aortic and mitral valve disease. *Am J Cardiol* 1975;35:221.
2. Smith N, McAnulty JH, Rahimtoola SH. Severe aortic stenosis with impaired left ventricular function and clinical heart failure: Results of valve replacement. *Circulation* 1978;58:255.
3. Braunwald E. Valvular heart disease. In: Braunwald E, ed. *Heart Disease: A Textbook of Cardiovascular Medicine*. Philadelphia: WB Saunders; 1992.

4. Osborn MJ. Mechanisms, incidence and prevention of sudden cardiac death. In: Bradenburg RO, Fuster V, Giuliani ER, McGoon DC. *Cardiology.* Year Book Medical Publisher; 1991.

5. Ross J, Braunwald E. Aortic stenosis. *Circulation* 1968;38(suppl 5):61.

6. Frank S, Johnson A, Ross J Jr. Natural history of valvular aortic stenosis. *Br Heart J* 1973;35:41.

7. Hakki AH, Kimbiris D, Iskandrian AS, et al. Angina pectoris and coronary artery disease in patients with severe aortic valvular disease. *Am Heart J* 1980;100:441.

8. Chizner MA, Pearled DL, DeLeon AC. The natural history of aortic stenosis in adults. *Am Heart J* 1980;99:419.

9. Campbell M. Calcific aortic stenosis and congenital bicuspid aortic valves. *Br Heart J* 1968;30:606.

10. Klein RC. Ventricular arrhythmias in aortic valve disease: Analysis of 102 patients. *Am J Cardiol* 1984;53:1079.

11. Flamm MM, Braniff BA, Kimball R, et al. Mechanism of effort syncope in aortic stenosis. *Circulation* 1967;35(suppl II):II-109.

12. Schwartz LS, Goldfischer J, Sprague GJ, et al. Syncope and sudden death in aortic stenosis. *Am J Cardiol* 1969;23:647.

13. Leake D. Effort syncope in aortic stenosis. *Br Heart J* 1959;21:289.

14. Dhingra RC, Amat-y-Leon F, Pietras RJ, et al. Sites of conduction disease in aortic stenosis.: Significance of valve gradient and calcification. *Ann Intern Med* 1977;87:275.

15. Acar J, Ducimetiere P, Cadilhac M, et al. Prognosis of surgically treated chronic aortic valve disease. Predictive indicators of early postoperative risk and long-term survival, based on 439 cases. *J Thorac Cardiovasc Surg* 1978;75:383.

16. McKay RG, Grossman W. Balloon valvuloplasty for treating pulmonic, mitral, aortic, and prosthetic valve stenoses. In: Braunwald E, ed. *Heart Disease: A Textbook of Cardiovascular Medicine, Update I.* Philadelphia: WB Saunders; 1988.

17. Levy D, Savage D. Prevalence and clinical features of mitral valve prolapse. *Am Heart J* 1987;113:1281.

18. Procacci PM, Savran SV, Schreiter SL, et al. Prevalence of clinical mitral-valve prolapse in 1169 young women. *N Engl J Med* 1976;294:1086.

19. Darsee JR, Mikolich JR, Nicoloff NB, et al. Prevalence of mitral valve prolapse in presumably healthy young men. *Circulation* 1979;59:619.

20. Jeresaty RM. Mitral valve prolapse: definition and implications in athletes. *J Am Coll Cardiol* 1986;7:231.

21. Kligfield P, Levy D, Devereux RB, et al. Arrhythmias and sudden death in mitral valve prolapse. *Am Heart J* 1987;113:1298.

22. Savage DD, Levey D, Garrison RJ, et al. Mitral valve prolapse in the general population. III. Dysrhythmias: the Framingham study. *Am Heart J* 1983;106:582.

23. Winkle RA, Lopes MG, Fitzgerald JW, et al. Arrhythmias in patients with mitral valve prolapse. *Circulation* 1975;52:73.

24. DeMaria AN, Amsterdam EA, Vismara LA, et al. Arrhythmias in the mitral valve prolapse syndrome: Prevalence, nature, and frequency. *Ann Intern Med* 1976;84:656.

25. Kligfield P, HochIeiter C, Kramer H, et al. Complex arrhythmias in MR with and without mitral valve prolapse: contrast to arrhythmias in mitral valve prolapse without MR. *Am J Cardiol* 1985;55:1545.

26. Bekheit SG, Ali AA, Deglin SM, et al. Analysis of QT interval in patients with idiopathic mitral valve prolapse. *Chest* 1982;61:82.

27. Pocock WA, Barlow JB. Etiology and electrocardiographic features of the billowing posterior mitral leaflet syndrome. *Am J Cardiol* 1971;51:731.

28. Devereux RB, Perloff JK, Reichek N, et al. Mitral valve prolapse. *Circulation* 1976;54:3.

29. Hancock EW, Cohn K. The syndrome associated with midsystolic click and late systolic murmur. *Am J Med* 1966;41:183.

30. Shappell SD, Marshall CE, Brown RE, et al. Sudden death and the familial occurrence of midsystolic click, late systolic murmur syndrome. *Circulation* 1973;48:1128.

31. Wei JY, Bulkley BH, Schaeffer AH, et al. Mitral-valve prolapse syndrome and recurrent ventricular tachyarrhythmias: A malignant variant refractory to conventional drug therapy. *Ann Intern Med* 1978;89:6.

32. Puddu PE, Pasternac A, Tubau JF, et al. QT interval prolongation and increased plasma catecholamine levels in patients with mitral valve prolapse. *Am Heart J* 1983;105:422.

33. Wit AL, Cranefield PF. Triggered activity in cardiac muscle fibers of the simian mitral valve. *Circ Res* 1976;38:85.

34. Nishimura RA, McGoon MD, Shub C, et al. Echocardiographically documented mitral valve prolapse: Long-term follow-up of 237 patients. *N Engl J Med* 1985;313:1305.

35. Jeresaty RM. Sudden death in the mitral valve prolapse-click syndrome. *Am Heart J* 1976;37:317.

36. Campbell RWF, Godman MG, Fiddler GI, et al. Ventricular arrhythmias in syndrome of balloon deformity of mitral valve: Definition of possible high risk group. *Br Heart J* 1976;38:1053.

37. Jeresaty RM. *Mitral Valve Prolapse.* New York: Raven Press; 1979;259.

38. Pocock WA, Bosman CK, Chesler E, et al. Sudden death in primary mitral valve prolapse. *Am Heart J* 1984;107:378.

39. Chesler E, King RA, Edwards JE. The myxomatous mitral valve and sudden death. *Circulation* 1983;67:632.

40. Leichtman D, Nelson R, Gobel FL, et al. Bradycardia with mitral valve prolapse: A potential mechanism of sudden death. *Ann Intern Med* 1976;85:453.

41. Goldschlager N, Pfeifer J, Cohn K, et al. The natural history of aortic regurgitation. *Am J Med* 1973;54:577.

42. Spagnuolo M, Kloth H, Taranta A, et al. Natural history of rheumatic aortic regurgitation: Criteria predictive of death, congestive heart failure and angina in young patients. *Circulation* 1971;44:368.

43. Johnson LW, Grossman W, Dalen JE, et al. Pulmonic stenosis in the adult: Long-term follow-up results. *N Engl J Med* 1972;287:1159.

44. Nugent EW, Freedom RM, Nora JJ, et al. Clinical course in pulmonary stenosis. *Circulation* 1977;56(suppl I):38.
45. Rahimtoola SH. Valvular heart disease: A perspective. *J Am Coll Cardiol* 1983;1:199.
46. Blackstone EH, Kirklin JW. Death and other time-related events after valve replacement. *Circulation* 1985;72:4.
47. Konoshi Y, Matsuda K, Nishiwaki N, et al. Ventricular arrhythmias late after aortic and/or mitral valve replacement. *Jpn Cir J* 1985;49:576.
48. Hoffmann A, Burckhardt D. Patients at risk for cardiac death late after aortic valve replacement. *Am Heart J* 1990;120:1142.

Chapter XII

Sudden Death in Long QT Syndrome

The QT interval may be prolonged as a manifestation of drug and electrolyte abnormalities or it may represent a congenital and familial expression of cardiovascular disease. In either condition, it represents a significant risk for the development of life-threatening arrhythmia. The QT interval is considered prolonged when it exceeds 115% of the predicted normal.[1] A corrected QT interval of more than 440 milliseconds is always categorized as abnormal. The clinical situations in which the QT interval becomes prolonged are summarized in Table 1.[2]

Idiopathic Long QT Syndrome

Idiopathic long QT syndrome is a rare familial disorder in which affected members have QT prolongation and a propensity to syncope and malignant ventricular arrhythmias.[3] Two congenital forms of long QT syndrome have been described. One is the Jervell-Lange-Nielsen syndrome,[4] which is associated with deafness and has an autosomal recessive pattern of inheritance. The other, the Romano-Ward syndrome,[5,6] occurs without deafness and is autosomal dominant with a varying degree of penetration. Recently, a DNA marker on the short arm of the chromosome 11 has been linked to idiopathic long QT syndrome.[7] Sporadic, nonfamilial forms of idiopathic long QT syndrome have also been described and represent approximately 10% of the reported cases. It is possible that new mutations in a sin-

From: S. Goldstein, A. Bayés-de-Luna, J. Guindo-Soldevila: *Sudden Cardiac Death.* Armonk, NY: Futura Publishing Co., Inc., © 1994.

Table 1

Principal Causes of QT$_c$ Prolongation

Idiopathic long QT syndrome
  Congenital:
    Jervell-Lange-Nielsen syndrome
    Romano-Ward syndrome
  Sporadic forms
Postmyocardial infarction
Central nervous system diseases
Psychotropic drugs
Hypothyroidism
Hypothermia
Hypocalcemia
Nutritional deficits
Intracoronary injection of contrast material
Antiarrhythmic drugs
Organophosphate intoxication
Severe bradycardia and atrioventricular block

gle genetic locus may be substantiated for this disorder. The underlying electrophysiological abnormality of the idiopathic long QT syndrome is thought to be due to a genetic alteration in the myocellular channel protein that regulates potassium flux during electrical repolarization.[3] It may be related to a congenital autonomic nervous system imbalance with predominance of the left sympathetic nerves, causing prolongation of the QT interval and modification of the T wave.[8,9]

The clinical course of idiopathic prolonged QT syndrome is quite variable. Symptoms can range from malignant ventricular arrhythmias, characteristically of the torsade de pointes with syncope or sudden death, to an asymptomatic course with a normal life span. Certain families have a particularly malignant expression of the disease process and manifest sudden death at a young age in multiple generations.[10]

The different clinical presentations of idiopathic long QT syndrome and its relative risk of syncope or sudden death are summarized in Table 2.[3] Approximately 30% of patients are identified during clinical evaluation of syncope of unknown origin or aborted

Table 2

Clinical Identification of Patients with Long QT Syndrome

Patient Subgroups	LQTS Patients (%)	Risk of Syncope/Sudden Death
Unexplained syncope	30	High (5%/year)
Family member of LQTS patient	60	Variable
History of syncope	10	High (5%/year)
No syncope	50	Low (0.5%/year)
Asymptomatic patient with incidental QT_c prolongation (e.g., routine ECG)	10	Very low ($< 0.5\%$/year)

ECG = electrocardiogram; LQTS = long QT syndrome. (From Moss and Robinson.[3])

sudden death. It is important to note that these patients, despite recurrent syncope, are frequently misdiagnosed as having benign syncope or a seizure disorder. Often the correct diagnosis of long QT syndrome is established only after a tragic cardiac arrest occurs in a family member. Occasionally, an electrocardiogram had been taken prior to an arrest, but QT prolongation was not correctly appreciated by the physician interpreting the tracing.[11] Approximately 60% of patients with idiopathic long QT syndrome are identified when family members of an affected individual with syncope or cardiac arrest, the proband, have a screening electrocardiogram. The remaining 40% are often identified in a routine ECG examination. The development of DNA genetic markers has provided additional aid in identifying at-risk family members.

The risk of syncope or sudden death varies widely.(Table 2). The rate of recurrent cardiac events, syncope or sudden death in patients with a history of syncope is approximately 5% per year (Fig. 1). In contrast, asymptomatic individuals with prolonged QT_c interval have an incidence of syncope of approximately 0.5% per year (Table 2). Moss et al[11] published a prospective study of 3343 individuals from 328 families (Fig. 2). By age 12, 50% of the probands were identified after a syncopal event, 8% of the affected family members with QT_c greater than 0.44 seconds, and 2% of unaffected family members with QT_c less than 0.44 seconds experienced a first cardiac event. After 10 years of prospective follow-up, 37% of probands, 5% of affected

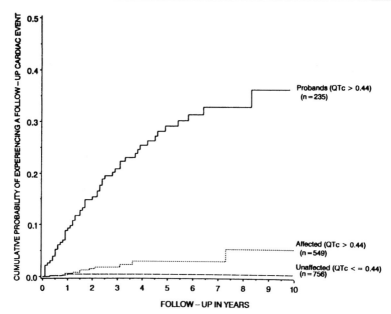

Figure 1. Cumulative probability of experiencing a follow-up cardiac event (syncope or probable LQTS-related death) using enrollment as the time origin for probands and affected and unaffected family members (from Moss et al.[11]).

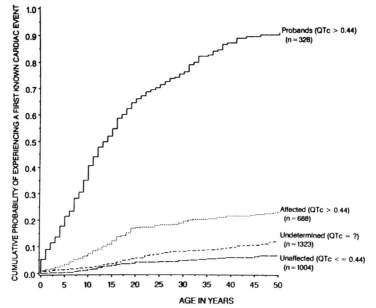

Figure 2. Cumulative probability of experiencing a first-known cardiac event (syncope or probable LQTS-related death) using birth for probands and affected, unaffected, and undetermined family members enrolled in the LQTS study (from Moss et al.[11]).

family members, and less than 1% of unaffected family members experienced a cardiac event.[11] Patients with documented recurrent sustained ventricular arrhythmias, T wave alterations, exaggerated QT_c prolongation (> 0.54 seconds), or atrioventricular block in the neonatal period are also associated with a significantly increased event rate.[10,11]

Symptoms, when they occur, generally begin in childhood or early adolescence. Syncope or sudden death often appear after an adrenergic stimuli. Moss et al.[11] reported that 47% of patients had one or more syncopal episodes occurring in association with intense emotions such as anger or fright; 41%, with vigorous physical activity exclusive of swimming; 19%, on awakening; 15%, while swimming; and 8%, on arousal by auditory stimuli such as the ringing of an alarm clock or a telephone or the sound of thunder (see Chapter VI).

Diagnosis is sometimes difficult since the length of the QT interval in the ECG varies. In families affected with the long QT syndrome, the QT interval may not be reliable. Using a QT of greater duration than 0.44 seconds, 11% of afflicted family members were misdiagnosed, whereas a QT of 0.47 in males and 0.48 in females included all cases but resulted in 40% of males and 20% of females with a false-negative diagnosis. DNA markers are, however, quite specific. Figure 3 shows the distribution of QT_c intervals in carriers and noncarriers of the long QT gene.[12] At any given moment it may be normal or slightly lengthened at rest, only to become prolonged during physical or mental stress. The QT_c interval may normalize with age in some affected individuals with prolonged QT syndrome.

Congenital prolonged QT syndrome is diagnosed in the presence of two major diagnostic criteria or one major and two minor criteria (Table 3).[13] Electrophysiological studies do not aid in the diagnosis. Programmed stimulation does not induce repetitive ventricular arrhythmias.[14] Ambulatory electrocardiographic recordings and exercise testing may be helpful in confirming the diagnosis and in evaluating its severity in a given patient. Ambulatory electrocardiographic recordings may reveal periods of profound bradycardia, runs of ventricular tachycardia, transient QT_c prolongation, or T alternation, all of which indicate an unfavorable prognosis. Autonomic dysfunction can be demonstrated in patients with a long QT interval, either by the inability to accelerate heart rate with exercise or after atropine,[15] or by the inability to adjust the QT interval induced by exercise or the Valsalva maneuver.[16] These dysfunctional phenom-

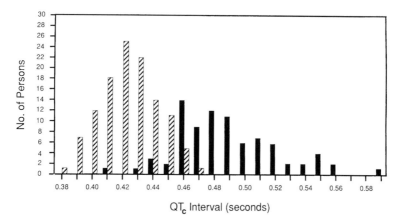

Figure 3. Distribution of QT_c intervals among carriers (solid bars) and noncarriers (hatched bars) of the long-QT gene in all three kindreds studied. The number of persons of either sex who had a given QT_c interval is shown. Spouses are not included (from Vincent, et al.[12]).

Table 3

Diagnostic Criteria of Congenital Long QT Syndrome

Major	Minor
Long QT interval (QT_c > 440 msec)	Congenital deafness
Syncope induced by stress	T wave alternance
Family history of long QT	Bradycardia (in children)
	Abnormal ventricular repolarization

From Schwartz PJ. Idiopathic long QT Syndrome: Progress and questions. *Am Heart J.* 1988; 109:399.

ena are not predictable in all patients, since different forms of presentation of autonomic nervous system imbalance can occur. Recent investigations suggest that an exaggerated QT prolongation in the recovery phase after exercise is the most characteristic finding in patients with long QT syndrome.[17,18]

Treatment with β-blockers and high-thoracic left sympathectomy are the most effective measures in the prevention of sudden death in these patients.[18] Data from the International Prospective Study demonstrate a dramatic improvement in survival as a result of treatment with β-blockers and highthoracic left sympathectomy when compared with other treatment (Fig. 4).[17] The three-year mortality after the first syncope was 6% in the group treated with these interventions and 26% in the group who received other treatment. Fifteen years after the first syncope event, the mortality rate in the two groups was 9% and 53%, respectively.[18] Data from approximately 800 patients[19] provided similar conclusions. In patients treated with β-blockers, the mortality rate was 6%, compared with 70% in the untreated group. The protective effect of β-blockers may be overestimated since approximately 20% of patients treated with these drugs continued to have syncopal episodes despite full-dose β-blockade. In those failures, a highthoracic left sympathectomy[19] was required.

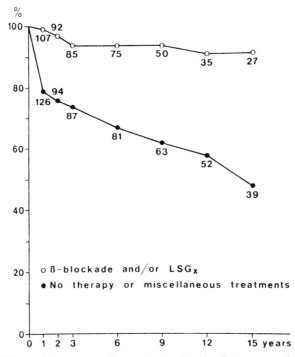

Figure 4. Effect of therapy on the survival, after the first syncopal episode, of 233 patients affected by the idiopathic LQTS. The protective effect of β-adrenergic blockade and of left stellectomy (LSGx) is evident. The mortality 3 years after the first syncope is 6% in the group treated differently or not treated. Fifteen years after the first syncope, the respective mortality rates are 9% and 53% (from Schwartz, et al.[17]).

High-thoracic left sympathectomy is indicated only when syncope recurs despite β-blocker therapy, when these drugs are contraindicated, or present side effects.[8,18–19] In 67 patients who failed to respond to high doses of β-blockers, the incidence of sudden death at five years after surgery was 8%.[18–20]

In those few patients who continue to have syncopal episodes despite the combination of high-thoracic left sympathectomy and β-blockers, other *experimental* therapies should be considered. In some cases the trigger of malignant ventricular arrhythmias depends on a reduction of heart rate. In this situation a cardiac pacemaker may be indicated.[20] In the remaining cases, an automatic implantable defibrillator may be the most rational approach. However, it should be remembered that in some patients with a long QT syndrome, malignant ventricular arrhythmias may recur frequently and an automatic defibrillator with its repeated defibrillations may cause severe psychological problems, particularly in young patients.

There is insufficient experience available with other experimental treatments. Complete denervation of the heart and calcium-entry blockers have both been proposed.[21] An unsuccessful case of autotransplant was recently reported.[18] However, good results have been reported with calcium-entry blockers, but experience is still very limited.

Finally, a frequent problem is the management of asymptomatic patients with long QT syndrome who are siblings or close relatives of symptomatic patients with a long QT syndrome. Present experience suggests that sudden death during the first syncopal episode is relatively uncommon, but it can occur. It is also well known that many asymptomatic patients will remain asymptomatic for life. Thus, we should carefully weigh the psychological consequences for a child or young person before starting complex treatment programs. The decision of whether or not to begin treatment should be individualized in each case (Fig. 5). Schwartz and coworkers[18] propose the following treatment approach to the asymptomatic patients:

1. patients with a long QT syndrome associated with congenital deafness, since their risk of sudden death is particularly high

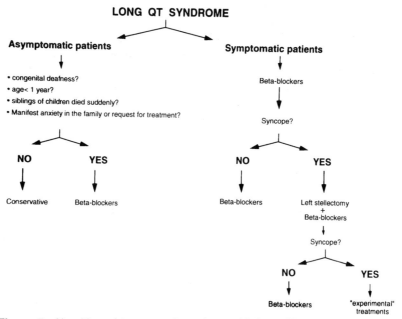

Figure 5. Algorithm of treatment in patients with long-QT syndrome (see text for explanation).

2. in neonates and during the first year of life because of the enhanced risk during this period
3. siblings of children who have had a sudden death experience
4. when there is a manifest anxiety in the family or an explicit request for treatment.

In the remaining situations, Schwartz et al. suggest instruction to the family members in cardiopulmonary resuscitation and follow a conservative approach.[18]

Acquired Neurogenic Long QT

The QT interval may also become prolonged in 32% of patients with intracranial hemorrhage, in 10% with intracranial aneurysms, in 7% with cerebral thrombosis and endocranial hypertension, and in less than 5% with cerebral metastasis and hypertensive encephalopathy.[22–24] That this electrocardiographic morphology appears after cryohypophysectomy for diabetes insipidus suggests that it may be due to a hypothalamic lesion, since it often occurs in subarachnoid hemorrhage. Recently torsade de pointes and ventricular flutter or fibrillation associated with QT_c intervals of greater than 0.55 seconds have been described in 4% of patients with subarachnoid hemorrhage.[24]

Drug-Induced Long QT

Ventricular arrhythmia of torsade de pointes has been described frequently in relation to long QT during treatment with antiarrhythmic drugs.[25] This is especially true for the class I antiarrhythmic drugs, quinidine, procainamide, disopyramide, flecainide, and aprindine. No antiarrhythmic drug, however, is free from risk of this arrhythmogenesis.[25–28] The appearance of torsade de pointes often coincides with a QT prolongation associated with a slow heart rate and hypokalemia. Any or all of these mechanisms can trigger early *afterpotentials,* which can account for the arrhythmia. That torsade de pointes cannot be induced by programmed electrical stimulation supports the existence of a metabolic mechanism other than reentry. In addition to electrolyte abnormalities and antiarrhythmic drugs, thioridazine[29] and other psychotropic drugs[30–33] and organophosphorus insecticides[34] are also associated with long QT interval, malignant ventricular arrhythmias, and sudden death.

Long QT and Ischemic
Heart Disease

In the first phase of acute experimental coronary occlusion there is a shortening of repolarization. After a few minutes of coronary occlusion and during the chronic phase of infarction, the QT_c lengthens. Prolongation of QT may signal a larger area of myocardial infarction,[35] or dispersion of the repolarization, which may be a potential marker of cardiac arrhythmogenesis. In the chronic phase of acute myocardial infarction,[36,37] a link between long QT and the incidence of ventricular arrhythmias has been observed in resuscitated cardiac arrest patients after ventricular fibrillation. In addition to a long QT_c (35% versus 18%, Haynes et al.[36] found more ST segment depression (46% versus 10%) and T wave abnormalities (52% versus 26%) were observed when cardiac arrest victims were compared to a control group. In 55 survivors of myocardial infarction followed for 7 years, Schwartz observed 28 sudden deaths, 18 of whom had a lengthened QT_c.[38] This study and others[39–42] suggest the possibility that the prolonged QT_c interval serves to define a subgroup of postinfarction patients at an increased risk of sudden death. These findings, however, have not been consistent (see Table 1, Chapter VII). The observation of a persistent QT prolongation recorded on serial electrocardiograms in postinfarction patients is more meaningful than an isolated measurement.[43] Serial measurements, rather than the evaluation of QT_c in a single basal ECG, obtained during normal daily activity using ambulatory electrocardiography may also be important for predicting the prognosis.[43] We recently measured QT_c using ambulatory electrocardiographic recordings at 5 measurements per hour in patients after a myocardial infarction. Patients with malignant ventricular arrhythmias had more frequent QT_c peaks over 500 milliseconds than the patients without malignant ventricular arrhythmias, regardless of their other clinical characteristics.[44,45] If these results are confirmed in larger series, measurement of the dynamic QT_c by ambulatory electrocardiographic recording may facilitate the stratification of postmyocardial infarction patients at risk of malignant ventricular arrhythmia.[45]

Long QT in Other Situations

Ventricular arrhythmias and sudden death in relation to long QT have also been reported in patients with hypocalcemia,[46] hypothyroidism,[47] in obese patients on severe weight reduction diets,[48] nutritional deficiencies associated with modified starvation diets, or postgastroplasty.[49,50] In addition, autonomic diabetic neuropathy may cause an imbalance in the sympathetic innervation of the heart, which can be associated with QT interval prolongation and an increased risk of sudden death.[51,52]

The QT zone of the electrocardiogram remains a fertile area of investigation. The multitude of electrophysiological phenomena hidden within this domain suggest that important mechanisms of arrhythmias lie here and are yet to be understood.

References

1. Tenth Conference on Optimal Electrocardiography. *Am J Cardiol* 1978;41:111.
2. Surawicz B, Knoebel SB. Long QT: Good, bad or indifferent? *J Am Cardiol Coll* 1984;4:398.
3. Moss AJ, Robinson J. Clinical features of the idiopathic long QT syndrome. *Circulation* 1992;85:I-140.
4. Jervell A, Lange-Nielson F. Congenital deaf-mutism, functional heart disease with prolongation of QT interval and sudden death. *Am Heart J* 1957;54:59.
5. Romano C. Congenital cardiac arrhythmia. *Lancet* 1965;1:658.
6. Ward OC. A new familial cardiac syndrome in children. *J Ir Med Assoc* 1964;54:103.
7. Keating M, Atkinson D, Dunn C, et al. Linkage of a cardiac arrhythmia, the long QT syndrome, and the Harvey *ras*-1 gene. *Science* 1991;252:704.
8. Milne JR, Ward DE, Spurrell RAJ, et al. The long QT syndrome: Effects of drugs and left stellate ganglion block. *Am Heart J* 1982;104:194.
9. Cinca J, Evangelista A, Montoyo J, et al. Electrophysiologic effects of unilateral right and left stellate ganglion block on the human heart. *Am Heart J* 1985;109:46.
10. Weintraub RG, Gow RM, Wilkinson JL. The congenital long QT syndromes in childhood. *J Am Coll Cardiol* 1990;16:674.
11. Moss AJ, Schwartz PJ, Crampton RS, et al. The long QT syndrome: Retrospective longitudinal study of 328 families. *Circulation* 1991;84:1136.
12. Vincent GM, Timothy KW, Leppert M, et al. The spectrum of symptoms and QT intervals in carriers of the gene for the long-QT syndrome. *N Engl J Med* 1992;327:846.
13. Schwartz PJ, Periti M, Milliani A. The long QT syndrome. *Am Heart J* 1975;89:378.
14. Bhandari AK, Shapiro WA, Morady F, et al. Electrophysiologic testing in patients with the long QT syndrome. *Circulation* 1985;71:63.
15. Curtiss EI, Heibel RH, Shaver JA. Autonomic maneuvers in hereditary QT interval prolongation (Romano-Ward syndrome). *Am Heart J* 1978;95:420.
16. Mitsutaka A, Takeshita A, Kuroiwa A, et al. Usefulness of the Valsalva maneuver in management of the long QT syndrome. *Circulation* 1981;63:1029.
17. Schwartz PJ, Locati E. The idiopathic long QT syndrome: Pathogenetic mechanisms and therapy. *Eur Heart J* 1985;6:103.
18. Schwartz PJ, Locati E, Priori SG, et al. The Long Q-T syndrome. In: Zipes DP, Jalife J, eds.*Cardiac Electrophysiology*. Philadelphia: WB Saunders Co; 1990;589.
19. Bhandari A, Scheinman MM, Moradi F, et al. Efficacy of left sympathectomy in the treatment of patients with long-QT syndrome. *Circulation* 1984;70:1018.

20. Eldar M, Griffin JY, Abbott JA, et al. Permanent cardiac pacing in patients with the long QT syndrome. *J Am Coll Cardiol* 1987;10:600.

21. Till AJ, Shinebourne EA, Pepper J, et al. Complete denervation of the heart in a child with congenital long QT and deafness. *Am J Cardiol* 1988;62:1319.

22. Surawicz B. The pathogenesis and clinical significance of primary T wave abnormalities. In: Schlant RC, Hurst JW, eds. *Advances in Electrocardiography.* New York: Grune & Stratton; 1972;377.

23. Surawicz B. Electrocardiographic pattern of cerebrovascular accident. *JAMA* 1966;197:913.

24. Di Pascuale G, Pilleni G, Andreoli A, et al. Torsade de pointes and ventricular flutter-fibrillation following spontaneous cerebral subarachnoid hemorrhage. *Int J Cardiol* 1988;18:163.

25. Velebit V, Podrid PJ, Cohen B, et al. Aggravation and provocation of ventricular arrhythmias by antiarrhythmic drugs. *Circulation* 1982; 65:886.

26. Keren A, Tzivoni D, Gavish D, et al. Etiology, warning signs and therapy of torsade de pointes. *Circulation* 1981;64;1167.

27. Sideris DA, Kontoyannis DA, Moulopuolos SD. Torsade de pointes and Aprindine. *Int J Cardiol* 1985;7:413.

28. Kennedy HL. Late proarrhythmia and understanding the time of occurrence. *Am J Cardiol* 1990;66:1139.

29. Kemper AJ, Dunlap R, Pietro DA. Thioridazine-induced torsade de pointes. *JAMA* 1983;249:2931.

30. Fowler N, McCall D, Chou TC, et al. Electrocardiographic changes and cardiac arrhythmias in patients receiving psychotropic drugs. *Am J Cardiol* 1976;37:323.

31. Crane GE. Cardiac toxicity and psychotropic drugs. *Dis Nerv Sys* 1970;31:534.

32. Weld FM, Bigger JT. Electrophysiological effects of imipramine on ovine cardiac Purkinje and ventricular muscle fibers. *Cir Res* 1980;46:167.

33. Rawling DA, Fozzard HA. Effects of imipramine on cellular electrophysiological properties of cardiac Purkinje fibers. *J Pharmacol Exp Ther* 1979;209:371.

34. Ludomirsky A, Klein HO, Sarelli P, et al. QT prolongation and polymorphous (torsadesde pointes): ventricular arrhythmias associated with organophosphorus insecticide poisoning. *Am J Cardiol* 1982; 49:1654.

35. Mirvis DM. Spatial variation of QT intervals in normal persons and patients with acute myocardial infarction. *J Am Coll Cardiol* 1985;5:625.

36. Haynes RE, Hallstrom AP, Cobb LA. Repolarization abnormalities in survivors of out-of-hospital ventricular fibrillation. *Circulation* 1978; 57:654.

37. Puddu PE, Bourassa MG, Leperance J, et al. Can the mode of death be predicted in patients with angiographically documented coronary artery disease? *Clin Cardiol* 1983;6:384.

38. Schwartz PJ, Wolf S. QT interval prolongation as predictor of sudden death in patients with myocardial infarction. *Circulation* 1978;57:1074.

39. Ahnve S, Helmers C, Lundman T, et al. QT$_c$ intervals in acute myocardial infarction: First-year prognostic implications. *Clin Cardiol* 1980; 3:303.

40. Moller M. QT interval in relation to ventricular arrhythmias and sudden cardiac death in postmyocardial infarction patients. *Act Med Scand* 1980;208:55.

41. Vedin A, Wilhelmsen L, Wedel H, et al. Predictor of cardiovascular deaths and non-fatal reinfarctions after myocardial infarction. *Acta Med Scand* 1977;201:309.

42. Puddu PE, Bourassa MG. Prediction of sudden death from QT$_c$ interval prolongation in patients with chronic ischemic heart disease. *J Electrocardiol* 1986;19:203.

43. Martí V, Bayés de Luna A, Arriola J, et al. Value of dynamic QT$_c$ in arrhthmology. *New Trend Arrhyth* 1988;4:683.

44. Martí V, Guindo J, Homs E, et al. Peaks of QT$_c$ lengthening measured in Holter recordings as a marker of life-threatening arrhythmias in postmyocardial infarction patients. *Am Heart J* 1992;124T:234.

45. Homs E, Viñolas X, Guindo J, et al. Automatic QT$_c$ lengthening measurement in Holter ECG as a marker of life-threatening arrhythmias in postmyocardial infarction patients. *J Am Coll Cardiol* 1992;21:274A.

46. Surawicz B. Relation between electrocardiogram and electrolytes. *Am Heart J* 1967;73:814.

47. Fredlund BO, Olsson SB. Long QT interval and ventricular tachycardia of torsade de pointes type in hypothyroidism. *Acta Med Scand* 1983;61:419.

48. O'Keefe JC, Butrous GS, Dymond DS, et al. Ventricular arrhythmias complicating weight reduction therapy in a patient with a prolonged QT interval. *Post Med J* 1985;61:319.

49. Isner JM, Sours HE, Paris AL, et al. Sudden, unexpected death in avid dieters using the liquid-protein-modified-fast diet: Observations in 17 patients and the role of the prolonged QT interval. *Circulation* 1979;60:1401.

50. Rassmussen LH, Andersen T. The relationship between QT$_c$ changes and nutrition during weight lost after gastroplasty. *Acta Med Scand* 1985;217:271.

51. Kahn JK, Sisson JC, Vinik AI. QT interval prolongation and sudden cardiac death in diabetic autonomic neuropathy. *J Clin Endocrinol Metab* 1987;64:751.

52. Bellavere F, Ferri M, Guarini L, et al. Prolonged QT period in diabetic autonomic neuropathy: A possible role in sudden cardiac death? *Br Heart J* 1988;59:379.

Chapter XIII

Preexcitation Syndromes and Sudden Death

Although ventricular arrhythmias are responsible for the vast majority of sudden cardiac deaths, the role of supraventricular arrhythmias in the genesis of sudden death is not well known. Recent studies suggest that supraventricular arrhythmias, particularly in the presence of an accessory conduction pathway, may cause sudden death in a small, but significant, number of cases.[1,2] Wang et al.[2] retrospectively evaluated 290 patients with aborted sudden death who were referred for invasive electrophysiological study. The importance of supraventricular tachycardia as a cause of sudden death was emphasized by the presence of 13 patients (4.5% in that series). Six of those patients had an accessory conduction pathway and either atrial fibrillation or atrioventricular reentrant tachycardia that degenerated into ventricular fibrillation. The remaining patients had atrioventricular (AV) reentrant tachycardia, atrial fibrillation, or enhanced AV node conduction which deteriorated into ventricular fibrillation (Fig. 1).

Wolff-Parkinson-White Syndrome and Sudden Death

It is common for patients with Wolff-Parkinson-White syndrome to experience episodes of paroxysmal atrial tachyarrhythmias.[3] Although the risk of sudden death is low, a small percentage of these patients may develop ventricular fibrillation and sudden death[4] (Fig. 2).

From: S. Goldstein, A. Bayés-de-Luna, J. Guindo-Soldevila: *Sudden Cardiac Death.* Armonk, NY: Futura Publishing Co., Inc., © 1994.

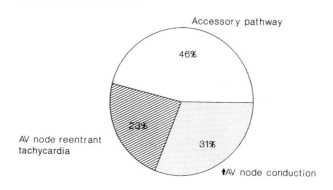

Accessory pathway

46%

AV node reentrant
tachycardia

23%

31%

↑AV node conduction

13/290 (4.5%) of aborted sudden death

Figure 1. Supraventricular tachyarrhythmias and sudden death (from Wang et al.[2]).

A review of the literature between 1938 and 1983 disclosed 87 reports of sudden death with Wolff-Parkinson-White syndrome.[5-33] The greatest risk of sudden death is in patients with atrial fibrillation with a rapid ventricular response. This is due to the existence of one or several anomalous pathways with a very short antegrade refractory period.[14,16,28,32,34-36] Because of the rarity of ventricular fibrillation in patients with Wolff-Parkinson-White syndrome, it is difficult to establish the principal risk factors for sudden death. In two large series that have examined electrophysiological and exercise testing or ambulatory recordings, a good sensitivity and negative predictive value for the identification of patients at high risk was achieved.[5,28] They have, however, a low specificity and positive predictive value.[37]

Klein et al.[28] examined the risk of ventricular fibrillation in patients with Wolff-Parkinson-White syndrome. They compared 31 patients with at least one episode of ventricular fibrillation to 73 patients who were studied for symptomatic Wolff-Parkinson-White arrhythmias, but without ventricular fibrillation. Of the 31 patients

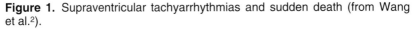

Figure 2. Ventricular fibrillation appeared during rapid atrial fibrillation in a patient with Wolff-Parkinson-White syndrome (Reproduced with permission from Bayés de Luna. *Textbook of Clinical Electrocardiography.* New York: Futura Publishing Company; 1993).

with ventricular fibrillation, 6 had identifiable causes unrelated to preexcitation. In the remaining 25 patients, ventricular fibrillation occurred following atrial fibrillation with a rapid conduction over the accessory pathways. The clinical characteristics of patients with and without ventricular fibrillation are shown in Table 1. A history of atrial fibrillation or reciprocating tachycardia was more common in patients with ventricular fibrillation. The two groups did not differ in sex, age, duration of symptoms, associated cardiac anomalies, or use of digitalis. Ventricular fibrillation occurred within 10 hours after acute administration of digoxin for treatment of atrial fibrillation in 6 patients. Electrophysiological studies reveal that there was a significantly greater incidence of multiple accessory atrioventricular

Table 1

Clinical Characteristics of Patients with Ventricular Fibrillation and the Wolff-Parkinson-White Syndrome

Characteristic	Ventricular Fibrillation n = 31	Control n = 73	P Value
Male (%)	68.0	65.8	NS
Age at onset of symptoms (yr)			
Mean	18.3	19.5	NS
Range	6–68	1–57	NS
Duration of symptoms (yr)			
Mean	9.4	12.1	NS
Range	0–42	0–50	
Age at study (yr)			
Mean	27.8	31.7	NS
Range	8–68	10–60	
Associated anomaly (%)	20.0	20.5	NS
Digoxin therapy (%)	48.0	37.0	NS
History of atrial fibrillation %	76.0	49.3	0.01
History of both atrial fibrillation and reciprocating tachycardia (%)	56.0	24.7	0.004

(From Klein et al.[28])

pathways in patients with ventricular fibrillation. The location of the accessory pathway, however, did not distinguish the ventricular fibrillation group from the control group. All patients in the ventricular fibrillation group were capable of antegrade conduction over the accessory pathway at cycle lengths of 300 milliseconds or less. They also had refractory periods of less than 350 milliseconds, although there was considerable overlap in the two groups. The R-R interval between preexcitation beats in the ventricular fibrillation group was significantly shorter than that in the control group (180 versus 240 milliseconds, ($P < 0.001$). The shortest R-R interval did not exceed 250 milliseconds in any patient with ventricular fibrillation. The researchers concluded that patients with Wolff-Parkinson-White syndrome who are prone to ventricular fibrillation have a history of atrial fibrillation or reciprocating tachycardia, demonstrate rapid conduction over an accessory pathway during atrial fibrillation, and have multiple accessory pathways.

The European Cooperative Study analyzed the clinical and electrophysiological data of 23 patients with Wolff-Parkinson-White syndrome from seven European centers.[5] All patients were resuscitated from ventricular fibrillation. The results were compared with 100 patients with Wolff-Parkinson-White syndrome and symptomatic supraventricular tachyarrhythmias, but without ventricular fibrillation. In 6 of the 23 patients (26%), ventricular fibrillation was the first manifestation of Wolff-Parkinson-White syndrome. Only 1 patient was taking antiarrhythmic drugs when ventricular fibrillation occurred. No significant differences were found between patients with and without ventricular fibrillation in age, complaints of palpitations, syncope, and presence of structural heart disease. The retrograde effective refractory period of the accessory pathway, the atrial refractory period, and the fastest atrial pacing rate with 1:1 antegrade conduction over the accessory pathway were similar in both groups. Significant differences were found for sex, permanent preexcitation on the electrocardiogram, type of documented supraventricular tachyarrhythmias, shortest R-R interval less than or equal to 220 milliseconds during spontaneous atrial fibrillation, inducibility of supraventricular tachyarrhythmias, ventricular effective refractory period of less than or equal to 190 milliseconds, mean shortest R-R interval during induced atrial fibrillation of less than or equal to 180 milliseconds and the presence of multiple accessory pathways (Table 2). After comparing the clinical data of patients with and without ventricular fibrillation, they suggested criteria of high and low

Table 2

Clinical Characteristics and Electrocardiographic Data of Patients with Wolff-Parkinson-White Syndrome

	VF	Control	P	% Sensitivity	% Specificity	% +PV	% −PV
	% of pts. n = 23	% of pts. n = 100					
Male	87	67	0.05	86	33	22	91
Syncope	17	7	NS				
Heart disease	39	17	NS				
ECG perm. WPW	100	77	0.01	100	23	24	100
Documented Spontaneous Arrhythmias							
CMT	43	23	NS				
AFL	22	2	0.01	21	98	71	84
AF	43	19	0.05	43	81	34	86
SH RR spont.							
AF ≤ 220 ms	100	58	0.05	100	42	47	100
AF or CMT	74	39	0.01	73	61	30	91
Doc. SVT	78	39	0.001	78	61	31	92
Doc. > 1 SVT	26	4	0.01	26	96	60	84

AF = atrial fibrillation; AFL = atrial flutter; CMT = circus movement tachycardia; Doc. SVT = documented supraventricular tachycardia; ECG perm. WPW = permanent preexcitation in available electrocardiograms; NS = not significant; + PV = positive predictive value; − PV = negative predictive value; SH = shortest; SVT = supraventricular tachycardia; VF = ventricular fibrillation. (From Torner P et al.[5])

risk for sudden death (Table 3). The most important conclusion of this study was that the characteristics of antegrade conduction of the anomalous pathway during atrial fibrillation is the major determinant of risk for ventricular fibrillation. In addition, the type of supraventricular tachyarrhythmia previously documented, the presence of more than one supraventricular tachycardia in the same patient, and two or more anomalous pathways were also important predictors. The presence of intermittent preexcitation on the surface ECG and RR interval of greater than 220 milliseconds during atrial fibrillation identified a group of patients at low risk of ventricular fibrillation. The lack of prognostic value of syncope and the importance of multiple accessory pathways as a risk factor for ventricular fibrillation in patients with Wolff-Parkinson-White syndrome has recently been confirmed by other researchers.[38–40]

In patients at high risk of sudden death it is possible to prevent the occurrence of arrhythmias by interrupting the anomalous pathway with surgery or ablation techniques[41–43] (Chapter XVIII). To carry out this type of treatment, a thorough electrophysiological study is necessary in order to determine the number of anomalous pathways and their anatomical position. It is important to know if the trigger is of intranodal or atrial origin, and with or without participation of the anomalous pathways. This is particularly important since it is necessary to suppress all the mechanisms responsible for the arrhythmias.

A large experience with surgery has been developed, most of which is confined to the endocardial approach.[44] The epicardial approach also can be used, particularly when there is a right anomalous pathway. The excellent results, however, reported with catheter ablation techniques[45] have almost totally supplanted surgery for Wolff-Parkinson-White syndrome.[46] The possibility for success with ablation techniques is greater than 95%. Catheter ablation has become the first option for symptomatic patients (Chapter XVIII). It is also the treatment of choice for asymptomatic patients who have a short antegrade refractory period of the accessory pathway and a high ventricular rate during induced atrial fibrillation.

Lown-Ganong-Levine Syndrome

Little data exists concerning the Lown-Ganong-Levine syndrome and sudden death.[47,48] However, in some patients with this phenomenon, atrial fibrillation, atrial flutter with 1:1 atrioventricu-

Table 3

Clinical and Electrophysiological Characteristics of High- and Low-Risk of VF in WPW Patients

	% Specificity	% Sensitivity
High Risk		
Clinical characteristics:		
1. Spontaneous documentation of more than 1 type of SVT	96	26
2. Spontaneous documentation of AFL	98	22
3. Spontaneous documentation of AFL + AF	98	13
Electrophysiological characteristics:		
1. Shortest RR induced AF ≤ 180 ms	96	60
2. More than 1 AP	96	27
3. Shortest paced CL 1:1 VA conduction AP ≤ 240 ms	87	66
Low Risk		
Clinical characteristics:		
1. Intermittent WPW on ECG, disappearance of WPW on exercise test, Holter monitoring, or after ajmaline administration	96	48
2. Intermittent WPW on ECG	100	23
3. Shortest RR spontaneous AF > 220 ms	100	42
Electrophysiological characteristics:		
1. Shortest RR induced AF > 280 ms	100	58
2. SVT not inducible	100	21
3. ERP of the ventricle ≤ 190 ms	91	42

(From Torner P., et al.[5]) SVT = supraventricular tachycardia; AFL = atrial flutter; AF = atrial fibrillation; AP = accessory pathway; CL = circle length; VA = ventriculoatrial; ERP = effective refractory period.

lar conduction, and atrioventricular reciprocating tachycardia involving retrograde conduction via an accessory pathway, can cause ventricular fibrillation. This is seen especially in the presence of co-existent organic heart disease.

With catheter ablation techniques, cardiologists have almost completely erased the presence of preexcitation syndrome in clinical cardiology. At the same time, this technology has been applied to other less lethal, but equally debilitating, arrhythmia syndromes such as accelerated supraventricular tachycardias. This technological advance is an example of how new technologies can completely change the course of clinical cardiology.

References

1. Anderson JL. Supraventricular tachyarrhythmias: Not always so benign. *J Am Coll Cardiol* 1991;18:1720.
2. Wang Y, Scheinman MM, Chien WW, et al. Patients with supraventricular tachycardia presenting with aborted sudden death: Incidence, mechanisms, and long-term follow-up. *J Am Coll Cardiol* 1991;18:1711.
3. Mantakas ME. Natural history of WPW syndrome discovered in infancy. *Am J Cardiol* 1978;41:1097.
4. Munger TM, Packer DL, Hammill SC, et al. A population study of the natural history of Wolff-Parkinson-White syndrome in Olmsted County, Minnesota, 1953–1989. *Circulation* 1993;87:866.
5. Torner P, Brugada P, Smeets J, et al. Ventricular fibrillation in the Wolff-Parkinson-White syndrome. *Eur Heart J* 1991;12:144.
6. Wood FC, Wolferth CC, Geckeler GD. Histologic demonstration of accessory muscular connections between auricle and ventricle in a case of short P-R interval and prolonged QRS complex. *Am Heart J* 1943;25:454.
7. Kimball JL, Burch G. The prognosis of the Wolff-Parkinson-White syndrome. *Ann Intern Med* 1947;27:239.
8. Fox TT, Weaver J, March HW. On the mechanism of the arrhythmias with aberrant atrioventricular conduction (Wolff-Parkinson-White). *Am Heart J* 1952;43:507.
9. Solsona J. Una Nueva aportación de síndrome de Wolff, Parkinson y White, típico, con estrechez mitral y muerte súbita. *Rev Esp Cardiol* 1961;14:854.
10. Westlake RB, Cohen W, Syracuse P, et al. Wolff-Parkinson-White syndrome and familiar cardiomegaly. *Am Heart J* 1962;64:314.
11. Touche M, Jouvet M, Touche S. Fibrillation ventriculaire au cours d'un syndrome de Wolff-Parkinson-White. Reduction par choc electrique externe. *Arch Mal Coeur* 1966;59:1122.
12. Okel BB. The Wolff-Parkinson-White syndrome. Report of a case with fatal arrhythmia and autopsy findings of myocarditis, interatrial lipomatous hypertrophy, and prominent right moderator band. *Am Heart J* 1968;75:673.

13. Puech P. Les formes graves du syndrome de Wolff-Parkinson-White. *Ann Cardiol Angéiol* 1968;17:25.
14. Kaplan MA, Cohen KL. Ventricular fibrillation in the Wolff-Parkinson-White syndrome. *Am J Cardiol* 1969;24:259.
15. Martin-Noel P, Denis B, Grundwald D, et al. Deux cas mortels de syndrome de WPW. *Arch Mal Coeur* 1970;63:1647.
16. Dreifus LS, Haiat R, Watanabe Y, et al. Ventricular fibrillation: A possible mechanism of sudden death in patients with Wolff-Parkinson-White syndrome. *Circulation* 1971;43:520.
17. Fontaine G, Bruhata M, Plagne A, et al. Le traitement des formes graves du syndrome de Wolff-Parkinson-White. *Coeur Med Int* 1972; 11:329.
18. Castillo-Fenoy A, Goupil A, Offenstadt G, et al. Syndrome de Wolff-Parkinson-White et mort subite. *Ann Med Interne* 1973;124:871.
19. James TN, Puech P. De subitaneis mortibus. IX. Type A Wolff-Parkinson-White syndrome. *Circulation* 1974;50:1264.
20. Coskey RL, Danzig R. Cardiac arrest due to extreme tachycardia with Wolff-Parkinson-White syndrome. *West J Med* 1974;120:319.
21. Lem CH, Toh CCS, Chia BL. Ventricular fibrillation in type B Wolff-Parkinson-White syndrome. *Aus NZ J Med* 1974;4:515.
22. Di Biase M, Calabrese P, Ciociola P, et al. Síndrome di preexcitazione e fibrillazione ventricolare. *Boll Soc Ital Cardiol* 1975;3:525.
23. Aquaro G, Idone P, Marra S, et al. Fibrillazione ventriculare nella sindrome di Wolff-Parkinson-White. *Min Cardioang* 1976;24:867.
24. Duvernoy WFC. Sudden death in Wolff-Parkinson-White syndrome. *Am J Cardiol* 1977;39:472.
25. Brechenmacher C, Coumel P, Fauchier JP et al. De subitaneis mortibus. XXII. Intractable paroxysmal tachycardias which proved fatal in type A Wolff-Parkinson-White syndrome. *Circulation* 1977;55:408.
26. Lipsitt LP, Sturner WQ, Oh W, et al. Wolff-Parkinson-White and sudden-infant-death syndromes. *N Engl J Med* 1979;300:1111.
27. Papa LA, Saia JA, Chung EK. Ventricular fibrillation in Wolff-Parkinson-White syndrome, type A. *Heart Lung* 1978;7:1015.
28. Klein GJ, Bashore TM, Sellers TD, et al. Ventricular fibrillation in the Wolff-Parkinson-White syndrome. *N Engl J Med* 1979;301:1080.
29. Márquez-Montes J, Esteve JJ, Rufilanchas JJ, et al. Arritmias Graves en el Síndrome de Wolff-Parkinson-White. *Rev Esp Cardiol* 1980;33:217.
30. Serrano S, Olias F, Estrada RV, et al. Graves complicaciones del síndrome de Wolff-Parkinson-White. *Rev Clin Esp* 1980;158:239.
31. Byrum CJ, Wahl RA, Behrendt DM, et al. Ventricular fibrillation associated with use of digitalis in a newborn infant with Wolff-Parkinson-White syndrome. *J Pediatr* 1982;101:400.
32. García-Cosío F, Benson DW, Anderson RW, et al. Onset of atrial fibrillation during antidromic tachycardia: Association with sudden cardiac arrest and ventricular fibrillation in a patient with Wolff-Parkinson-White syndrome. *Am J Cardiol* 1982;50:353.
33. Gulamhusein S, Ko P, Klein GJ. Ventricular fibrillation following verapamil in the Wolff-Parkinson-White syndrome. *Am Heart J* 1983; 106:145.

34. Wellens HJJ, Bar RW, Farré J, et al. Sudden death in the Wolff-Parkinson-White syndrome. In: Kulbertus HE, Wellens HJJ, eds. *Sudden Death.* London: Martinus Nijhoff; 1980;392.

35. Wellens HJJ, Durrer D. "Wolff-Parkinson-White" and atrial fibrillation: relation between refractory period of the accessory pathways and ventricular rate during atrial fibrillation. *Am J Cardiol* 1974;34:777.

36. Castellanos A, Myerburg RJ, Craparo K, et al. Factors regulating ventricular rates during atrial flutter and fibrillation in the preexcitation (Wolff-Parkinson-White) syndrome. *Br Heart J* 1973;35:811.

37. Sharma AJ, Yee R, Guiraudon G, et al. Sensitivity and specificity of invasive and noninvasive testing for risk of sudden death in Wolff-Parkinson-White syndrome. *J Am Coll Cardiol* 1987;10:373.

38. Auricchio A, Klein H, Trappe HJ, et al. Lack of prognostic value of syncope in patients with Wolff-Parkinson-White syndrome. *J Am Coll Cardiol* 1991;17:152.

39. James TN. Syncope and sudden death in the Wolff-Parkinson-White syndrome. *J Am Coll Cardiol* 1991;17:159.

40. Teo SW, Klein GJ, Guiraudon GM, et al. Multiple accessory pathways in the Wolff-Parkinson-White syndrome as a risk factor for ventricular fibrillation. *Am J Cardiol* 1991;67:889.

41. Guiraudon GM, Klein GJ, Sharma AD, et al. Surgery for the Wolff-Parkinson-White syndrome: The epicardial approach. In: Zipes DP, Jalife J, eds. *Cardiac Electrophysiology: From Cell to Bedside.* Philadelphia: WB Saunders; 1990;978.

42. Borggrefe M, Budde T, Poczeck A, et al. High frequency alternating current ablation of accessory pathway in humans. *J Am Coll Cardiol* 1987;10:576.

43. Jackman WM, Wang X, Friday K, at al. Catheter ablation of accessory atrioventricular pathways (Wolff-Parkinson-White syndrome) by radiofrequency current. *N Engl J Med* 1991;324:1605.

44. Ferguson TB Jr, Cox JL. Surgical treatment for the Wolff-Parkinson-White syndrome: The endocardial approach. In: Zipes DP, Jalife J, eds. *Cardiac Electrophysiology: From Cell to Bedside.* Philadelphia: WB Saunders; 1990;978.

45. Warin JF, Haissaguerre M, Lemetayer P, et al. Catheter ablation of accessory pathways with a direct approach: Results in 35 patients. *Circulation* 1988;78:800.

46. Kuck KH, Geiger M, Schlüter M, et al. The radio-frequency current approach to successful catheter ablation of accessory pathways. *Eur Heart J* 1990;11:324A.

47. Bendit DG, Pritchett LC, Smith WM, et al. Characteristics of atrioventricular conduction and the spectrum of arrhythmias in Lown-Ganong-Levine syndrome. *Circulation* 1978;57:454.

48. Castellanos A, Bayés de Luna A, Zaman L, et al. Risk factors for ventricular fibrillation in the preexcitation syndromes. *Practical Cardiol* 1983;9:167.

Chapter XIV

Sudden Death in Congenital Heart Disease

There are multiple mechanisms of sudden death in the pediatric and adolescent age group. Driscoll[1] reviewed 13 studies involving 61 children and adolescents who had died suddenly. He found that about one-half of the patients had hypertrophic cardiomyopathy, one-fourth had anomalous origin of the left coronary artery, and the remaining patients had aortic stenosis, cystic medial necrosis, and sinus node artery obstruction. The cause of sudden death was unknown in 3% of the cases. Other causes of sudden cardiac death in pediatric population include rupture of the aorta in patients with Marfan's syndrome, Kawasaki's disease with coronary artery involvement, Ebstein's anomaly, primary pulmonary hypertension, and the postoperative stage of tetralogy of Fallot, interventricular septal defect, complete atrioventricular canal, transposition of the great vessels, interatrial septal defect, and coarctation of the aorta. In one analysis of five pediatric studies, acute myocarditis accounted for 9% of sudden pediatric deaths.[2] Mitral valve prolapse, long QT syndrome, and Wolff-Parkinson-White syndrome are other important causes of sudden death in the young.

Sudden death occurs in 1.3 to 8.5 pediatric patients per 100,000 patients per year.[3] This accounts for 600 deaths per year in the United States. Sudden death is more common in males than females (1.7 versus 0.64 deaths per 100,000 patients per year).[4] In patients aged 1 to 20 years, sudden nontraumatic death accounts for 2% to 20% of deaths.[5,6]

From: S. Goldstein, A. Bayés-de-Luna, J. Guindo-Soldevila: *Sudden Cardiac Death.* Armonk, NY: Futura Publishing Co., Inc., © 1994.

Congenital Coronary Artery Anomalies

Congenital coronary anomalies are an uncommon cause of sudden death. It is, however, the second most common cause of sudden death in young athletes and usually occurs during physical stress (Chapter XVI). Anomalous origin of the left coronary artery from the right sinus of Valsalva[7-9] is the coronary anatomy most often associated with sudden death. In this position, the left main coronary artery abruptly turns toward the left ventricle and passes between the pulmonary root and the aorta (Fig. 1). Sudden death during exercise is thought to be due to kinking at the origin of the left main trunk or to compression of the left coronary artery between the trunks of the pulmonary artery and aorta, due to the increased systolic volume and pressure occurring during exercise. Together with the increased myocardial oxygen requirement that occurs during exercise, there is a resultant imbalance between oxygen supply and demand. This imbalance is thought to facilitate the appearance of malignant ventricular arrhythmias and sudden death. Other coronary artery anomalies are also associated with sudden death (Fig. 2). Angiography has been required to identify these structural abnormalities. Recently Fernandes et al.,[10] using transesophageal echocardiography, described the relationship between the coronary vessels

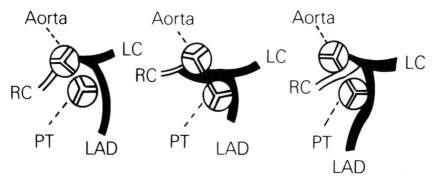

Figure 1. The anomalous origin of the left coronary artery on the right Valsalva sinus and of the right coronary artery on the left coronary sinus, compared to the normal origin of both coronary arteries. LAD = left anterior descending coronary artery; LC = left coronary; PT = pulmonary trunk; RC = right coronary. (Reproduced with permission from Maron et al. Causes of sudden death in competitive athletes. *J Am Coll Cardiol* 1986;7:204.)

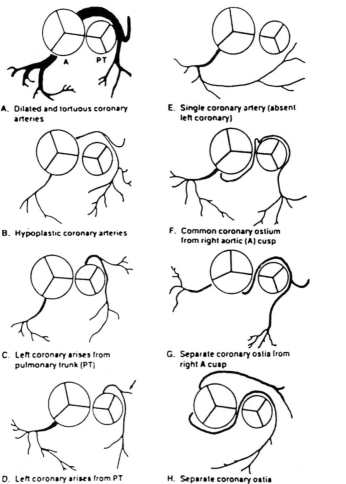

A. Dilated and tortuous coronary arteries

B. Hypoplastic coronary arteries

C. Left coronary arises from pulmonary trunk (PT)

D. Left coronary arises from PT with hypoplastic left circumflex

E. Single coronary artery (absent left coronary)

F. Common coronary ostium from right aortic (A) cusp

G. Separate coronary ostia from right A cusp

H. Separate coronary ostia from non-coronary A cusp

Figure 2. The different congenital anomalies of the coronary arteries that can be associated with sudden death. (From Toki E, McClellan JJ. *Med Sport.* 1971;5:1.)

and great vessels in better detail than can be obtained with angiography (Fig. 3).

Ebstein's Disease

In an international cooperative study of sudden cardiac death in children, 6% were due to Ebstein's disease,[11], 20% occurring in the

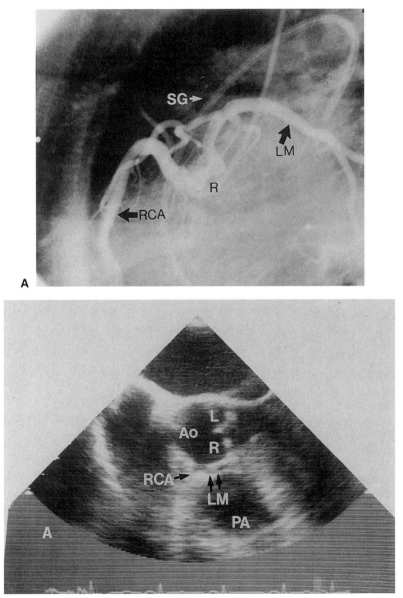

Figure 3. Angiographic (A) and transesophageal echocardiographic (TEE) (B) evaluation of an anomalous origin of the left coronary artery arising from a common right aortic sinus. Transesophageal echocardiography shows the abnormal course of the left main coronary artery between the aorta and pulmonary trunk. Ao = aorta; LM = left main coronary artery; PA = pulmonary artery; R = right coronary cusp; RCA = right coronary artery; SG = Swan-Ganz catheter (from Fernandes F et al.[10]).

first year of life.[12] Ebstein's disease is often associated with a variety of cardiac arrhythmias including paroxysmal supraventricular tachycardia, atrial fibrillation or flutter, nodal reentry tachycardias, Wolff-Parkinson-White syndrome, and ventricular arrhythmias. It is assumed that sudden death was a consequence of one of those arrhythmias in children.

Primary Pulmonary Hypertension and Eisenmenger's Syndrome

Primary pulmonary hypertension and Eisenmenger's syndrome are responsible for 17% of deaths in the international cooperative study of infant sudden death carried out by Lambert et al.[11] Sudden death is the main cause of mortality, presumably due to a cardiac arrhythmia.[13]

Postoperative Stage of Different Congenital Heart Disease

Although cardiac surgery for congenital heart disease has improved the long-term morbidity and mortality of children, there is a significant increase in the risk of sudden death in the postoperative stage of a variety of congenital heart diseases.[14] In general, the risk of arrhythmias and sudden death is greatest in those patients with poor hemodynamic results. Patients at risk are those who are symptomatic and have severe limitation of activity, cardiac enlargement, or arrhythmias.

Sudden death occurs in 2% to 10% of patients who have undergone surgery for tetralogy of Fallot.[15,16] After repair, 95% of patients develop right bundle branch block and 9% with additional left superior-anterior hemiblock. Although sudden death was initially attributed to advanced atrioventricular block,[14] recent studies indicate that the main cause of sudden death in these patients was ventricular tachyarrhythmia[16,17] which is frequently observed after surgery.[15–19] Ventricular arrhythmias are more common in older patients and in those patients with elevated right ventricular systolic and end-diastolic pressures after surgery.[19] The incidence of sudden death rises to 30% to 38% in patients with correction of tetralogy of

Fallot in whom ventricular premature beats are present on conventional ECG, ambulatory electrocardiographic recording, or during exercise testing.[15–17] Electrophysiological studies and programmed electrical stimulation have been used to identify patients at high risk.[20–23] Signal-averaged ECG also may be useful for risk stratification after repair of tetralogy of Fallot. In one series ventricular late potentials were detected in 53% of patients.[24] In a study by Stelling et al.[25] late potentials had a high sensitivity and negative predictive value for inducible ventricular tachycardia.

Some studies[19] suggest that treatment of ventricular arrhythmias results in a decrease in sudden death. Ventricular arrhythmia on routine electrocardiogram occurred in 100% of patients who later died suddenly, compared with 12% of those who did not die ($P < 0.01$). Sudden death did not occur in any of the 44 patients who were successfully treated with antiarrhythmic agents including phenytoin, propranolol, quinidine, dysopyramide, mexiletine, or amiodarone, compared to 39% in whom ventricular arrhythmias were untreated or who were unsuccessfully treated ($P < 0.01$).[19]

In patients operated on for transposition of the great vessels, the incidence of postoperative sudden death is 2% to 8%.[26,27] A significant number of patients develop arrhythmias after the Mustard or Senning procedures. Several studies have shown that 60% to 80% of patients were not in sinus rhythm six years after surgery.[28,29] Many patients have bradyarrhythmias and 10% to 15% have tachyarrhythmias, predominantly atrial flutter. Following the Mustard repair operation, sudden death has been attributed to sick sinus syndrome[30–32] and atrial flutter.[33] Other congenital heart diseases that have led to sudden death are interatrial and interventricular septal defects,[11] complete atrioventricular canal,[34] and coarctation of the aorta.[35,36] Dissection or rupture of the ascending aorta is the presumed cause of sudden death in patients with coarctation.

Congenital Advanced Atrioventricular Block

Children with complete atrioventricular block, whether acquired or congenital, are known to die suddenly. It is particularly common in the postoperative phase of various heart diseases, including corrected transposition of the great arteries,[37,38] ventriculoseptal defect, tetralogy of Fallot, and complete atrioventricular canal.[39] The incidence of sudden death increases to 60% to 80%[34,40,41] in patients with complete postoperative atrioventricular block who are not paced. The incidence of sudden death is lower [42] in patients who are unpaced with congenital complete atrioventricular block occurring as a unique phenomenon.

Congenital heart disease of itself may be associated with arrhythmias, in part due to purely anatomical reasons, but also due to pathophysiology of the disease. It is particularly frustrating to have life-threatening arrhythmias appear after the correction of congenital defects. A greater awareness of this problem has led to greater care being taken by operating surgeons and increased arrhythmic surveillance in the postoperative period.

References

1. Driscoll DJ, Edwards WD. Sudden unexpected death in children and adolescents. *J Am Coll Cardiol* 1985;5:118B.
2. Denfield SW, Garson A. Sudden death in children and young adults. *Pediatr Clin North Am* 1990;37:215.
3. Silka MJ, Kron J, Walance CG, et al. Assessment and follow-up of pediatric survivors of sudden cardiac death. *Circulation* 1990;82:341.
4. Gillette PC, Garson AJ. Sudden cardiac death in the pediatric population. *Circulation* 1992;85:I-64.
5. James TN. 15th Bethesda Conference report: Sudden cardiac death. *J Am Coll Cardiol* 1985;5:1B.
6. Molander N. Sudden natural death in later childhood and adolescence. *Arch Dis Child* 1982;57:572.
7. Liberthson RR, Dinsmore RE, Fallon JT. Aberrant coronary artery origin from the aorta. *Circulation* 1979;59:748.
8. Cheitlin MD, DeCastro CM, McAllister HA. Sudden death as a complication of anomalous left coronary origin from the anterior sinus of Valsalva: A not so minor congenital anomaly. *Circulation* 1974;50:780.
9. Kimbiris D, Iskandrian AS, Segal BL, et al. Anomalous aortic origin of coronary arteries. *Circulation* 1978;58:606.
10. Fernandes F, Alam M, Smith S, et al. The role of transesophageal echocardiography in identifying anomalous coronary arteries. *Circulation* 1993;88:2532.
11. Lambert EC, Menon VA, Wagner HR, et al. Sudden unexpected death from cardiovascular disease in children: A cooperative international study. *Am J Cardiol* 1974;34:89.
12. Watson H. Natural history of Ebstein's anomaly of tricuspid valve in childhood and adolescence: An international cooperative study of 505 cases. *Br Heart J* 1974;36:417.
13. Grossman W, Braunwald E. Pulmonary hypertension. In: Braunwald E, ed. *Heart Disease: A Textbook of Cardiovascular Medicine*. Philadelphia: WB Saunders; 1992;790.
14. Wolff GS, Rowland TW, Ellison RC. Surgically induced right bundle branch block with left anterior hemiblock. *Circulation* 1972;46:587.
15. Quattlebaum TG, Varghese PJ, Neill CA, et al. Sudden death among postoperative patients with tetralogy of Fallot. *Circulation* 1976;54:289.

16. Gillette PC, Yeoman MA, Mullins CE, et al. Sudden death after repair of tetralogy of Fallot. *Circulation* 1977;56:566.
17. James FW, Kaplan S, Chou T. Unexpected cardiac arrest in patients after surgical correction of tetralogy of Fallot. *Circulation* 1975;52:691.
18. Rosing DR, Borer JS, Kent KM, et al. Long-term hemodynamic and electrocardiographic assessment following operative repair of tretalogy of Fallot. *Circulation* 1977;58:I-209.
19. Garson A, Randall DC, Gillette PC, et al. Prevention of sudden death after repair of tetralogy of Fallot: Treatment of ventricular arrhythmias. *J Am Coll Cardiol* 1985;6:221.
20. Horowitz LN, Vetter VL, Harken AH, et al. Electrophysiologic characteristics of sustained ventricular tachycardia occurring after repair of tetralogy of Fallot. *Am J Cardiol* 1980;46:446.
21. Garson A, Porter C, Gillette PC, et al. Induction of ventricular tachycardia during electrophysiologic study after repair of Tetralogy of fallot. *J Am Coll Cardiol* 1983;1:1492.
22. Kugler JD, Mooring PH, Pinsky WW, et al. Sustained ventricular tachycardia following repair of tetralogy of Fallot: New electrophysiologic findings. *Am J Cardiol* 1982;49:998.
23. Chandar JS, Wolff GS, Garson A, et al. Ventricular arrhythmias in postoperative tetralogy of Fallot. *Am J Cardiol* 1990;65:655.
24. Zimmermann M, Friedli B, Adamec R, et al. Frequency of ventricular late potentials and fractioned right ventricular electrograms after operative repair of tetralogy of Fallot. *Am J Cardiol* 1987;59:448.
25. Stelling JA, Danford DA, Kugler JD, et al. Late potentials and inducible ventricular tachycardia in surgically repaired congenital heart disease. *Circulation* 1990;82:1690.
26. Saalouke MG, Rios J, Perry LW, et al. Electrophysiologic studies after Mustard's operation for transposition of the great vessels. *Am J Cardiol* 1978;41:1104.
27. Champsaur GL, Sokol DM, Trusler GA, et al. Repair of transposition of the great arteries in 123 pediatric patients. *Circulation* 1973;47:1032.
28. Duster MC, Bink-Boelkens MTE, Wampler D, et al. Long-term follow-up of dysrhythmias following the Mustard precedure. *Am Heart J* 1985;109:1323.
29. Haynes CJ, Gersony WM. Arrhythmias after the Mustard operation for transposition of the great arteries: A long-term study. *J Am Coll Cardiol* 1986;7:133.
30. Gillette PC, El-Said GM, Silvarjan N, et al. Electrophysiological abnormalities after Mustard operation for transposition of the great arteries. *Br Heart J* 1974;36:186.
31. Gillette PC, Kugler JD, Garson A, et al. Mechanisms of cardiac arrhythmias after the Mustard operation for transposition of the great arteries. *Am J Cardiol* 1980;45:1225.
32. Bharati S, Molthan ME, Veasy G, et al. Conduction system in two cases of sudden death two years after the Mustard procedure. *J Thorac Cardiovasc Surg* 1979;77:101.
33. Garson A, Bink-Boelkens M, Hesslien PS, et al. Atrial flutter in the young: A collaborative study of 380 cases. *J Am Coll Cardiol* 1985;6:871.

34. Levy MJ, Cuello L, Tuna N, et al. Atrioventricular communis. *Am J Cardiol* 1964;14:587.
35. Forfang K, Rostad H, Sorland S, et al. Late sudden death after surgical correction of coarctation of the aorta. *Acta Med Scand* 1979;206:375.
36. Reifenstein GH, Levine SA, Gross RE. Coarctation of the aorta: A review of 104 autopsied cases of the "adult type," 2 years of age or older. *Am Heart J* 1947;33:146.
37. Friedberg DZ, Nadas AS. Clinical profile of patients with cogenital corrected transposition of the great vessels. *N Engl J Med* 1970;282:1053.
38. Walker WJ, Cooley DA, McNamara DG, et al. Corrected transposition of the great vessels, atrioventricular heart block and ventricular septal defect: A clinical triad. *Circulation* 1958;17:249.
39. Godman MJ, Roberts NK, Izukawa T. Late postoperative conduction disturbances after repair of ventricular septal defect and tetralogy of Fallot. *Circulation* 1974;49:214.
40. Lillehei CW, Sellers RD, Bonnabeau RC, et al. Chronic postsurgical complete heart block. *J Thorac Cardiovasc Surg* 1963;46:436.
41. Stanton RE, Lindesmith GG, Meyer BW. Pacemaker therapy in children with complete heart block. *Am J Dis Child* 1975;129:484.
42. Michaelsson M, Engle MA. Congenital complete heart block: An international study of the natural history. In: Engle MA, ed. *Pediatric Cardiology*. Philadelphia: FA Davis; 1972;85.

Chapter XV

Sudden Infant Death Syndrome

Sudden death is generally considered to be a problem unique to the adult population. While this is generally true, sudden infant death syndrome, or crib death, remains an important clinical problem in apparently healthy children during the first year of life. This syndrome has been defined as the death of infants with no previous clinical history and in whom a thorough postmortem examination fails to demonstrate a cause of death.[1-3]

Epidemiology

Sudden infant death syndrome has a peak incidence between the second and fourth months of life and then declines progressively to become almost uncommon after the sixth month.[4] During the first two weeks of life, when infant mortality is increased due to other causes, sudden infant death is not usually observed (Fig. 1).

Sudden infant death syndrome represents the main cause of death in the first year of life in the United States, involving approximately 10,000 infants each year.[5] Incidence varies widely from country to country, and even within the same country[4,6-25] (Table 1). It appears that temperate countries have a higher incidence of sudden infant death than do those with warmer climates. The incidence in Alaska, for example, is approximately 6/1000 live births, while in California it is only 1.5/1000. In Spain and other Mediterranean countries the incidence is much lower, varying between 0.01 and

From: S. Goldstein, A. Bayés-de-Luna, J. Guindo-Soldevila: *Sudden Cardiac Death.* Armonk, NY: Futura Publishing Co., Inc., © 1994.

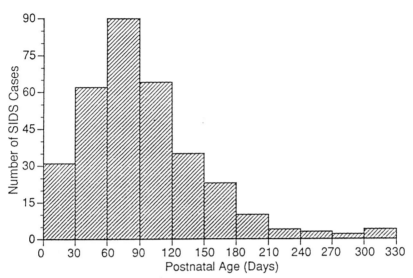

Figure 1. Age distribution of victims of sudden infant death in King County, Washington, 1969–1977 (from Petersen[4]). SIDS = sudden infant death syndrome.

0.24/1000 live births. The incidence of sudden infant death also appears to have a seasonal variability and is more frequent in winter.[26]

In addition to the geographic and environmental factors, sudden infant death has been related to other factors. Poor social conditions, associated with minimal prenatal medical care, fewer medical follow-ups during the first year of life, and lower intellectual level of the mother contribute to the risk of sudden death. Smoking during pregnancy doubles the risk of sudden infant death.[27] The incidence of crib death in infants of narcotic-dependent mothers is 20.9/1000 live births, six times greater than that of infants born of non-narcotic-dependent mothers.[28] In these cases, as in women with a low socioeconomic level, the increased incidence should be interpreted with caution. Many of these pregnancies are unwanted and some may actually be homicidal deaths in infants of narcotic-dependent mothers.[28–30]

Pathogenesis

The etiology and mechanisms responsible for this syndrome are controversial. It is currently presumed that the mechanism of sudden infant death syndrome is due to an autonomic nervous system disorder that affects the regulation of the cardiovascular and

Table 1

Worldwide Geographic Comparisons of Sudden Infant Death Syndrome: Crude Incidence Rates

Location	Period	Rate/1000 live birth
Canada		
Ontario	1964–1974	3.0
United States		
California	1968	1.5
Cuyahoga County, OH	1965–1974	2.5
Dade County, FL	1965–1974	1.5
Hennepin County, MN	1965–1974	1.5
King County, WA	1965–1974	2.5
Philadelphia County, PA	1965–1974	2.1
Shelby County, TN	1965–1974	2.1
Upper New York State	1974	1.4
Olmsted County, MN	1946–1965	1.2
North Carolina	1972–1974	2.1
Collaborative Perinatal Project	1959–1966	2.3
Czechoslovakia		
Middle Bohemia	1967	0.8
Denmark		
Copenhagen	1956–1971	0.9
Great Britain		
Northern Ireland	1965–1967	2.3
Oxford	1965–1970	2.8
Glasgow	1970	2.7
Netherlands	1969–1971	0.6
Sweden		
Stockholm	1968–1972	0.6
Japan		
Hokkaido & Kyushu	1974	1.2
New Zealand		
Aukland	1970–1972	1.9
Southern Australia	1965–1970	1.7
Tasmania	1970–1976	2.9
Western Australia	1973	2.2
France	1980–1985	1.03–1.61
Germany	1980–1985	1.05–1.58
Portugal	1980–1985	0.01–0.12
Italy	1980–1983	0.02–0.05
Spain	1980–1983	0.13–0.24

(Adapted from Peterson DP[4] and Camarasa F.[23])

respiratory systems,[31] which leads to apnea, cardiac rhythm disorders, and sudden death. Few deaths are due to heart disease.[32] Several researchers suggest the possibility that some may be due to long QT syndrome.[33–37] Schwartz et al.[37] analyzed the electrocardiograms of 5000 presumably healthy newborn infants. Among them, three were later victims of sudden infant death syndrome, and all three had a prolonged QT interval at the time of a neonatal electrocardiogram. Other investigators have failed to confirm this finding. It is possible that the long QT syndrome could account for 10% to 15% of the cases of infant sudden death. Wolff-Parkinson-White syndrome and other arrhythmias have also been associated with sudden death in infants.[38] Southall[5] was not able to correlate arrhythmias detected during a 24-hour electrocardiogram to sudden infant death syndrome. They prospectively recorded 24-hour ECGs and respiratory movement in 6914 full-term and 2337 pre-term infants or infants of low-birth weight. Forty recordings were made in 29 infants (11 full-term, 12 preterm) who subsequently suffered sudden infant death syndrome. None of the 29 infants had prolonged apnea with cessation of breathing movements for more than 20 seconds. Only one preterm infant had multiple parasystolic ventricular premature complexes. None of the infants had evidence of the preexcitation syndrome. Compared with recordings obtained in control infants, there was no evidence of abnormal prolongation of the QT_c interval. In this study, sudden infant death syndrome could not be predicted by either prolonged apnea or cardiac arrhythmias.[5]

Autopsy studies have shown mild cardiovascular and respiratory abnormalities. These findings, however, do not explain the sudden death of the infants. Endocardial thickening[39] and abnormal luminal narrowing of the sinus node[40] and atrioventricular node arteries[41] have been reported, as well as changes in the atrioventricular node and the bundle of His branches.[42–44] An observed increase in the smooth muscle of the pulmonary arteries could be attributed to chronic hypoxia.[45,46] Abnormalities affecting the central vagal nucleus[47] and some of the melanized fibers of the cervical vagus[48] have also been found. Disorders of the autonomic nervous system were detected in some infants who suffered an aborted sudden death event.[49–52] Kahn et al.[50] elicited an enhanced vagal response to ocular compression in the form of prolonged asystoles. Shannon and Kelly[31] detected disturbances in the heart rate and RR variability in infants with aborted sudden death syndrome.

Prevention

There is an unfortunate inability to predict sudden infant death syndrome. However, there are several groups of infants at greatest risk of crib death. They include infants who have undergone a near-miss sudden infant death syndrome, siblings of infants who died suddenly, and infants with prolonged apneas. Special apnea monitors with alarms that are activated when prolonged apneic periods occur are now available.[53,54] They may, however, cause considerable family anxiety and are not always totally reliable.

References

1. Guntheroth WG. *Crib Death: Sudden Infant Death Syndrome.* New York: Futura Publishing Company; 1989.
2. Culberston JL, Krous HF, Bendell RD. *Sudden Infant Death Syndrome: Medical Aspects and Psychological Management.* Baltimore: Johns Hopkins University Press; 1988.
3. Schwartz PJ, Southall DP, Valdés-Dapena M. The sudden infant death syndrome: Cardiac and respiratory mechanisms and interventions. *Ann NY Ac Sci* 1988;533:1.
4. Peterson DR. Evolution of the epidemiology of sudden infant death syndrome. *Epidemiologic Rev* 1980;2:97.
5. Southall DP, Richards JM, de Swiet M, et al. Identification of infants destined to die unexpectedly during infancy: Evaluation of predictive importance of prolonged apnea and disorders of cardiac rhythm or conduction. First report of a multicentred prospective study into the sudden infant death syndrome. *Br Med J* 1983;286:1092.
6. Kraus AS, Steele R, Langworth JT. Sudden unexpected death in infancy in Ontario. Part I. Methodology and findings related to the host. *Can J Public Health* 1967;58:359.
7. Kraus JF, Borhani NO. Post-neonatal sudden unexplained death in California: A cohort study. *Am J Epidemiol* 1972;95:497.
8. Peterson DR, Chinn NM. Sudden infant death trends in six metropolitan communities. *Pediatrics* 1979;60:75.
9. Standfast SJ, Jereb S, Janerich DT. The epidemiology of sudden infant death in upstate New York. *JAMA* 1979;241:1121.
10. Fitzgibbon JP, Nobrega FT, Ludwig J, et al. Sudden, unexpected, and unexplained death in infants. *Pediatrics* 1969;43:980.
11. Blok JH. The incidence of sudden infant death syndrome in North Carolina's cities and counties: 1972–1974. *Am J Public Health* 1978; 68:367.
12. Naeye RL, Ladis B, Drage JS. Sudden infant death syndrome: A prospective study. *JAMA* 1976;130:1207.

13. Bergman AB, Beckwith JB, Ray CG. Part II. Epidemiology. Sudden infant death syndrome: Proceedings of the Second International Conference on Causes of Sudden Death in Infants. Seattle: University of Washington Press; 1970;25.

14. Biering-Sorensen F, Jorgensen T, Hilden J. Sudden infant death in Copenhagen 1956–1971: I. Infant feeding. *Acta Paediatr Scand* 1978;17:129.

15. Peterson DR, Beckwith JB, Benson EA. The sudden infant death syndrome in hospitalized babies. *Pediatrics* 1974;54:644.

16. Fredrick J. Sudden unexpected death in infants in the Oxford Record Linkage Area. *Br J Prev Soc Med* 1974;27:93.

17. Richards IDG, McIntosh HT. Confidential inquiry into 226 consecutive infant deaths. *Arch Dis Child* 1972;47:697.

18. Robinson RR. SIDS 1974. Proceedings of the Francis E. Camps International Symposium on sudden and unexpected deaths in infancy. Toronto: The Canadian Foundation for the Study of Infant Deaths; 1974;91.

19. Naito J. Study on infants' sudden death: Infants' sudden death in Hokkaido and Kyushu: Report of the studies of the Nippon Auku Research Institute, No 12; 1976;83.

20. Beal S. Sudden infant death syndrome. *Med J Aust* 1972;2:1223.

21. Grice AC, McGlashan ND. Sudden death in infancy in Tasmania, 1970–1976. *Med J Aust* 1978;2:177.

22. Hilton JMN, Turner KJ. Sudden death in infancy syndrome in Western Australia. *Med J Aust* 1976;1:427.

23. Camarasa i Piquer F. La síndrome de la mort sobtada del lactant (SMSL). *Ann Med* (Barc) 1989;75:223.

24. Vidal Bota J. Síndrome de la muerte súbita del lactante y episodios inexplicados de apnea. Visiín actual del problema. *An Esp Pediatr* 1988;29(S32):258.

25. Medina Ramos N, Huguet P, Toran N. Muerte súbita en la infancia. Aportación de 95 casos autópsicos. *Rev Esp Pediat* 1975;31:813.

26. Bosner RS, Knight BH, West RR. Sudden infant death syndrome in Cardiff: association with epidemic influenza and with temperature–1955–1974. *Int J Epidemiol* 1978;7:335.

27. Malloy MH, Kleinman JC, Land GH, et al. The association of maternal smoking with age and cause of infant death. *Am J Epidemiol* 1988;128:46.

28. Rajegowda BK, Kandall SR, Faciglia H. Sudden unexpected death in infants of narcotic-dependent mothers. *Early Human Dev* 1978;2:219.

29. Meadow R. Not so sudden infant death. *Arch Dis Child* 1989;64:1216.

30. Anonymous. Sudden infant death and suffocation. *Br Med J* 1989; 299:455.

31. Shannon DC, Kelly DH. SIDS and near-SIDS. *N Engl J Med* 1982; 306:959.

32. Valdés-Dapena MA. Sudden infant death syndrome: A review of the medical literature 1974–1979. *Pediatrics* 1980;66:597.

33. Maron BJ, Clark CE, Goldstein RE, et al. Potential role of QT interval prolongation in sudden infant death syndrome. *Circulation* 1976; 54:423.

34. Kelly DH, Shannon DC, Liberthson RR. The role of the QT interval in the SIDS. *Circulation* 1977;55:633.

35. Steinschneider A. Sudden infant death syndrome and prolongation of the QT interval. *Am J Dis Child* 1978;132:688.

36. Schwartz PJ, Montemerlo M, Facchini M. The QT interval throughout the first six months of life: A prospective study. *Circulation* 1982;66:496.

37. Schwartz PJ. Cardiac sympathetic innervation and sudden infant death syndrome. *Am J Med* 1976;60:167.

38. Keeton BR, Southall E, Rutter N. Cardiac conduction disorders in six infants with near-miss sudden infant deaths. *Br Med J* 1977;2:600.

39. Williams RB, Emery JL. Endocardial fibrosis in apparently normal hearts. *Histopathology* 1978;2:283.

40. Kozakewich HPW, McManus BM, Vawter GF. The sinus node in sudden infant death syndrome. *Circulation* 1982;65:1242.

41. Anderson KR, Hill RW. Occlusive lesions of cardiac conduction tissue arteries in sudden infant death syndrome.*Pediatrics* 1982;69:50.

42. James TN. Sudden death in babies: New observations in the heart. *Am J Cardiol* 1968;22:479.

43. Valdés-Dapena MA, Greene M, Basavanard N, et al. The myocardial conduction system in sudden death in infancy. *N Engl J Med* 1973;289:1179.

44. Lie JT, Rosenberg HS, Erickson EE. Histopathology of the conduction system in the sudden infant death syndrome. *Circulation* 1976;53:3.

45. Williams A, Vawter G, Reid L. Increased muscularity of the pulmonary circulation in victims of sudden infant death. *Pediatrics* 1979;63:18.

46. Naeye RL, Whalen P, Ryser M, et al. Cardiac and other abnormalities in the sudden infant death syndrome. *Am J Pathol* 1976;82:1.

47. Tadkashima S, Armstrong D, Becker L, et al. Cerebral hypoperfusion in the sudden infant death syndrome: Brainstem gliosis and vasculature. *Ann Neurol* 1978;4:257.

48. Sachis PN, Armstrong DL, Becker LE, et al. The vagus nerve and sudden infant death syndrome: A morphometric study. *J Pediatr* 1981;98:278.

49. Schwartz PJ. Cardiac sympathetic innervation and the sudden infant death syndrome: A possible pathologic link. *Am J Med* 1967;60:167.

50. Kahn A, Riazi J, Blum D. Oculocardiac reflex in near-miss for sudden infant syndrome infants. *Pediatrics* 1983;71:49.

51. Salk L, Grellong BA, Dietrich J. Sudden infant death: normal cardiac habituation and poor autonomic control. *N Engl J Med* 1974;291:219.

52. Guilleminault C, Ariagno R, Souquet M, et al. Abnormal polygraphic findings in near-miss sudden infant death. *Lancet* 1976;1:1326.

53. Davis PA, Milner AD, Silverman M, et al. Monitoring and sudden infant death syndrome: An update. Report from the Foundation for study of infant deaths and the British paediatric respiratory group. *Arch Dis Child* 1990;65:238.

54. Samuels MP, Poet CF, Southall DP. Monitoring and sudden infant death syndrome. *Arch Dis Child* 1990;65:913.

Chapter XVI

Sudden Death in Other Cardiovascular Diseases

Sudden Death in Apparently Healthy People: Primary Ventricular Fibrillation

In the absence of heart disease or other known causal factors, sudden cardiac death is exceptional. Even when ventricular premature impulses and modulating factors exist, the absence of vulnerable myocardium makes the appearance and perpetuation of malignant arrhythmias difficult. However, sudden death occurs without detectable heart disease. A definite cardiovascular etiology is absent in up to 8% of patients who die suddenly.[1,2] In 233 victims of sudden death who died while wearing an ambulatory electrocardiographic recorder, 5% of patients had no known cardiac disorder[3,4] (Fig. 1). Idiopathic ventricular fibrillation represents about 1% of all cases of resuscitated out-of-hospital cardiac arrest.[5,6] Between 3% to 9% of ventricular fibrillation episodes are not related to acute myocardial infarction.[6,7] In patients under 40 years of age, 14% of ventricular fibrillation episodes occur in the absence of definable heart disease.[8,9]

Viskin and Belhassen[10] reviewed 54 patients with idiopathic ventricular fibrillation occurring in patients without known heart disease reported between 1948 and 1990. Data on age and gender were available in 45 patients, of whom 33 were males and 12 were females, aged 9 to 68 years (mean 36 ± 16) years. Fifty (93%) pa-

From: S. Goldstein, A. Bayés-de-Luna, J. Guindo-Soldevila: *Sudden Cardiac Death*. Armonk, NY: Futura Publishing Co., Inc., © 1994.

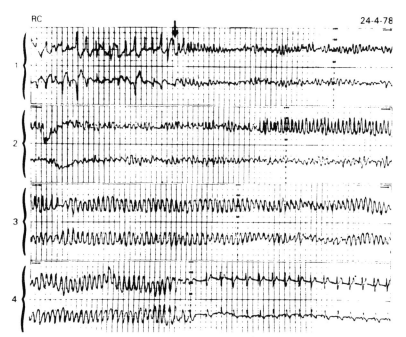

Figure 1. Idiopathic ventricular fibrillation with spontaneous reversion recorded on Holter ECG. (Reproduced with permission from Dubner et al. *Am Heart J* 1983;105:691.)

tients were resuscitated from ventricular fibrillation, while syncope due to documented nonsustained ventricular fibrillation occurred in four. Prodromal symptoms of syncope and palpitations were noted in 28% and 15% of patients, respectively. Episodes of documented ventricular fibrillation occurred invariably during the daytime. Psychological stress preceded ventricular fibrillation in 22% of patients, while physical exertion was involved in 15%. Electrophysiologic study without antiarrhythmic treatment was available in 36 patients. Sustained ventricular tachyarrhythmias were induced in 69% of cases. The inducible arrhythmia was ventricular fibrillation in 7 patients, sustained polymorphic ventricular tachycardia in 11, sustained monomorphic ventricular tachycardia in 1, and sustained ventricular tachycardia of unrecorded morphology in 6 patients.

The possibility exists, however, that subclinical or latent heart disease may not have been recognized while the patient was alive or appreciated at the time of postmortem study. Routine clinical examination may not disclose abnormalities in patients with malignant ventricular arrhythmias. Endomyocardial biopsy may demonstrate histologic lesions with interstitial fibrosis, cellular hypertrophy or, in rare cases, myocarditis, which can explain a sudden death.[11–13] In the study of Viskin and Belhassen,[10] histologic abnormalities[10] were observed in 11 patients, 4 of whom demonstrated nonspecific or granulomatous myocarditis. With improved diagnostic techniques, the number of patients with "no apparent heart disease" or "primary ventricular arrhythmias" may decrease.

The prognosis of patients with idiopathic ventricular fibrillation is not favorable.[10,14,15] During a follow-up from 2 months to 14 years in 37 patients, 4 died suddenly within a year of diagnosis.[10] Five additional patients experienced recurrent nonfatal ventricular fibrillation or ventricular tachycardia and 1 had recurrent syncope. Thus, in this retrospective study there was a 25% recurrence of malignant ventricular tachyarrhythmias. In 15 patients treated with a type IA antiarrhythmic drug, neither sudden death nor recurrent syncope occurred. In contrast, there were 2 sudden deaths and 3 nonfatal recurrences among 12 patients treated with beta-blocking agents.[10]

Other studies confirm the unfavorable prognosis of patients with idiopathic ventricular fibrillation.[14,15] Recurrence rate of ventricular fibrillation was observed in 33% of the patients not treated with antiarrhythmic agents.[14] Recurrent sudden death occurred in 22% of patients treated with antiarrhythmic drugs. The conclusion of these studies suggests that automatic implantable cardioverter defibrillator should be considered as the treatment of choice in survivors of cardiac arrest without organic heart disease (Chapter XVIII).

Most of these observations regarding idiopathic ventricular fibrillation are based on isolated case reports or retrospective studies. Conclusions based on these studies should be made with some caution. A prospective international registry, the Unexplained Cardiac Arrest Registry of Europe (UCARE), is presently underway.[16] This official project of the Working Group on Arrhythmias of the European Society of Cardiology may improve our knowledge on idiopathic ventricular fibrillation.

Sudden Death in Athletes

Since Pheidippides died in Athens in 490 B.C. after announcing the victory in Marathon over the Persians,[17] cases of sudden death occurring during or immediately after exercise have been reported.

The incidence of sudden death has increased in the last few years, coinciding with the popularity of active sports, particularly jogging, squash, and swimming. Sudden death in athletes usually occurs as a result of cryptic cardiovascular diseases.[18–20] Other abnormalities have also been reported to cause occasional sudden death, such as subarachnoid hemorrhage,[21] acute gastrointestinal bleeding,[22] or traffic accidents.[23]

Sudden cardiac death of an athlete during training or competition attracts enormous attention since it affects young, apparently healthy subjects. The true incidence is difficult to estimate. Despite these difficulties, attempts have been made to evaluate the statistical risk of sudden death during athletic activities. In football players, Opie[18] estimated that sudden death occurs once in every 50,000 hours of football play or once in every 3000 hours of refereeing. Koplan[24] calculates that 1/100,000 joggers die suddenly every year while running. A more recent study of the incidence of sudden death in joggers reported an incidence of sudden death 17 times higher than that estimated by Koplan.[23]

Until 1983, 109 cases of sudden death in athletes were published.[25] Fifty-one deaths occurred during or immediately after running, 32 in football players, 9 in basketball players, 4 in tennis players, and 13 in other sports. In the last few years, an increased incidence of sudden death in squash players has attracted special attention,[26–28] Northcote et al.[28] collected 60 cases of sudden death in squash players, 59 males and 1 female, between the ages of 22 and 66. Death was due to cardiac disease in 58 cases; 51 with ischemic events, 4 due to valvular heart disease, 2 in individuals with a history of arrhythmias, and 1 with hypertrophic myocardial heart disease. Only 2 deaths were of noncardiac origin. Forty-five of the victims had prodromal symptoms, the most frequent being chest pain, and 22 had known coronary risk factors, usually hypertension.

The cardiovascular anomalies most commonly associated with death in athletes[29–31] are highly conditioned by the subject's age. In young athletes under 35, sudden death occurs fundamentally in patients with cardiomyopathy, usually, but not exclusively, of the hypertrophic variety[29] (Fig. 2). Other less common disorders are congenital anomalies of the coronary arteries, aortic rupture, idiopathic left ventricular hypertrophy, and coronary atherosclerosis. Less frequent sudden death is due to myocarditis, mitral valve prolapse, aortic valvular stenosis, and sarcoidosis. In contrast, sudden

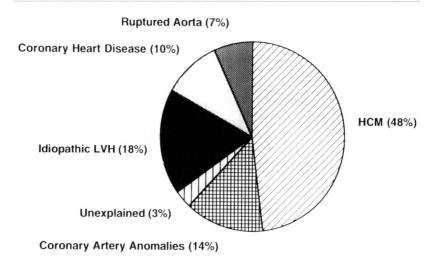

Ruptured Aorta (7%)

Coronary Heart Disease (10%)

HCM (48%)

Idiopathic LVH (18%)

Unexplained (3%)

Coronary Artery Anomalies (14%)

< 35 YEARS OLD

Figure 2. Disease associated with sudden death in young athletes (from Maron et al.[29]). HCM = hypertrophic cardiomegaly; LVH = left ventricular hypertrophy.

death in athletes over 35[29] (Fig. 3) is due to coronary heart disease in 80% of victims. Other forms of heart disease such as hypertrophic cardiomyopathy, mitral prolapse, and acquired valvular heart disease explain an additional 15%, and in approximately 5% of cases, no organic heart disease can be identified.

In athletes who have significant risk factors, a thorough study of cardiac factors including ECG, stress test, ambulatory ECG, signal-averaged ECG, echocardiogram, electrophysiological study, and even a coronary angiography is necessary. In athletes with Wolff-Parkinson-White syndrome, esophageal atrial stimulation has also been recommended in order to trigger tachyarrhythmias and to understand atrial conduction mechanisms in individual patients.[32] If an athlete has Wolff-Parkinson-White syndrome and paroxysmal supraventricular arrhythmias during exercise, radiofrequency ablation of the accessory pathway is often recommended.

In patients with heart disease without symptoms or ECG abnormalities during the stress test, close follow-up is recommended and athletic activity should be guided by severity of the disease. In general, competitive sports are not recommended in these patients.

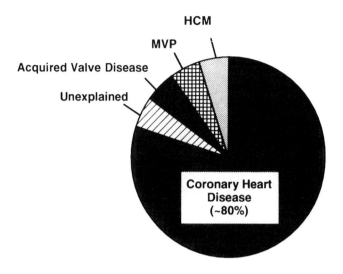

≥ 35 YEARS OLD

Figure 3. Disease associated with sudden death in athletes over 35 (from Maron et al.[29]). HCM = hypertrophic cardiomyopathy; MVP = mitral valve prolapse.

Borderline cases do exist in which the decision may be individualized. This could apply to patients with mitral valve prolapse without mitral insufficiency, or mild aortic insufficiency. In those situations, if all the tests are negative, the decision to participate in the sport should be made with the athlete, considering the advantages and risks of the athletic activity. The American College of Cardiology recently published guidelines on this subject.[33] We believe that it is important for competitive athletes to be examined by a cardiologist in order to evaluate the clinical situation of each individual and decide whether or not a particular activity is advisable and safe.

Electrolyte Imbalance

Electrolyte imbalance can precipitate malignant ventricular arrhythmia, particularly when ventricular premature impulses and vulnerable myocardium coexist. We have previously discussed the role of electrolyte imbalance in the genesis of sudden death[34,35] (Chapter II).

The quality of the water supply has also been proposed as a cause of both ischemic heart disease and sudden death. Hard water is considered to be protective, while soft water contributes to mortality due to ischemic heart disease[36–39] (Chapter V). The key determinant for the increased mortality associated with soft water appears to be a magnesium deficiency. A number of studies relate hypomagnesemia to ventricular arrhythmias.[40] Diuretics can also cause magnesium depletion. An increased incidence of arrhythmias has been observed in patients with low magnesium levels.[41–43] Both hypokalemia and hypomagnesemia increase cardiac sensitivity to digoxin, even when blood digoxin levels are normal.[44] Treatment with magnesium sulfate has been shown to be effective in the treatment of ventricular tachycardias of the torsade de pointes type.[45,46]

Hypomagnesemia has also been related to increased reactivity of the vascular smooth muscle structure and it is suspected that magnesium depletion may facilitate coronary spasm.[47,48] Chadda et al.[47] demonstrated experimentally in dogs that after 100 days of a low-magnesium diet, ergonovine can induce coronary spasm and ischemic sudden death associated with ventricular fibrillation.

Magnesium depletion can occur in the setting of an acute myocardial infarction.[38,49–51] Flink et al.[52] suggested that lipolysis induced by catecholamines increases the release of free fatty acids that bind magnesium and causes hypomagnesemia in the first hours after infarction. These observations may explain the increased electrical instability present in the first hours of myocardial infarction. Magnesium sulfate has been demonstrated to be effective in the treatment of ventricular arrhythmias in the acute phase of myocardial infarction.[45]

Obesity

Obesity itself is an important predictor of sudden death as a coronary risk factor (Chapter V). Treatment of obesity with high-protein liquid slimming diets has also led to sudden death.[53–56] This usually occurs in young women after rapid weight loss averaging 35% of basal weight in five months.[53,54] The electrocardiograms of these patients demonstrate prolongation of the QT interval, nonspecific repolarization changes, and low-voltage QRS complexes (Chapter XII). Death usually is a result of a malignant ventricular arrhythmia. In addition, instances of advanced atrioventricular block have been described.[56] Postmortem study of these individuals exposed to rapid weight loss exhibit signs of prolonged fasting characterized by thinning of myocardial fibers and increased myocardial lipofuscin pigmentation. Mononuclear myo-carditis was observed in two patients and in one, ganglionitis and neuritis similar to that seen in victims of sudden death with an idiopathic long QT syndrome[53,55] was reported.

Cardiac Tumors

Intracardiac tumors, either benign or malignant, can cause syncope and sudden death.[57] The mechanism of death is usually physical obstruction of the blood flow in the cardiac chamber. Occasionally cardiac tumors may cause ventricular tachyarrhythmias or different types of bradyarrhythmias. The most common primary cardiac tumor, atrial myxoma, causes syncope in approximately 20% of cases and almost 15% of patients with atrial myxomas die suddenly.[58]

Aortic Dissection

Dissection of the aorta is also a consideration in patients who dies suddenly.[59] In young patients, it is often associated with Marfan's syndrome, which explains 7% of the cases of sudden death in athletes under 35 (Fig. 2). In elderly patients it is usually associated with hypertension of long duration.

Massive Pulmonary Emoblism

Massive pulmonary embolism can also result in sudden death.[60] It is usually due to thromboembolism, although fat emboli occurring after orthopedic surgery, or amniotic emboli during childbirth,[61,62] may also cause acute pulmonary embolism.

Arterial Hypertension

Several studies suggest that patients with arterial hypertension are at increased risk of ventricular arrhythmias and sudden death.[63–65] The Framingham study demonstrated that left ventricular hypertrophy is a powerful risk factor for sudden death, congestive heart failure, acute myocardial infarction, and stroke (Chapter

V). In addition recent data suggest that elevated resting heart rate in hypertensive patients (> 90 beats per minute is also an important independent prognostic factor for sudden cardiac death.[65] The results of the trial indicate that beta blockers, but not diuretics, reduce the risk of sudden death in patients with hypertension (Chapter XVII).

This varied picture of sudden death adds a degree of uncertainty to the puzzle of these events. Although the vast number of sudden death events are due to ischemia and coronary heart disease, an intriguing variety of unknown and poorly understood phenomena may initiate a sudden fatal arrhythmic event.

References

1. Reichenbach DD, Moss NS, Meyer E. Pathology of the heart in sudden cardiac death. *Am J Cardiol* 1977;39:865.
2. Raymond JR, van den Berg EK, Knapp MJ. Nontraumatic prehospital sudden death in young adults. *Arch Intern Med* 1988;148:303.
3. Bayés de Luna A, Guindo J, Rivera I. Ambulatory sudden death. *J Ambul Holter Mon* 1988;2:3.
4. Bayés de Luna A, Coumel Ph, Leclercq JF. Ambulatory sudden death: Mechanisms of production of fatal arrhythmia on the basis of data from 157 cases. *Am Heart J* 1989;117:151.
5. Myerburg RJ, Conde CA, Sung RJ, et al. Clinical, electrophysiologic and hemodynamic profile of patients resuscitated from prehospital cardiac arrest. *Am J Med* 1980;68:568.
6. Cobb LA, Baum RS, Alvarez H, et al. Resuscitation from out-of-hospital ventricular fibrillation: 4-years' follow-up. *Circulation* 1975;51:III-223.
7. Swerdlow CD, Bardy GH, McAnulty J, et al. Determinants of induced sustained arrhythmias in survivors of out-of-hospital ventricular fibrillation. *Circulation* 1987;76:1053.
8. Reich P, DeSilva RA, Lown B, et al. Acute psychological disturbances preceding life-threatening ventricular arrhythmias. *JAMA* 1981;246:223.
9. Morady F, Scheinman MM, Hess DH, et al. Clinical characteristics and results of electrophysiologic testing in young adults with ventricular tachycardia or ventricular fibrillation. *Am Heart J* 1983;106:1306.
10. Viskin S, Belhassen B. Idiopathic ventricular fibrillation. *Am Heart J* 1990;120:661.
11. Strain JE, Grose RM, Factor SM, et al. Results of endomyocardial biopsy in patients with spontaneous ventricular tachycardia but without apparent structural heart disease. *Circulation* 1983;68:1171.
12. Vignola PA, Kazutaka A, Swayne PS, et al. Lymphocytic myocarditis presenting as unexplained ventricular arrhythmias. *J Am Coll Cardiol* 1984;4:812.

13. Sugrue DD, Holmes DR, Gersh BJ, et al. Cardiac histologic findings in patients with life-threatening ventricular arrhythmias of unknown origin. *J Am Coll Cardiol* 1984;4:952.
14. Siebels J, Schneider MAE, Geiger M, et al. Unexpected recurrences in survivors of cardiac arrest without organic heart disease. *Eur Heart J* 1991;(suppl);12:86. Abstract.
15. Wever E, Hauer R, Oomen A, et al. Unfavorable outcome in patients with primary electrical disease who survived unexpected cardiac arrest. *Eur Heart J* 1991;(Suppl);12:86. Abstract.
16. Priori SG, Borggrefe M, Camm AJ, et al. Unexplained cardiac arrest. The need for a prospective registry. *Eur Heart J* 1992;13:1445. Editorial.
17. Herodotus; De Selincourt A, Trans. *The Histories.* New York: Penguin Books Inc;1954;397.
18. Opie LH. Sudden death and sport. *Lancet* 1975;i:263.
19. Vuori I, Makarainen N, Jaaskelainen A. Sudden death and physical activity. *Cardiolgy* 1978;63:287.
20. Jokl E, McLellan JT. *Exercise and Cardiac Death.* Baltimore: University Park Press; 1971.
21. Lynch P. Soldiers, sports and sudden death. *Lancet* 1980;i:1235.
22. National Safety Council Accident Facts. Chicago: NSC; 1981.
23. Thompson PD, Funk EJ, Carleton RA, et al. Incidence of death during jogging in Rhode Island from 1975 through 1980. *JAMA* 1982;274:2535.
24. Koplan JP. Cardiovascular deaths while running. *JAMA* 1979;242:2578.
25. Northcote RJ, Ballantyne D. Sudden cardiac death in sport. *Br Med J* 1983;287:1357.
26. Fowler AW. Cause of death on squash courts. *On Call* 1980;14:7.
27. Northcote RJ, Evans ADB, Ballantyne D. Sudden death in squash players. *Lancet* 1984;i:148.
28. Northcote RJ, Flannigan C, Ballantyne D. Sudden death and vigorous exercise: A study of 60 deaths associated with squash. *Br Heart J* 1986;55:198.
29. Maron BJ, Epstein SE, Roberts WC. Causes of sudden death in competitive athletes. *J Am Coll Cardiol* 1986;7:204.
30. Maron BJ, Roberts WC, McAlliser HA, et al. Sudden cardiac death in young athletes. *Circulation* 1980;62:218.
31. Waller BF, Roberts WC. Sudden death while running in conditioned runners aged 40 years or over. *Am J Cardiol* 1980;45:1292.
32. Furlanello F, Vergara G, Berttini R, et al. Progress in the study of Wolff-Parkinson-White syndrome of the athletes: The transesophageal atrial pacing during bycicle exercise. *J Sports Card* 1984;1:102.
33. Mitchell JH, Maron BJ, Epstein SE. 16th Bethesda Conference: Cardiovascular abnormalities in the athlete: Recommendations regarding elegibility for competition. *J Am Coll Cardiol* 1985;6:1186.
34. Hollenberg NK, Hollifield JW. Potassium/Magnesium depletion: Is your patient at risk of sudden death? *Am J Med* 1987;82:3A.
35. Birkenhäger WH, Solomon RJ, Wills MR. Electrolyte disturbances and cardiac risks. *Drugs* 1984;28(suppl 1):1.

36. Crawford T, Crawford MD. Prevalences and pathological changes of ischemic heart disease in hard water and in a soft water area. *Lancet* 1967;i:229.
37. Schroeder HA. Municipal drinking water and cardiovascular death rates. *JAMA* 1966;95:125.
38. Anderson TW, LeRiche WH, Hewitt D, et al. Magnesium water hardness and heart disease. In: Cantin M, Seelig MS, eds. *Magnesium in Health and Disease.* New York: Spectrum Books;1980;565.
39. Anderson TW, Neri LC, Schreiber GB, et al. Ischemic heart disease, water hardness, and myocardial magnesium. *Canadian Med Assoc J* 1975;113:199.
40. Lauler DP. Magnesium deficiency: Pathogenesis, prevalence, and strategies for repletion. *Am J Cardiol* 1989;63:1G.
41. Wester PO, Dyckner T. Diuretic treatment and magnesium losses. Paper presented by the Swedish Society of Cardiology: Electrolytes and Cardiac Arrhythmias. Stockholm: 1980;194.
42. Dyckner T. Serum magnesium in acute myocardial infarction. *Acta Med Scand* 1980;207:59.
43. Dyckner T, Wester PO. Magnesium and potassium in serum and muscle in relation to disturbances of cardiac rhythm. In: Cantin M Seelig MS, eds. *Magnesium in Health and Disease.* New York: Spectrum Books; 1980;551.
44. Iseri LT, Chung P, Tobis J. Magnesium therapy for intractable ventricular tachyarrhythmias in normomagnesemic patients. *West J Med* 1983;138:215.
45. Abraham AS, Rosenmann D, Kramer M, et al. Magnesium in prevention of lethal arrhythmias in acute myocardial infarction. *Arch Intern Med* 1987;147:753.
46. Tzivoni D, Banai S, Schuger C, et al. Treatment of torsade de pointes with magnesium sulfate. *Circulation* 1988;77:392.
47. Chadda K, Schultz N, Hamby R. Coronary spasm and magnesium deficiency: Possible role in sudden coronary death. *Circulation* 1981;64 (suppl.IV): 321.
48. Altura B. Sudden death ischemic heart disease and dietary magnesium intake: Is the target site coronary vascular smooth muscle? *Med Hypoth* 1979;5:843.
49. Iseri LT, Alexander LC, McCaughey RS, et al. Water and electrolyte content of cardiac and skeletal muscle in heart failure and myocardial infarction. *Am Heart J* 1952;43:215.
50. Heggtveit HA, Tanser P, Hunt BJ. Magnesium content of normal and ischemic human heart. Proceedings of the 7th International Congress of Clinical Pathology. Montreal: 1969;53.
51. Ebel H, Gunther T. Role of magnesium in cardiac disease. *J Clin Chem Clin Biochem* 1983;21:249.
52. Flink EB, Brick JE, Shane SR. Alterations of long chain free fatty acid and magnesium concentrations in acute myocardial infarction. *Arch Intern Med* 1981;141:441.
53. Isner JM, Sours HE, Paris AL, et al. Sudden, unexpected death in avid dieters using the liquid-protein-modified-fast diet: Observations in

17 patients and the role of the prolonged QT interval. *Circulation* 1979;60:1401.

54. Singh BN, Gaarder TD, Kanegae T, et al. Liquid protein diets and torsades de pointes. *JAMA* 1978;240:115.

55. Siegel RJ, Cabeen WR, Roberts WC. Prolonged QT interval-ventricular tachycardia syndrome from massive rapid weight with sinus node ganglionitis and neuritis. *Am Heart J* 1981;102:121.

56. Lantigua RA, Amatruda JM, Biddle TL, et al. Cardiac arrhythmias associated with a liquid protein diet for the treatment of obesity. *N Engl J Med* 1980;303:735.

57. Colucci WS, Braunwald E. Primary tumors of the heart. In: Braunwald E, ed. *Heart Disease: A Textbook of Cardiovascular Medicine.* Philadelphia: WB Saunders; 1992;1451.

58. Fisher J. Cardiac myxoma. *Cardiovasc Rev Rep* 1983;9:1195.

59. Eagle KA, De Sanctis RW. Diseases of the aorta. In: Braun-wald E, ed. *Heart Disease: A Textbook of Cardiovascular Medicine.* Philadelphia: WB Saunders; 1992;1528.

60. Goldhaber SZ, Braunwald E. Pulmonary embolism. In: Braunwald E, ed. *Heart Disease: A Textbook of Cardiovascular Medicine.* Philadelphia: WB Saunders; 1992;1558.

61. Morgan M. Amniotic fluid embolism. *Anaesthesia* 1979;34:20.

62. Aronson ME, Nelson PK. Fatal air embolism in pregnancy resulting from an unusual sexual act. *Obstet Gynecol* 1967;30:127.

63. Meserli FH, Soria F. Hypertension, left ventricular hypertrophy, ventricular ectopy, and sudden death. *Am J Med* 1992;93:2A-21S.

64. Bayés de Luna A, Viñolas X, Guindo J. Ventricular arrhythmias in left ventricular hypertrophy and heart arrhythmias in left ventricular hypertrophy and heart failure. *Eur Heart J* 1993;14:62J.

65. Wannamethee G, Shaper AG, Perry IJ. Hypertension, heart rate, and sudden cardiac death. *J Hypertension* 1992;l0:1435.

Chapter XVII

Prevention of Sudden Cardiac Death:
A Pharmacological Approach

Prevention of sudden death is one of the foremost challenges to modern cardiology because of its dramatic presentation and its socioeconomic repercussions. Many of its victims are relatively young, in their productive years, and have an acceptable quality of life in spite of heart disease. Because of this, a variety of investigations have been carried out in an attempt to develop primary and secondary approaches to the prevention of sudden death.

Primary and Secondary Correction of Coronary Risk Factors

Since ischemic heart disease is the main cause of sudden death, any reduction in the incidence of ischemic disease may have a favorable effect on sudden death. The correction of coronary risk factors including lipid disorders, hypertension, smoking, obesity, diabetes, sedentary lifestyle, and stress are important areas of primary prevention.

Although a decreased trend in the incidence of total and sudden death has been detected in primary prevention studies (Table 1), it is not possible to demonstrate that correction of any specific factor explains the reduction in cardiac mortality or sudden death.[1]

From: S. Goldstein, A. Bayés-de-Luna, J. Guindo-Soldevila: *Sudden Cardiac Death.* Armonk, NY: Futura Publishing Co., Inc., © 1994.

Table 1

Sudden Cardiac Death and Nonsudden Death Associated with Coronary Artery Disease in Studies of Primary Prevention

Studies	Interv.	No. of subjects	SCD		NSD + CAD	
			Interv.	Control	Interv.	Control
Treatment of hypercholesterolemia:						
Los Angeles Veterans Administration	Diet	846	18	27	23	23
Helsinki Mental Hospital	Diet	922	(Undetermined)		6	12
WHO-Clofibrate	Clofibrate	10,627	23	17	35	34
LCR-CPPT	Cholesterol	3,806	(Undetermined)		30	38
Multifactorial treatment:						
Oslo	Cholesterol tobacco	1,232	3	11	3	3
MRFIT	Multiple	12,866	54	58	61	66
WHO-MRFIT	Multiple	60,881	(Undetermined)		83	64
Total		91,180	98	113	241	240
			(77)	(88)	(53)	(53)

Interv. = intervention; LCR-CPPT = Lipid Research Clinics Primary Prevention Trials; MRFIT = Multiple Risk Factor Intervention Trial; NSD + CAD = nonsudden death associated with coronary artery disease; SCD = sudden cardiac death; WHO = World Health Organization.

Placebo-controlled studies in hypertension using thiazide diuretic regimens mostly demonstrated a reduction in overall mortality. This reduction is, however, mainly due to a mortality reduction in stroke and renal failure. No clear effect on coronary mortality has been demonstrated in these studies.[2] In the Multiple Risk Factor Intervention Trial (MRFIT)[3] and the Medical Research Council Study,[4] in which diuretics were used to reduce blood pressure, an actual increase in cardiac mortality was noted. This increase was associated with an increased incidence of ventricular arrhythmias. In contrast, the mortality results of the Metoprolol Atherosclerosis Prevention in Hypertensives (MAPHY) Study that compared metoprolol to diuretics in the treatment of arterial hypertension showed that metoprolol reduced both total cardiac mortality and sudden death.[5] In a mean follow-up of 42 months, total mortality was significantly lower (65/1609) in patients randomized to metoprolol than in the patients randomized to diuretics (83/1625) ($P = 0.028$). Sudden cardiac death constituted 78% of all cardiovascular mortality. There were 32 sudden deaths in the metoprolol group and 45 in the diuretic group ($P = 0.017$) (Fig. 1). The observed reduction in sudden death in the

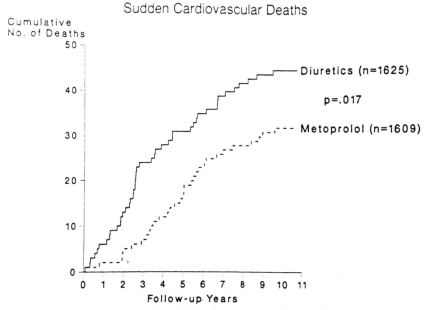

Figure 1. The comparison of the effect on sudden death of diuretic and metoprolol therapy for hypertension (from Olsson et al.[5]).

metoprolol group should be interpreted with caution since the difference observed in the MAPHY trial could be due to an increased rate of sudden cardiovascular death in thiazide-treated patients.

Trials in hypertensive patients using calcium entry blocking agents and angiotensin converting enzyme inhibitors, in addition to measuring mortality, also examine their effect on ventricular mass and ventricular arrhythmias. However, it is not clear if these factors can be used as surrogates for mortality.

In other primary prevention studies, no significant decrease in sudden death has been achieved with control of cholesterol or blood pressure.[6,7] In contrast, there is substantial evidence that cessation of smoking before or after acute myocardial infarction has an important salutary influence on subsequent mortality. Postmyocardial infarction patients who continue smoking have twice the risk of death compared to those who stop.[8]

The introduction of new drugs for the treatment of hyperlipidemia has the potential to modify both total and sudden death mortality. Gemfibrozil, a drug that inhibits cholesterol synthesis, for instance, demonstrated a significant reduction in new infarctions over a relatively short five-year follow-up, without influencing mortality.[9] Two trials in progress are evaluating the efficacy of Lovastatin and Simvastatin, HMG Co-A reductase inhibitors, on mortality in patients with known ischemic heart disease.[10]

Although most studies attempt to reduce mortality by modifying only one specific risk factor at a time, some multifactorial intervention studies have been initiated. Hämäläinen et al.[11] used a multifactorial approach toward secondary prevention and reduced the risk of sudden cardiac death. They studied 375 postmyocardial infarction patients randomly allocated to a multifactorial intervention or control group. The intervention program began a few weeks after acute myocardial infarction and consisted of optimal medical care, physical activity, antismoking and dietary advice, and discussions of psychosocial problems. Patients in the control group were followed by their own doctors and did not participate in any organized rehabilitation programs. The incidence of sudden death during the 10 years after follow-up was 12.8% in the intervention group compared to 23% in the controls ($P = 0.006$) (Fig. 2). Coronary mortality was 35.1% and 47.1%, respectively ($P = 0.03$). The difference between groups was highly significant during the first three years and remained unchanged during the rest of the follow-up.

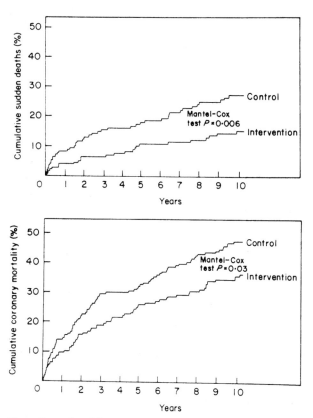

Figure 2. The effect of multifactor intervention on cumulative sudden death and coronary mortality after acute myocardial infarction (from Hämäläinen et al.[11]).

Thrombolytic Agents

Revascularization of patients with acute ischemia using fibrinolytic therapy, percutaneous transluminal coronary angioplasty, and surgery has influenced both immediate and long-term mortality. Several studies reported that thrombolysis reduced the incidence of sudden death in postmyocardial infarction patients[12–15] (see Table 1, Chapter IX). The incidence of sudden death in patients receiving thrombolysis ranged between 1% to 2% during the first year after hospital discharge[12–17] but without comparisons in a randomized controlled study.

Thrombolysis is reported to reduce the incidence of ventricular arrhythmias during ambulatory electrocardiographic recording,[10,18,19] ventricular late potentials,[19-22] and the incidence of sustained ventricular arrhythmias induced by programmed electrical stimulation.[23-25] This salutary effect was observed even in patients with depressed left ventricular dysfunction.[26] Farrell et al.[27] observed that the frequency of ventricular arrhythmias, signal-averaged late potentials, and ejection fraction less than 40% were more frequent in patients who did not receive thrombolytic therapy. The incidence of arrhythmic deaths at two years was 4.5% in patients treated with thrombolytic agents and 10.6% in controls ($P < 0.001$).

From these studies, it appears that the changes in the natural history of postmyocardial infarction patients occurring as a result of the widespread use of thrombolytic agents requires a reevaluation of previously accepted methods of risk stratification.

Antithrombotic Drugs

Platelet-inhibiting drugs have also been used to reduce the incidence of sudden cardiac death in both primary and secondary prevention programs. The administration of sulfinpyrazone, dipyridamole, ticlopidine, and aspirin have demonstrated varying results.[12] Only aspirin therapy demonstrates a consistent efficacy, particularly in the acute phase of myocardial infarction and unstable angina.[16,28-30]

Aspirin therapy as primary prevention of ischemic heart disease was investigated in two large randomized primary studies.[31] The United States Physicians' Health Study[32] and the British Doctors' Trial[33] reported an overall 33% reduction in nonfatal myocardial infarction ($P < 0.0002$) without affecting mortality. Associated with this benefit, an increased risk of hemorrhagic strokes was observed in the aspirin group.

In patients with unstable angina, aspirin significantly reduced the incidence of reinfarction[34-36] and total mortality.[35] In acute myocardial infarction, the ISIS-2 study[16] reported a beneficial effect of aspirin similar to that of streptokinase. Together, the two drugs produced an additive effect. Aspirin is now routinely used in patients with suspected and acute myocardial infarction.

In postmyocardial infarction patients, a meta-analysis of 31 randomized trials of a variety of antiplatelet therapies indicated a reduction in cardiovascular mortality of 13%, in recurrent nonfatal reinfarction of 31%, and in nonfatal strokes of 42%.[37] It has not been demonstrated, however, that antiplatelet drugs have a unique effect on sudden death in postmyocardial infarction patients. The initial reports of the Anturane Reinfarction Trial[38] suggested a 74% reduction in risk of sudden death at seven months in patients treated with sulfinpyrazone. However, important methodological problems emerged which led the United States Food and Drug Administration (FDA) to deny the claim that the drug reduced the risk for sudden death in postmyocardial infarction patients.[39] A subsequent study, the Anturane Reinfarction Italian Study Group,[40] was unable to demonstrate any reduction in the sudden death in patients treated with sulfinpyrazone.

The benefit of aspirin therapy was also evaluated in patients undergoing cardiac surgery. Patients with stable angina pectoris undergoing coronary bypass surgery who received aspirin and dipyridamole had fewer myocardial infarctions (5% versus 12%, $P = 0.05$) and new coronary lesions (23% versus 35%, $P = 0.04$), than those treated with a placebo.[41] Stroke and transient cerebral ischemia were also significantly reduced but there was, however, no difference in total mortality or cardiac death.

Several trials have examined the value of anticoagulant therapy after acute myocardial infarction.[12] (Table 2). The most recent and most convincing study, the Warfarin Reinfarction Study (WARIS),[42] demonstrated a significant reduction in mortality (24%) and reinfarction (34%) during a follow-up of 37 months (Fig. 3).

β-Adrenergic Blocking Agents

β-adrenergic blocking agents have earned a major role in the prevention of total mortality and sudden cardiac death. They have been observed to reduce infarct size and decrease mortality when administered in the acute phase of myocardial infarction, and to reduce both total and sudden cardiac death in patients who have survived the early phase of myocardial infarction.

Both metoprolol[43] and atenolol[44] were observed to improve survival when administered in the acute phase of myocardial infarction. The TIMI II-B study[45] examined the benefit of immediate versus deferred metoprolol administration following thrombolytic therapy. It was concluded that immediate intravenous administration of metoprolol (5 mg doses at two-minute intervals over six minutes), followed by 50 mg orally every 12 hours in the first 24 hours, and 100

Table 2

Results of Some Long-Term Trials of Anticoagulants After Myocardial Infarction

Trial (Year)	No. of Pts.	Mortality		Reinfarction		Embolic Events	
		Drug (%)	Placebo (%)	Drug (%)	Placebo (%)	Drug (%)	Placebo (%)
Medical Research Council Trial (1964)	383	15	21	17	43*	1	4*
Veterans Administration Cooperative Trial (1965)	747	31	33	16	21	4	8*
German Austrian Aspirin Trial (1980)	946	12	10	5	8	1	2*
Sixty Plus Reinfarction Study (1980)	878	6	11*	5	13*	1	3*
Warfarin Reinfarction Study (1990)	1214	15	20*	13	20*	3	7*

* = statistically significant difference.

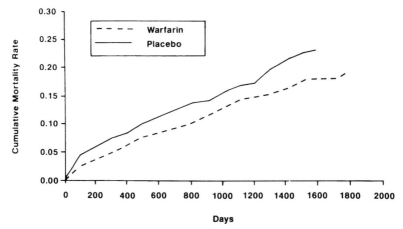

Figure 3. Cumulative rates of death from all causes, according to treatment with placebo or warfarin (from Smith et al.[42]).

mg orally every 12 hours thereafter, offered no benefit over late oral administration (50 mg/12 hours on day six, followed by 100 mg/12 hours thereafter) in improving ventricular function and mortality, but did decrease reinfarction and angina.

The administration of β-adrenergic blocking agents two to three weeks after a myocardial infarction was shown to improve survival.[46–51] Table 3 summarizes the main trials. The largest body of information is reported by the Norwegian Timolol[47] and the β-Blocker Heart Attack Trials.[48] Ten milligrams of Timolol were administered twice daily, and propranolol was given in doses of 180 to 240 mg daily. These two studies showed that, when either timolol or propranolol were administered within two to three weeks after myocardial infarction, a decrease in mortality of between 25% and 36% in the first two years could be achieved, as compared with placebo-control patients (Figs. 4 and 5). In addition, a significant reduction in reinfarction and sudden death was also observed in the actively treated timolol group.[47] Recently, Olsson et al.[52] pooled five available randomized double-blind studies of postmyocardial infarction trials of 5474 patients treated twice daily with 100 mg of metoprolol or matching placebo and followed between three months to three years. In addition to a significant decrease in total mortality, there was a highly significant reduction in sudden death (104 in placebo group and 62 in metroprolol group, $P = 0.002$) (Fig. 6).

Table 3

Selected Results of Long-Term β Blocker Trials for Secondary Prevention After Acute Myocardial Infarction (MI)

Trial/Year	No. of Pts.	β-Blocker	Entry Time From MI (d)	Mean Follow-up (mo)	Mortality		Reinfarction	
					Drug (%)	Placebo (%)	Drug (%)	Placebo (%)
Multicentre International Study (1975)	3053	Practolol	1.0	24	6.3	8.2*	4	4
Julian et al. (1980)	1456	Sotalol	8.3	12	7.3	8.9	3	4
Norwegian Multicenter Study (1981)	1884	Timolol	11.5	17	10.4	16.2*	10	14*
β-Blocker Heart Attack Trial (1982)	3738	Propranolol	13.8	25	7.2	9.8*	4	5*
Taylor et al. (1982)	1103	Oxprenolol	14 mo	48	9.5	10.2	11	12
Boissel et al. (1990)	607	Acebutolol	2–22	10	5.7	11.0	2	1.3

* = statistically significant difference.

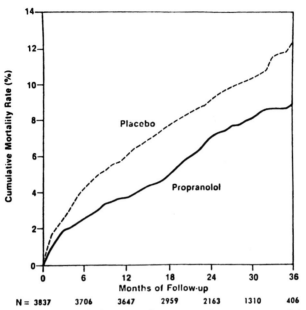

Figure 4. Life table cumulative mortality curves for groups receiving propranolol hydrochloride or placebo. N indicates total number of patients followed up through each time period (from β-Blocker Heart Attack Trial Research Group[48]).

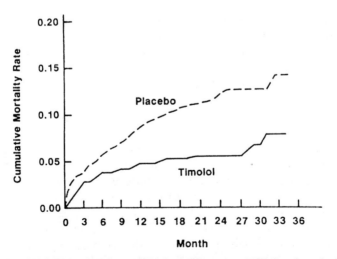

Figure 5. Effect of timolol on mortality from all causes.[47] (Reproduced with permission from Norwegian Study Group. Timolol-induced reduction in mortality and reinfarction in patients surviving acute myocardial infarction. *N Engl J Med* 1981;304:801.)

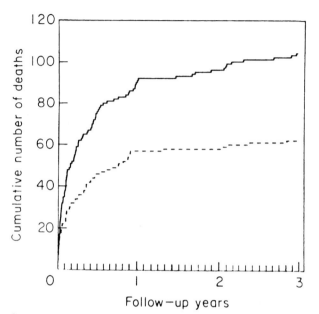

Figure 6. Cumulative number of sudden deaths reported in the five postinfarction trials. Solid line = placebo (n = 2721). P = 0.002; broken line = metoprolol (n = 2753). (From Olsen H, et al.[52])

The actual beneficial magnitude of these agents depends on the subgroup of treated postinfarction patients. Patients at an intermediate risk with an ejection fraction of 30% to 50% are the most appropriate candidates for treatment. In high-risk patients with evidence of heart failure, β-adrenergic blocking agents are beneficial but must be administered with great care. Since low-risk patients already have a low mortality rate, the benefit is only marginally important.

Analysis of patients with mild to moderate heart failure in the β-Blocker Heart Attack Trial[53] demonstrated that patients treated with oral propranolol experienced a 47% decrease in sudden death (Fig. 7). The effect of propranolol was also examined for its ability to suppress postmyocardial infarction ventricular ectopy. Although propranolol was effective in decreasing ventricular premature beats[54] (Fig. 8), a marginal benefit on sudden death mortality was observed when propranolol was compared in patients with complex ventricular premature beats to those with single premature beats[54] (Fig. 9). Although these studies indicate a major benefit of β-adrenergic

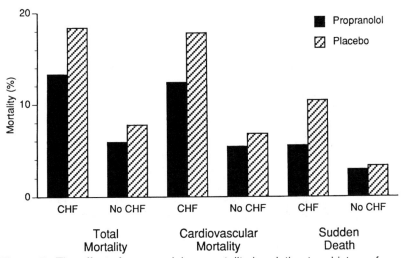

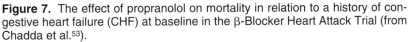

Figure 7. The effect of propranolol on mortality in relation to a history of congestive heart failure (CHF) at baseline in the β-Blocker Heart Attack Trial (from Chadda et al.[53]).

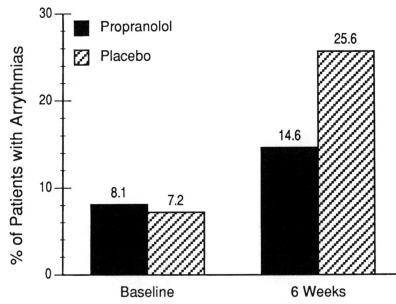

Figure 8. The effect of propranolol on the presence of ventricular arrhythmia six weeks after treatment in patients with acute myocardial infarction (from Friedman et al.[54]).

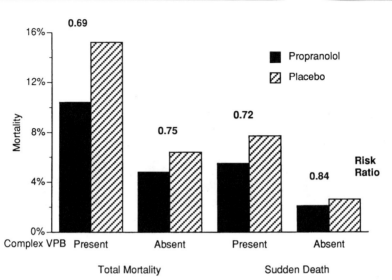

Figure 9. The effect of propranolol on total and sudden death mortality in relation to the presence or absence of complex ventricular premature beats (VPB). Risk ratio reflects the relative effect of propranolol on mortality rate in regard to complex VPB (from Friedman et al.[54]).

blocking agents when administered to patients after an acute transmural myocardial infarction, their benefits in non-Q wave infarction are not as certain.[55] Gheorghiade et al.[55] suggested that a question still remains as to the benefit of these agents in non-Q wave infarction.

The mechanism by which β-blockers affect mortality is not well understood. Possible mechanisms include an anti-ischemic effect or antiarrhythmic effect. Others have suggested that the effect of the drugs is related to the degree of bradycardia achieved (Fig. 10). In view of the results of our study[56,57] of ambulatory electrocardiographic recordings in patients dying suddenly which demonstrated an increase in heart rate prior to malignant arrhythmia, it is possible that heart rate suppression is its major mechanism of sudden death prevention.

Calcium Antagonists

Neither verapamil, diltiazem, nor nifedipine have demonstrated reduction in either total or sudden cardiac death in postmyocardial infarction patients. In the Diltiazem Reinfarction Study Group,[58,59]

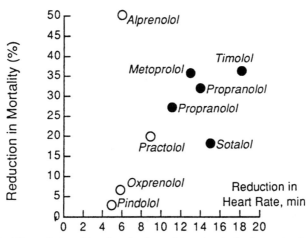

Figure 10. The relationship of reduction of heart rate to the reduction in mortality in β-blocker trials. (Reproduced with permission from Kjekshus JK. Importance of heart rate in determining β-blocker efficacy in acute and long-term myocardial infarction trials. *Am J Cardiol* 1986;57:43F.)

576 patients with acute nontransmural infarction were evaluated. Diltiazem was effective in reducing the rate of reinfarction and recurrent angina pectoris during a two-week period. When diltiazem was tested in postinfarction patients, however, no benefit was observed. Subgroup analysis of patients with heart failure and low ejection fraction showed that diltiazem increased mortality in patients with ejection fractions of less than 40% or with heart failure and pulmonary congestion (Fig. 11).

The Danish Verapamil Infarction Trial I (DAVIT I)[60] and the DAVIT II[61] suggested that verapamil may also be useful in the prevention of major events, death, or reinfarction in postmyocardial infarction patients without heart failure (Fig. 12). In contrast, verapamil could be safely administered in patients with decreased left ventricular function, but without any significant effect on mortality. Overall, there was no benefit observed with verapamil therapy in patients with heart failure, but benefit was observed in the nonheart failure group (Fig. 13). Many studies examined the role of nifedipine in postinfarction patients,[62] and all have demonstrated a negative or a neutral effect on mortality. There is little benefit associated with the use of calcium channel blocking agents, with the exception of verapamil, in the secondary prevention of mortality after an acute myocardial infarction.

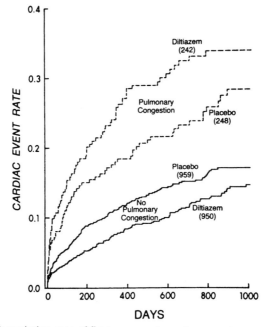

Figure 11. Cumulative rate of first recurrent cardiac events, according to treatment in patients with and without pulmonary congestion. Diltiazem-treated patients with pulmonary congestion had a higher rate of cardiac events than patients receiving placebo; diltiazem-treated patients without pulmonary congestion had a lower rate of cardiac events than patients receiving placebo. The values in parenthesis are number of patients. (Reproduced with permission from Multicenter Diltiazem Post-Infarction Trial Research group. *N Engl J Med* 1988;319:385.)

Vasodilators

Since poor ventricular function significantly increases the risk of sudden death, effective treatment or prevention of heart failure could be beneficial. Several trials of vasodilator therapy have been carried out in an attempt to prevent and treat heart failure and improve postmyocardial infarction mortality.[63] The results of the Vasodilator Heart Failure Trial (V-HeFT I)[64] showed that treatment with hydralazine (300 mg/day) and isosorbide dinitrate (160 mg/day) significantly prolonged survival of patients with congestive heart failure (Fig. 14) when compared to prazosin or a placebo. In the first year of follow-up, the mortality of the group treated with hydralazine

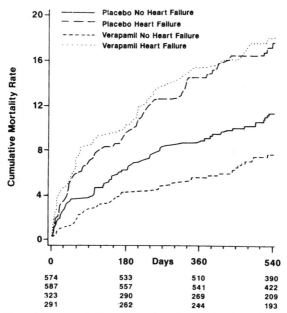

Figure 12. Cumulative mortality rates according to treatment in patients who have had heart failure and those who have not ($P = 0.02$). Bottom axis shows the number of patients at risk (placebo, no heart failure, n = 574; verapamil, no heart failure, n = 587; placebo, heart failure, n = 323; verapamil, heart failure, n = 291. (The Danish Study Group on Verapamil in Myocardial Infarction.[61])

and nitrate was 38% less than that of the placebo group. At three years of follow-up, the reduction in mortality was 36%. The effect of these drugs on the incidence of sudden death was not reported.

Retrospective examination of several short-term trials suggests that angiotensin-converting enzyme inhibitors, including captopril, enalapril, and lisinopril, may reduce mortality.[65] The Cooperative North Scandinavian Enalapril Survival Study (CONSENSUS)[66] used 2.5 to 40 mg/day of enalapril for the treatment of patients with severe congestive heart failure and demonstrated a reduction of 31% in mortality (Fig. 15). However, the reduction in mortality was due to the progression of congestive heart failure only, not to the incidence of sudden death. The effect of enalapril on survival in patients with congestive heart failure with ejection fraction of less than 35% was examined in the Studies of Left Ventricular Dysfunction (SOLVD).[67] Patients receiving conventional treatment were randomly assigned to receive enalapril (2.5 to 20 mg/day) or placebo. Ap-

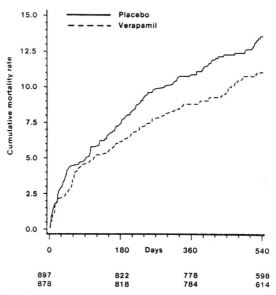

Figure 13. Cumulative mortality rate, according to treatment (P 5 0.11). The number of patients at risk are shown at the bottom (placebo, n 5 897; verapamil, n 5 878). (Reproduced with permission from The Danish Study Group on Verapamil in Myocardial Infarction.[61])

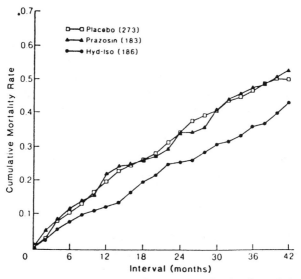

Figure 14. Veterans Administration Cooperative Study. Cumulative mortality from the time of randomization in the three treatment groups (from Cohn et al.[64]).

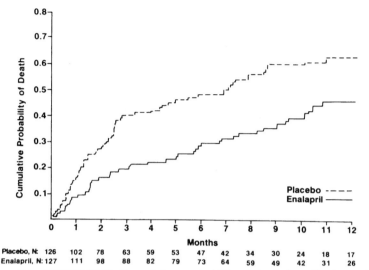

Figure 15. CONSENSUS. Cumulative probability of death in patients treated with placebo or enalapril (from CONSENSUS Trial Study Group[66]).

proximately 90% of patients were in NYHA class II or III. After a mean follow-up of 41.4 months, 510 deaths occurred in the placebo group (39.7%) and 452 in the enalapril group (35.2%) (16% of risk reduction; $P = 0.0036$). There was no effect on arrhythmic death in this study. The largest benefit was found in the prevention of death attributed to progressive heart failure. Thus, the results of CONSENSUS and SOLVD both indicated that enalapril is useful in the prevention of cardiac mortality not only in patients with advanced congestive heart failure (NYHA class IV), but also in patients with mild to moderate heart failure (NYHA class II and III). In both studies, however, no effect was observed on the reduction of sudden cardiac death.

The V-HeFT II[68] compared enalapril (20 mg/day) with hydralazine-isosorbide dinitrate (360 mg of hydralazine plus 160 mg of isosorbide dinitrate daily) in patients with mild to moderate heart failure. The two-year mortality in the enalapril group was significantly lower than in those patients treated with hydralazine and isosorbide dinitrate ($P = 0.016$) (Fig. 16). In the V-HeFT II study, enalapril significantly reduced the incidence of ventricular tachycardia; this reduction parallels the reduction of sudden death.[68] In this instance, however, the lower mortality in the enalapril group was attributable almost entirely to a reduction in the incidence of

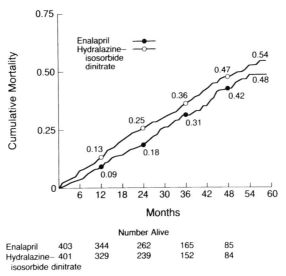

Figure 16. Cumulative mortality in the enalapril and hydralazine- isosorbide dinitrate treatment arms over the entire follow-up period. Cumulative mortality rates are shown after each 12-month period. For the comparison of the treatment arms after two years and overall, $P = 0.016$ and $P = 0.08$, respectively (log-rank test). The number of patients alive after each year is shown below the graph (from Cohn et al.[68]).

sudden cardiac death. This beneficial effect was most prominent in patients with mild congestive heart failure. Similar observations were made in patients evaluated for heart transplant. Fonarow et al.[69] observed that captopril, compared to hydralazine-isosorbide dinitrate therapy, decreased the incidence of sudden cardiac death. Sudden death occurred in 3 of 44 patients randomized to captopril and 18 of 62 patients receiving hydralazine-isordil ($P = 0.006$).

Although there are some contradictory results, it appears that angiotensin- converting enzyme inhibitors are consistently useful in the prevention of death in patients with heart failure. It is possible that these agents decrease cardiac death by decreasing peripheral vasoconstriction. Sudden death reduction may be affected by decreasing neurohumoral activation which occurs as a result of decreased cardiac output.[70] Whether or not vasodilators are useful in preventing cardiac death and sudden death in asymptomatic or mildly symptomatic patients with depressed left ventricular dysfunction has been investigated in three clinical trials: the Survival and Ventricular Enlargement (SAVE) trial[71] with captopril, the prevention arm of the SOLVD trial (SOLVD-II)[72] with enalapril, and the Acute Infarction Ramipril Efficacy (AIRE) trial.[73] The results of the SOLVD-II trial[72] indicate that early vasodilator treatment in asymptomatic patients with left ventricular dysfunction reduced the number of hospital admissions and myocardial infarctions and had a marginal effect on mortality. In SAVE, the administration of captopril to patients for 3 to 16 days after an acute myocardial infarction improved survival and reduced morbidity and mortality due to major cardiovascular events.[71] These benefits were observed regardless of the use of aspirin, thrombolytic, or β-blocker therapy. Captopril reduced cardiovascular deaths by 19% ($P = 0.015$) and congestive heart failure deaths by 34% ($P = 0.04$). The drug tended to reduce all types of cardiovascular death. The risk of sudden death was reduced by 19%.[74] In the AIRE study,[73] ramipril was administered for 3 to 10 days after an acute myocardial infarction to patients who had clinical evidence of heart failure at any time after the acute event. Mortality from all causes was reduced by 27% ($P = 0.002$). Ramipril reduced both sudden and presumed arrhythmic death and progression to severe failure.[75] The benefit of ramipril appeared during the first month of treatment.

Antiarrhythmic Drugs

An important aspect of the prevention of sudden death centers on the effectiveness of antiarrhythmic agents. Many uncontrolled studies, using different drugs, suggested that a reduction in mortality was possible in patients with ventricular arrhythmias. The therapeutic methodology used included acute drug test,[76] programmed electrical stimulation,[77-79] adjustment of plasma levels,[80] and empirical therapy.[81-87]

Graboys et al.[76] suggested that antiarrhythmic treatment, guided by acute drug testing combining ambulatory electrocardiography with exercise testing, significantly reduced mortality in patients with malignant ventricular arrhythmias. In 123 patients treated with this algorithm, without control comparison, annual mortality decreased from 41% to 2.3% in patients with grade 4B and 5 ventricular arrhythmias. When the drugs were withdrawn after several years of therapy, malignant ventricular arrhythmias recurred, associated with an increase in sudden death events. Of 24 patients who discontinued treatment, 12 (50%) experienced recurrence of malignant ventricular arrhythmias, 9 with cardiac arrest. In 11 (46%), the ventricular arrhythmia had the same severity as prior to treatment. These and similar observations created a climate of opinion during the 1970s and 1980s that antiarrhythmic therapy was an essential component of postmyocardial infarction therapy.

A number of nonrandomized studies reported the efficacy of programmed electrical stimulation in the prevention of sudden death in patients with malignant ventricular arrhythmias.[77–79] The patients in whom drug treatment prevented the electrophysiological induction of sustained ventricular tachycardia or ventricular fibrillation appeared to benefit from this approach. The first year mortality was 9% versus 43% of patients in whom the arrhythmia could not continue and could be inducible. Both the acute drug test and programmed electrical stimulation have significant drawbacks.[88] Acute drug testing can be performed only in patients with frequent ventricular arrhythmias. Criteria for drug efficacy have been determined intuitively, with little statistical support, and few controls. Programmed electrical stimulation is even more expensive and complex than acute drug testing. As well as being invasive, it also limits its repeated use in patients. Moreover, there is no uniform stimulation protocol and the true significance of the arrhythmias induced artificially in the laboratory is not clear. Whether they correlate with the patient's spontaneous arrhythmias is still unknown. Furthermore, certain antiarrhythmic agents such as amiodarone are poorly tested during electrophysiological testing, and yet are presumed to be highly effective in chronic treatment. There are few comparative studies of the acute drug test and programmed electrical stimulation.[89–91] Mitchell et al.[89] suggested that programmed electrical stimulation may offer better results than the acute drug test. On the contrary, the results of the ESVEM trial indicate that ambulatory monitoring may be better than programmed electrical stimulation for guiding antiarrhythmic therapy.[90,91] A comparison between the administration of metoprolol to electrophysiologically guided therapy in symptomatic patients with sustained ventricular tachycardia was carried out by Steinbeck et al.[92] Although suppression of arrhythmia during electrophysiological study identified low-risk patients, there was no difference in the outcome of this guided therapy to metoprolol administration.

The entire concept of what constitutes an antiarrhythmic drug has been challenged by Nattel and Waters.[93] In a concept statement, they emphasize the importance of understanding the pathological substrate and its role in the genesis of life-threatening arrhythmias.

Myerburg et al.[80] reported that plasma levels of antiarrhythmics are an important guide to the efficacy of antiarrhythmic treatment. They observed, in a small study, that the maintenance of stable plasma levels within therapeutic limits produced an important reduction in mortality in patients with malignant ventricular arrhythmia who survived out-of-hospital cardiac arrest. Patients who achieved therapeutic plasma levels had a 15% recurrence of cardiac arrest in the first year compared to 31% whose treatment was discontinued. Other studies examining the relationship of blood levels to arrhythmia suppression have been less supportive of this theory.

Empiric treatment with amiodarone was found to be effective in reducing the incidence of sudden death in patients with malignant ventricular arrhythmias.[81–85] In 32 patients with malignant ventricular arrhythmias, treated empirically with amiodarone and followed for 16.9 months, the incidence of sudden death was 25%[82] (Table 4). Amiodarone was effective in most patients with sustained ventricular tachycardia and ventricular fibrillation whose ejection fraction was over 30%. In contrast, in patients with ventricular fibrillation and ejection fraction under 30%, the mortality rate was higher in spite of amiodarone treatment. Nademanee et al.[81] reported the effect of amiodarone in 72 out-of-hospital patients resuscitated after cardiac arrest. The incidence of sudden death was 8%, 12%, and 27% at one, two, and four years, respectively. Using historical comparisons, amiodarone was thought to be effective in individuals with an

Table 4

Mortality According to the Type of Malignant Ventricular Arrhythmia and the Left Ventricular Ejection Fraction (EF)

	n	Deaths	Survivors	p
VF and EF < 30%	5	5*	0	
VF and EF ≥ 30%	6	0	6	$P < 0.05$
VT and EF < 30%	8	2**	6	
VT and EF ≥ 30%	9	1*	8	$P = NS$

VF = ventricular fibrillation; VT = ventricular tachycardia; * = sudden death; ** = death due to heart failure.

ejection fraction over 30%. Similar results were obtained by Olson et al.[86] In this study, amiodarone was effective in patients with an ejection fraction greater than or equal to 40%. In contrast, patients with an ejection fraction of less than 40% remained at high risk for sudden death, and should be considered for additional or alternative therapy.

The CASCADE study[84,87] was designed to compare the empiric administration of amiodarone to therapy with other antiarrhythmic drugs guided by electrophysiological testing and Holter recording in survivors of cardiac arrest. This study demonstrated that empiric therapy with amiodarone was more effective than conventional drugs in preventing recurrence of total or near-fatal arrhythmias (Fig. 17). Survival free of cardiac death, resuscitated ventricular fibrillation, or syncopal defibrillator shock at two years for amiodarone and conventional therapy was 82% versus 69%, at four years 66% versus 52%, and, at six years, 53% versus 40% ($P = 0.007$) (Fig. 17). However, amiodarone was associated with a higher incidence of serious side effects.

It is clear that in asymptomatic postmyocardial infarction patients, frequent and complex ventricular arrhythmias are markers

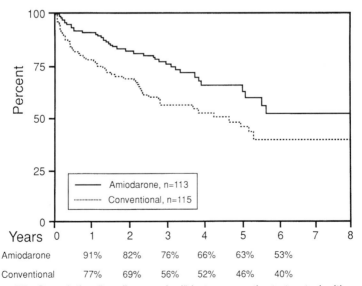

Figure 17. Cumulative "cardiac survival" between patients treated with amiodarone or conventional treatment (from The CASCADE Investigators[87]).

of a poor prognosis. However, suppression of these arrhythmias has not only failed to be beneficial, but may also increase mortality[94–102] (Table 5). Until the Cardiac Arrhythmia Suppression Trial (CAST),[103–106] a randomized placebo study of ventricular premature beat suppression had not been carried out. The CAST compared flecainide, encainide, and moricizine with placebo, substituting one drug for another, based upon ventricular premature beat suppression using ambulatory electrocardiography. Once ventricular premature beat suppression was observed, patients were randomized to that drug, causing suppression, or to a placebo. CAST-I found that patients treated with encainide or flecainide had an excess of arrhythmic death and fatal myocardial infarction[104,105] (Fig. 18). Moricizine, studied in a similar manner (CAST-II), was also stopped due to its lack of efficacy[106] (Fig. 19). Because of these find-

Table 5

Results of the Long-term Antiarrhythmic Trials in Postmyocardial Infarction Patients

Study	Antiarrhythmic	Mortality		Follow-up (Mo)
		Control	Treated	
Collaborative group[94]	Phenytoin	9.1%	8.1%	12
Kosowsky[95]	Procainamide	2.6%	10.3%	36
Peter[96]	Phenytoin	18.4%	24.3%	24
Ryden[97]	Tocainide	8.9%	8.9%	6
Bastian[98]	Tocainide	4.1%	5.6%	6
Chamberlain[99]	Mexiletine	11.7%	13.3%	4
IMPACT[100]	Mexiletine	4.8%	7.6%	9
Gottlieb[101]	Aprindine	22.0%	17.0%	12
CAPS[103]	Enc, Fle, Mor, Im	2.0%	1.2%	12
CAST-I[104,105]	Enc, Fle	3.0%	7.7%	12
STSD-I[108]	Amiod/Metop	7.7%	3.5%/15.4%	36
BASIS[109]	Amiodarone	5.0%	13.0%	12

Amoid = Amiodarone; Enc = encainide; Fle = Flecainide; Im = imipramine; Metop = metaprolol; Mor = moricizine.

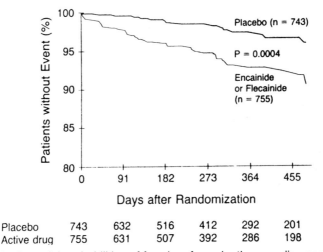

| Placebo | 743 | 632 | 516 | 412 | 292 | 201 |
| Active drug | 755 | 631 | 507 | 392 | 286 | 198 |

Figure 18. Actuarial probabilities of freedom from death or cardiac arrest due to arrhythmia in the CAST study. (Reproduced with permission from Echt et al.[105])

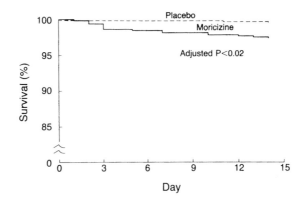

No. at risk (% surviving)

| Placebo | 660 (100) | 659 (99.9) | 658 (99.7) |
| Moricizine | 665 (100) | 655 (98.5) | 608 (97.7) |

Figure 19. Survival of patients during the first 14 days of treatment with moricizine or placebo. The end point was death or nonfatal cardiac arrest from any cause. The adjusted P value is based on the log-rank statistic and adjusted for sequential monitoring. Fifty patients who began immediate titration with moricizine completed titration, and their data were censored before 14 days (from the Cardiac Arrhythmia Suppression Trial II Investigators[106]).

ings, most of the class Ic antiarrhythmic agents have been with-drawn from therapy. At the same time, the suppression hypothesis widely proposed by Lown has been discredited, at least with these three drugs.

The Spanish Trial on Sudden Death-I (STSD-I)[107,108] compared three groups of postmyocardial infarction patients stratified accord-ing to ejection fraction and the presence or absence of potentially ma-lignant ventricular arrhythmias. In the STSD, treatment was not conditioned by the ambulatory electrocardiographic findings. Pa-tients with ejection fraction between 20% to 45% and frequent or complex ventricular premature complexes were randomized to amio-darone, metoprolol, or placebo. After three years of follow-up, only 30 of the 368 patients randomized died (8.1%), half of whom died sud-denly (Table 5). Mortality of patients given amiodarone (3.5% ± 4.2) was significantly lower than that of patients given metoprolol (15.4% ± 3.5, $P = 0.006$), although it was not significantly different from controls (7.7 ± 2.5) (Fig. 20).

The Basel Antiarrhythmic Study of Infarct Survival (BA-SIS)[109,110] suggested that amiodarone may prevent cardiac mortality in high-risk postmyocardial infarction patients with Lown class III

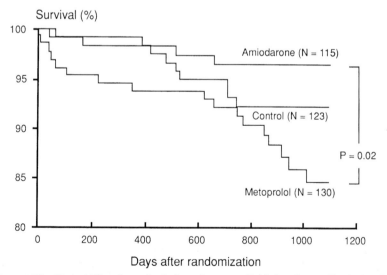

Figure 20. Probability of survival of postmyocardial infarction patients treated with metoprolol, amiodarone or placebo (from Navarro-Lopez et al.[108]).

or IVb. Between 1981 and 1987, 312 patients were randomized to amiodarone (n = 98), individualized antiarrhythmic treatment (n = 100), or placebo (n = 114). After a one-year follow-up, patients treated with amiodarone had a greater probability of survival and a lower risk of arrhythmic events (Fig. 21). Moreover, long-term follow-up of patients included in this study suggests that the beneficial effect of amiodarone on survival persists for several years despite discontinuation of the drug after one year.[110]

The results of the Canadian Amiodarone Myocardial Infarction Arrhythmia Trial (CAMIAT) Pilot Study suggest that amiodarone[111] in moderate dosage is tolerated and may be effective in reducing sudden death. The final results of this study and the results of a current large-scale European trial (EMIAT) may provide a more definitive answer to the real efficacy of amiodarone in prevention of sudden death after acute myocardial infarction.

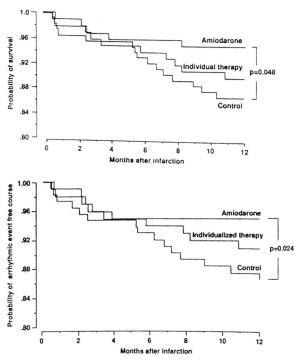

Figure 21. Probability of 12-month survival in the three treatment groups of patients with asymptomatic complex ventricular arrhythmias after myocardial infarction (from Burkart et al.[109]).

The pharmacological approach to the prevention of sudden death has been marked by unsuspected successes and some notorious failures. The inability to achieve a benefit and the demonstration of lethality of acute antiarrhythmic drug therapy in CAST has seriously chastised the cardiology community and challenged the concept of arrhythmia suppression. Preliminary comparison of ambulatory electrocardiographic-guided therapy, as used in CAST with electrophysiological drug therapy, failed to support the presumed benefit of this later approach. It is possible that pleuri-potential drugs such as amiodarone may be beneficial. β-adrenergic blocking agents, which have multiple physiological effects, stand almost alone in decreasing sudden death mortality in patients with ischemic heart disease, with and without ventricular ectopy, whereas calcium blocking agents, which held great promise, failed to have any positive effect on mortality. The role of angiotensin- converting enzyme inhibitors requires further investigation. The most pedestrian of all drugs, aspirin, has found a central role in modifying mortality by its apparent effect on platelet function. This, together with the observations in regard to β-adrenergic blocking agents, suggests that the path to prevention of sudden death in patients with both ischemic and nonischemic heart disease lies in modifying the pathophysiology of the disease process, and not in the superficial suppression of the ventricular ectopic beat.

References

1. Oliver MF. Lack of impact of prevention on sudden cardiac death. *J Am Coll Cardiol* 1985;5:150-B.
2. MacMahon JW, Cutler JA, Furberg C, et al. The effect of drug treatment for hypertension on morbidity and mortality from cardiovascular disease: A review of randomized controlled trials. *Prog Cardiovasc Dis* 1986;24:I-99.
3. Multiple Risk Factor Intervention Trial Research Group. Multiple Risk Factor Intervention Trial: Risk factor changes and mortality results. *JAMA* 1982;248:1465.
4. Medical Research Council Working Party on Mild to Moderate Hypertension. Ventricular extrasystoles during thiazide treatment. *Br Med J* 1983;287:1249.
5. Olsson G, Tuomilehto J, Berglund G, et al., for the MAPHY Study Group. Primary prevention of sudden cardiovascular death in hypertensive patients. Mortality results from the MAPHY study. *Am J Hypertens* 1991;4:151.

6. The Coronary Drug Project Research Group. Clofibrate and niacin in coronary heart disease. *JAMA* 1975;231:360.

7. Elveback LR, Connolly DC, Kurland LT. Coronary heart disease in residents of Rochester, Minnesota. II. Mortality, incidence and survivorship 1950–1975. *Mayo Clin Proc* 1981;56:665.

8. Mulcahy R. Influence of cigarette smoking on morbidity and mortality after myocardial infarction. *Br Heart J* 1983;49:410.

9. Frick MH, Elo O, Haapa K, et al. Helsinki Heart Study: Primary prevention trial with gemfibrozil in middle-aged men with dyslipemia. *N Engl J Med* 1987;317:1237.

10. Jones PH. Lovastatin and Simvastatin prevention studies. *Am J Cardiol* 1990;66:39B.

11. Hämäläinen H, Luurila OJ, Kallio V, et al. Long-term reduction in sudden death after a multifactorial intervention program in patients with myocardial infarction: 10-year results of a controlled investigation. *Eur Heart J* 1989;10:55.

12. Fuster V, Verstreate M, eds. *Thrombosis in Cardiovascular Disorders.* Philadelphia: WB Saunders; 1992.

13. Gruppo Italiano Per Lo Studio Della Streptochi-Nasi Nell'Infarcto Miocardico (GISSI). Long-term effects of intravenous thrombolysis in acute myocardial infarction: Final report of the GISSI study. *Lancet* 1987;2:871.

14. The TIMI II Study Group. Comparison of invasive and conservative strategies after treatment with intravenous tissue plasminogen activator in acute myocardial infarction: Results of the Thrombolysis in Myocardial Infarction (TIMI) Phase II trial. *N Engl J Med* 1989;320:618.

15. Califf RM, Topol EJ, George BS, et al. and the TAMI study group. One-year outcome after therapy with tissue plasminogen activator: Report from the Thrombolysis and Angioplasty in Myocardial Infarction Trial. *Am Heart J* 1990;119:777.

16. ISIS-2 Collaborative Group. Randomized trial of intravenous streptokinase, oral aspirin, both or neither among 17,187 cases of suspected acute myocardial infarction: ISIS-II. *Lancet* 1988;2:349.

17. AIMS Trial Study Group. Effect of intravenous APSAC on mortality after acute myocardial infarction: Preliminary report of a placebo-controlled clinical trial. *Lancet* 1988;1:545.

18. Theroux P, Morissette D, Juneau M, et al. Influence of fibrinolysis and percutaneous transluminal coronary angioplasty on frequency of ventricular premature complexes. *Am J Cardiol* 1989;63:797.

19. Turitto G, Risa AL, Zanchi E, et al. The signal-averaged electrocardiogram and ventricular arrhythmias after thrombolysis for acute myocardial infarction. *J Am Coll Cardiol* 1990;15:1270.

20. Breithardt G, Borggrefe M, Karbenn U. Late potentials as predictors of risk after thrombolytic treatment? *Br Heart J* 1990;64:174.

21. Gang ES, Lew AS, Hong M, et al. Decreased incidence of ventricular late potentials after successful thrombolytic therapy for acute myocardial infarction. *N Engl J Med* 1989;321:712.

22. Moreno FL, Karagounis L, Ipsen S, et al. Thrombolysis-related early reperfusion reduces ECG late potentials after acute myocardial infarction. *J Am Coll Cardiol* 1991;17:312A.

23. Kersschot IE, Brugada P, Ramentol M, et al. Effects of early reperfusion in acute myocardial infarction on arrhythmias induced by programmed stimulation: A prospective, randomized study. *J Am Coll Cardiol* 1986;7:1234.

24. McComb JM, Gold HK, Leinbach RC, et al. Electrically induced ventricular arrhythmias in acute myocardial infarction treated with thrombolytic agents. *Am J Cardiol* 1988;62:186.

25. Bourke JP, Young AA, Richards DAB, et al. Reduction of incidence of ventricular tachycardia after myocardial infarction by treatment with streptokinase during infarct evolution. *J Am Coll Cardiol* 1990; 16:1703.

26. Sager T, Perlmutter RA, Rosenfeld LA, et al. Electrophysiological effects of thrombolytic therapy in patients with a transmural myocardial infarction complicated by left ventricular aneurysm formation. *J Am Coll Cardiol* 1988;12:19.

27. Farrell T, Bashir Y, Poloniecki J, et al. The effects of thrombolysis on risk stratification for arrhythmic events in post infarction patients. *J Am Coll Cardiol* 1991;17:17A.

28. Willard JE, Lange RA, Hillis LD. The use of aspirin in ischemic heart disease. *N Engl J Med* 1992;327:175.

29. Fuster V, Badimon L, Cohen M, et al. Insights into the pathogenesis of acute ischemic syndromes. *Circulation* 1988;77:1213.

30. Freedman LM. Platelet active agents in the prevention of sudden cardiac death. In: Morganroth J, Horowitz LN, eds. *Sudden Cardiac Death.* Orlando: Grune & Stratton; 1985;257.

31. Hennekens CH, Peto R, Hutchinson GB, et al. An overview of the British and American aspirin studies. *N Engl J Med* 1988;318:923.

32. The Steering Committee of the Physicians' Health Study Research Group. Final report on the aspirin component of the ongoing Physicians' Health Study. *N Engl J Med* 1989;321:129.

33. Peto R, Gray R, Collins R, et al. A randomized trial of the effects of prophylactic daily aspirin among male British doctors. *Br Med J* 1988;296:313.

34. Lewis HD, Davis JW, Archibald DG, et al. Protective effects of aspirin against acute myocardial infarction and death in men with unstable angina: Results of a Veterans Administration Cooperative Study. *N Engl J Med* 1983;309:396.

35. Cairns J, Gent M, Singer J, et al. Aspirin, sulfinpyrazone or both in unstable angina. Results of a Canadian Multicenter Trial. *N Engl J Med* 1985;313:1369.

36. Theroux P, Ouimet H, McCans J, et al. Aspirin, heparin or both to treat acute unstable angina. *N Engl J Med* 1988;319:1105.

37. Antiplatelet Trialists' Collaboration. Secondary prevention of vascular disease by prolonged antiplatelet therapy. *Br Med J* 1988;296:320.

38. The Anturane Reinfarction Trial Research Group. Sulfinpyrazone in the prevention of sudden death after myocardial infarction. *N Engl J Med* 1980;302:250.

39. Anturane Reinfarction Trial Policy Committee. The Anturane Reinfarction Trial: Reevaluation of Outcome. *N Engl J Med* 1982;306:1005.

40. Report from the Anturan Reinfarction Italian Study. Sulfinpyrazone in post-myocardial infarction. *Lancet* 1982;1:237.

41. Chesebro JH, Webster MWI, Smith HC, et al. Antiplatelet therapy in coronary artery disease progression: Reduced infarction and new lesion formation. *Circulation* 1989;80:II-266.
42. Smith P, Arnesen H, Holme I. The effect of warfarin on mortality and reinfarction after myocardial infarction. *N Engl J Med* 1990; 323:147.
43. Hjalmarson A, Elmfeldt D, Herlitz J, et al. Effect on mortality of metoprolol in acute myocardial infarction: A double-blind randomized trial. *Lancet* 1981;2:823.
44. ISIS-I (First Interventional Study of Infarct Survival) Collaborative Group. Randomized trial of intravenous atenolol among 16,027 cases of suspected acute myocardial infarction: ISIS-I. *Lancet* 1986;2:57.
45. Roberts R, Rogers WJ, Mueller HS, et al. for the TIMI Investigators. Immediate versus deferred β-blockade following thrombolytic therapy in patients with acute myocardial infarction: Results of the TIMI II-B Study. *Circulation* 1991;83:422.
46. Permanyer Miralda G, Galve Basilio E. Prophylactic β-blocking treatment after myocardial infarction. In: Bayés de Luna A, Betriu A, Permanyer G, eds. *Therapeutics in Cardiology*. Dordrecht: Kluwer Academic Publishers; 1988.
47. The Norwegian Multicenter Study Group. Timolol-induced reduction in mortality and reinfarction in patients surviving acute myocardial infarction. *N Engl J Med* 1981;304:801.
48. β-Blocker Heart Attack Trial Research Group. A randomized trial of propranolol in patients with acute myocardial infarction: Mortality results. *JAMA* 1982;247:1707.
49. Taylor SH, Silke B, Ebbut A, et al. Long-term prevention study with oxprenolol in coronary heart disease. *N Engl J Med* 1982;307:1293.
50. Julian DG, Prescott RJ, Jackson FS, et al. Controlled trial of sotalol for one year after myocardial infarction. *Lancet* 1982;1:1142.
51. Boissel JP, Leizorovicz A, Picolet H, et al. Efficacy of acebutolol after acute myocardial infarction. *Am J Cardiol* 1990;66:24C.
52. Olsson G, Wikstrand J, Warnold I, et al. Metoprolol-induced reduction in postinfarction mortality: Pooled results from five double-blind randomized trials. *Eur Heart J* 1992;13:28.
53. Chadda K, Goldstein S, Byington R, et al. Effect of propranolol after acute myocardial infarction in patients with congestive heart failure. *Circulation* 1986;73:503.
54. Friedman LM, Byington RP, Capone RJ, et al., for the β-Blocker Heart Attack Trial Research Group. Effect of propranolol in patients with myocardial infarction and ventricular arrhythmia. *J Am Coll Cardiol* 1986;7:1.
55. Gheorghiade M, Schultz L, Tilley B, et al. Effects of propranolol in non-Q-wave myocardial infarction in the β-Blocker Heart Attack Trial. *Am J Cardiol* 1990;66:129.
56. Bayés de Luna A, Guindo J, Rivera J. Ambulatory sudden death. *J Ambulat Monitor* 1989;2:3.
57. Bayés de Luna A, Coumel PH, Leclercq JF. Ambulatory sudden death: Mechanisms of production of fatal arrhythmia on the basis of data from 157 cases. *Am Heart J* 1989;117:154.

58. Gibson RS, Boden WE, Theroux P, et al. Diltiazem and reinfarction in patients with non-Q-wave myocardial infarction: Results of a double-blind, randomized, multicenter trial. *N Engl J Med* 1986; 315:423.

59. The Multicenter Diltiazem Postinfarction Trial Research Group. The effect of diltiazem on mortality and reinfarction after myocardial infarction. *N Engl J Med* 1988;319:385.

60. The Danish Study Group on Verapamil in Myocardial Infarction. Verapamil in acute myocardial infarction. *Eur Heart J* 1984;5:516.

61. The Danish Study Group on Verapamil in Myocardial Infarction. Effect of verapamil on mortality and major events after acute myocardial infarction (The Danish Verapamil Infarction Trial - DAVIT II). *Am J Cardiol* 1990;66:779.

62. Sirnes PA, Overskeid K, Pedersen TR, et al. Evolution of infarct size during the early use of nifedipine in patients with acute myocardial infarction. The Norwegian Nifedipine Multicenter Trial. *Circulation* 1984;70:638.

63. Guindo J, Bayés de Luna A, Torner P, et al. Treatment of heart failure: Impact on sudden death. In: Bayés de Luna A, Brugada P, Cosin J, Navarro-Lopez F, eds. *Sudden Cardiac Death.* Dordrecht: Kluwer Academic Publisher; 1991.

64. Cohn JN, Archibald DG, Zeiesche S, et al. Effect of vasodilator therapy on mortality in chronic congestive heart failure: Results of a Veterans Administration Cooperative Study. *N Engl J Med* 1986;314:1547.

65. Furberg CD, Yusuf S. Effect of drug therapy on survival in chronic congestive heart failure. *Am J Cardiol* 1988;62:41A.

66. The CONSENSUS Trial Study Group. The effects of enalapril on mortality in severe congestive heart failure: Results of the Cooperative North Scandinavian Enalapril Survival Study (CONSENSUS). *N Engl J Med* 1987;316:1429.

67. The SOLVD Investigators. Effect of enalapril on survival in patients with reduced left ventricular ejection fraction and congestive heart failure. *N Engl J Med* 1991;325:293.

68. Cohn JN, Johnson G, Ziesche S, et al. A comparison of enalapril with hydralazine-isosorbide dinitrate in the treatment of chronic congestive heart failure. *N Engl J Med* 1991;325:303.

69. Fonarow G, Chellimsky-Fallick C, Stevenson LW, et al. Impact of vasodilator regimen on sudden death in advanced heart failure: A randomized trial of angiotensin-converting enzyme inhibition and direct vasodilation. *J Am Coll Cardiol* 1991;17:92A.

70. Braunwald E. Ace inhibitors: A cornerstone of the treatment of heart failure. *N Engl J Med* 1991;325:351.

71. Pfeffer MA, Braunwald E, Moye LA, et al., on behalf of the SAVE Investigators. Effect of captopril on mortality and morbidity in patients with left ventricular dysfunction after myocardial infarction. *N Engl J Med* 1992;327:669.

72. The SOLVD Investigators. Effect of enalapril on mortality and the development of heart failure in asymptomatic patients with reduced left ventricular ejection fractions. *N Engl J Med* 1992;327:685.

73. The Acute Infarction Ramipril Efficacy (AIRE) Study Investigators. Effect of ramipril on mortality and morbidity of survivors of acute myocardial infarction with clinical evidence of heart failure. *Lancet* 1993;342:821.

74. Packer M, Davis BR, Hamm P, et al. Effect of captopril on cause-specific mortality in patients with left ventricular dysfunction after acute myocardial infarction: Results of the SAVE Trial. *Circulation* 1992; 86:I-250.

75. Cleland JGF, Erhardt L, Hall AS, Winter C, Ball SG. Validation of primary and secondary outcomes and classification of mode of death among patients with clinical evidence of heart failure after myocardial infarction: A report from the Acute Infarction Ramipril Efficacy (AIRE) Study Investigators. *J Cardiovasc Pharmacol* (in press).

76. Graboys TB, Lown B, Podrid PH, et al. Long-term survival of patients with malignant ventricular arrhythmia treated with antiarrhythmic drugs. *Am J Cardiol* 1982;50:437.

77. Prystowsky EN. Electrophysiologic-electropharmacologic testing in patients with ventricular arrhythmias. *PACE* 1988;11:225.

78. Wellens HJJ, Brugada P, Stevenson WG. Programmed electrical stimulation of the heart in patients with life-threatening ventricular arrhythmias: What is the significance of induced arrhythmias and what is the correct stimulation protocol? *Circulation* 1985;72:1.

79. Josephson ME, Horowitz LN, Spielman SC, et al. Electrophysiologic and hemodynamic studies in patients resuscitated from cardiac arrest. *Am J Cardiol* 1980;46:948.

80. Myerburg RJ, Zaman L, Kessler K, et al. Evolving concepts of management of stable and potentially lethal arrhythmias. *Am Heart J* 1982;103:615.

81. Nademanee K, Hendrickson JA, Cisnom DS, et al. Control of refractory life-threatening ventricular tachyarrhythmia by amiodarone. *Am Heart J* 1981;101:759.

82. Dominguez de Rozas JM, Garcia J, Guindo J, et al. Amiodarone as a drug of first choice in the prevention of sustained ventricular tachycardia and/or fibrillation. In: Bayés de Luna A, Betriu A, Permanyer G, eds. *Cardiovascular Therapy*. Dordrecht: Martinus Nijhoff; 1988.

83. Nademanee K, Stevenson W, Weiss J, et al. The role of amiodarone in the survivors of sudden deaths. In: Singh BNN, ed. *Control of Cardiac Arrhythmias by Lengthening Repolarization*. Armonk: Futura Publishing Company; 1988.

84. The CASCADE Investigators. Cardiac arrest in Seattle: Conventional versus Amiodarone Drug Evaluation (the CASCADE Study). *Am J Cardiol* 1991;67:578.

85. Myers M, Peter T, Weiss D, et al. Benefit and risks of long-term amiodarone therapy for sustained ventricular tachycardia/fibrillation: Minimum of three-year follow-up in 145 patients. *Am Heart J* 1990;119:8.

86. Olson PJ, Woelfel A, Simpson RJ, et al. Stratification of sudden death risk in patients receiving long-term amiodarone treatment for sustained ventricular tachycardia or ventricular fibrillation. *Am J Cardiol* 1993;71:823.

87. The CASCADE Investigators. Randomized antiarrhythmic drug therapy in survivors of cardiac arrest (the CASCADE Study). *Am J Cardiol* 1993;72:280.

88. Podrid PJ. Treatment of ventricular arrhythmia: Applications and limitations on noninvasive vs. invasive approach. *Chest* 1985;88:121.

89. Mitchell LB, Duff HJ, Manyari DE, et al. A randomized clinical trial of the noninvasive and invasive approaches to drug therapy of ventricular tachycardia. *N Engl J Med* 1987;317:1681.

90. Mason JW for the ESVEM investigators. A comparison of electrophysiologic testing with Holter monitoring to predict antiarrhythmic-drug efficacy for ventricular tachyarrhythmias. *N Engl J Med* 1993; 329:445.

91. The ESVEM Investigators. Determinants of predicted efficacy of antiarrhythmic drugs in the Electrophysiologic Study versus Electrocardiographic Monitoring Trial. *Circulation* 1993;87:323.

92. Steinbeck G, Andresen D, Bach P, et al. A comparison of electrophysiologically guided antiarrhythmic drug therapy with β-blocker therapy in patients with symptomatic, sustained ventricular tachyarrhythmias. *N Engl J Med* 1992;327:987.

93. Nattel S, Waters D. What is an antiarrhythmic drug? From clinical trials to fundamental concepts. *Am J Cardiol* 1990;66:96.

94. Collaborative Group. Phenytoin after recovery from myocardial infarction: Controlled trial in 568 patients. *Lancet* 1971;2:1055.

95. Kosowsky BD, Taylor J, Lown B, et al. Long-term use of procainamide following acute myocardial infarction. *Circulation* 1973;47:1204.

96. Peter T, Ross D, Duffield A, et al. Effect on survival after myocardial infarction of long-term treatment with phenytoin. *Br Heart J* 1978; 40:1356.

97. Ryden L, Arnman K, Conradson TB, et al. Prophylaxis of ventricular tachyarrhythmias with intravenous and oral tocainide in patients with and recovering from acute myocardial infarction. *Am Heart J* 1980;100:1006.

98. Bastian BC, Macfarlane PW, McLauchlan JH, et al. A prospective randomized trial of tocainide in patients following myocardial infarction. *Am Heart J* 1980;100:1017.

99. Chamberlain DA, Jewitt DE, Julian DG, et al. Oral mexiletine in high-risk patients after myocardial infarction. *Lancet* 1980;2:1324.

100. IMPACT Research Group. International Mexiletine and Placebo Antiarrhythmic Coronary Trial. Report on arrhythmia and other findings. *J Am Coll Cardiol* 1984;6:1148.

101. Gottlieb SM, Achuff SC, Mellitis ED, et al. Prophylactic antiarrhythmic therapy of high risk survivors of myocardial infarction: Lower mortality at 1 month but not at 1 year. *Circulation* 1987;75:792.

102. Moosvi AR, Goldstein S, VanderBurg Medendorp S, et al. Effect of empiric antiarrhythmic therapy in resuscitated out-of-hospital cardiac arrest victims with coronary artery disease. *Am J Cardiol* 1990;65:1192.

103. The Cardiac Arrhythmia Pilot Study (CAPS) Investigators. Effects of encainide, flecainide, imipramine, and moricizine on ventricular arrhythmias during the year after acute myocardial infarction: The CAPS. *Am J Cardiol* 1988;61:501.

104. The Cardiac Arrhythmia Suppression Trial (CAST) Investigators. Preliminary Report: Effect of encainide and flecainide on mortality in a randomized trial of arrhythmia suppression after myocardial infarction. *N Engl J Med* 1989;321:406.

105. Echt DS, Liebson PR, Mitchell LB, et al., and the CAST Investigators. Mortality and morbidity in patients receiving encainide and flecainide, or placebo. *N Engl J Med* 1991;324:781.

106. The Cardiac Arrhythmia Suppression Trial II (CAST) II Investigators. Effect of the antiarrhythmic agent moricizine on survival after myocardial infarction. *N Engl J Med* 1992;327:227.

107. Grupo de Investigadores del EEMS. Estudio Espanol de Muerte Subita. *Rev Esp Cardiol* 1989;42:77.

108. Navarro-Lopez F, Cosin J, Marrugat J, et al. Comparison of the effects of amiodarone versus metoprolol on the frequency of ventricular arrhythmias and on mortality after acute myocardial infarction. *Am J Cardiol* 1993;72:1243.

109. Burkart F, Pfisterer M, Kiowski W, et al. Effect of antiarrhythmic therapy on mortality in survivors of myocardial infarction with asymptomatic complex ventricular arrhythmias: Basel Antiarrhythmic Study of Infarct Survival (BASIS). *J Am Coll Cardiol* 1990;16:1711.

110. Pfisterer ME, Kiowski W, Bosnner H, et al. Long-term benefit of one-year amiodarone treatment for persistent complex ventricular arrhythmias after myocardial infarction. *Circulation* 1993;87:309.

111. Cairns JA, Connolly SJ, Gent M, et al. Post-myocardial infarction mortality in patients with ventricular premature depolarizations: Canadian Amiodarone Myocardial Infarction Arrhythmia Trial Pilot Study. *Circulation* 1991;84:550.

Chapter XVIII

Prevention of Sudden Death:
Nonpharmacological Approach

A series of nonpharmacological procedures have been developed recently that have the potential to prevent sudden death in high-risk patients for whom drug therapy is considered ineffective. These techniques can be divided into three main groups: implantable electrical devices, cardiac surgery, and catheter ablation techniques. All of them are invasive and hold a certain morbidity and mortality. Their use should therefore always be individualized after careful evaluation of the benefit and risk relationship for each case. Since these techniques usually require specialized training and are at present under continued research and development, their use should be restricted to centers of excellence.

Nonpharmacological treatment is usually indicated when a patient with a high risk of sudden death continues to express malignant arrhythmias in spite of adequate treatment with antiarrhythmic drugs. It is also possible that the risk of these procedures may become so low and their efficacy so predictable that they will supplant pharmacological therapy in certain conditions. Occasionally, nonpharmacological techniques may be the method of first choice as in symptomatic patients with Wolff-Parkinson-White syndrome. Catheter ablation of the anomalous pathway is the treatment of choice.

From: S. Goldstein, A. Bayés-de-Luna, J. Guindo-Soldevila: *Sudden Cardiac Death.* Armonk, NY: Futura Publishing Co., Inc., © 1994.

Implantable Electrical Devices

Pacemakers for Bradyarrhythmias

Before describing these techniques in detail, the important role of pacemakers in the prevention of sudden death due to bradyarrhythmias should be emphasized. Although the principal mechanism of sudden death is ventricular fibrillation, brady-arrhythmia, often triggered by sustained ventricular tachycardia, can be responsible for as many as 20% of cardiac arrest events (see Chapter III). Advanced atrioventricular block as a cause of sudden death occurs in approximately 7% of ambulatory sudden deaths. Bradyarrhythmias are usually due to a depression of automatic rhythm centers, generally accompanied by electromechanical dissociation. They are not usually the expression of isolated sinus disease, but the last manifestation of an end-stage cardiac disease. Patients with advanced atrioventricular block or sinus node disease can often be identified and treated at an early stage by pacemaker implantation.

After pacemaker implantation, sudden death still remains an unsolved problem, since it occurs in approximately 20% to 30% of paced patients. Severe heart disease indicated by the presence of bifascicular and trifascicular block is the strongest predictor of sudden death[1] in these patients.

In some cases bradycardia, due to dispersion of ventricular refractory periods, favors the appearance of ventricular arrhythmias. In this situation rapid pacing can suppress the development of such arrhythmias.[2] Thus, when the sustained ventricular tachycardia or ventricular fibrillation are bradycardia-dependent, prophylactic use of pacemakers can be beneficial. Temporary overdrive pacing has also been useful in the prevention of malignant ventricular arrhythmias in the setting of long QT syndrome and torsade de pointes.[3]

Patients with malignant ventricular arrhythmias often have concomitant conduction disturbances with variable degrees of heart block and/or depression of the sinus rhythm. Implantable pacemakers may be useful in stabilizing the sinus rhythm as one adds antiarrhythmic drugs. In our series of 136 patients with malignant ventricular arrhythmias treated with amiodarone, almost 20% of patients required pacemaker implantation during the follow-up.

In summary, pacemaker implantation in patients with malignant ventricular arrhythmias may be indicated to prevent severe bradyarrhythmia and its sequelae.

Pacing for the Termination of Tachyarrhythmia

Asynchronous paced stimuli can successfully terminate episodes of sustained ventricular and supraventricular tachycardia. The majority of ventricular and supraventricular tachycardias are due to a reentrant phenomenon. The physiological mechanism by which the premature paced extrastimulus stops the reentrant rhythm is due to the collision during the excitable gap, with the propagating wavefront in both the antegrade and retrograde directions. The invasion of this excitatory gap extinguishes and terminates the tachycardia[4] (Fig. 1). The first example of an implantable transvenous pacemaker use is shown in Figures 2A and B in which supraventricular tachycardia occurring in a patient with Wolff-Parkinson-White syndrome was reverted to sinus rhythm. The use of programmed electrical stimulation is widely used to both trigger and terminate ventricular tachycardias in the electrophysiology laboratory.[5] Many forms of electrical stimulation have been examined. It is believed that pacing-adaptive modalities using bursts or premature extrastimuli determined as a percentage of sensed tachycardia cycle length are superior to those with predetermined coupling intervals or pacing cycle lengths. It has also been demonstrated that the use of multiple extrastimuli or bursts are superior to one or two extrastimuli.[6] The most consistently effective termination mode is a brief burst of ventricular pacing of 4 to 20 beats at rates of 20% to 40% faster than tachycardia.[7] New pacing techniques are presently being developed with ultrarapid and subthreshold pacing. A single ventricular capture at the end of the ventricular refractory period is the most effective timing for the termination of sustained uniform ventricular tachycardias.

Efficacy and the risk of complications with antitachycardia devices are dependent on the rate of the tachycardia. Fisher[8] observed that when the tachycardia rate was greater than 250 beats per minute, or the patient was hypotensive, 17% of episodes were successfully terminated. This compares to 93% when the ventricular tachycardia rate was less than 250 beats per minute. Roy et al.[9] ob-

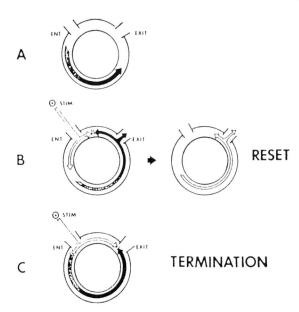

Figure 1. (A) Representation of a reentrant circuit is illustrated with separate entrance (ENT) and exit sites. The tachycardia wavefront propagating within the circuit is represented by the arrow, with the black portion being fully refractory tissue and the stippled portion partially refractory tissue. The area between the head and tail of the arrow is the fully excitable gap. (B) A premature stimulus (STIM) results in a wavefront of depolarization (white arrow) that propagates into the circuit and conducts in both an antegrade and retrograde direction. Although the premature wavefront collides retrogradely with the already propagating tachycardia wavefront, it is able to conduct antegradely through fully excitable tissue. When the premature wavefront exits the circuit, the next tachycardia beat is advanced, that is, resetting occurs. In C, the premature wavefront (white arrow) results from a more premature extrastimulus (STIM) and not only collides retrogradely with the already propagating tachycardia wavefront but encounters refractory tissue antegradely. The premature wavefront is thus extinguished within the circuit and tachycardia termination occurs.(Reproduced with permission from Rosenthal et al. *Am J Cardiol* 1988;61:770.)

tained similar results with an efficacy of 50% in tachycardias at a rate greater than 200 beats per minute and of 95% when tachycardia episodes were less than 200 beats per minute. Efficacy also depends upon the mode, the number of pacing stimuli, and the rate of pacing trains. By applying a single extrastimulus, 18% to 57% of tachycardias can be interrupted, compared to overdrive pacing trains where efficacy varies between 54% and 90%.

The main limitation of pacemakers for the termination of tachycardia is the risk of induction of recurrent ventricular tachycardias

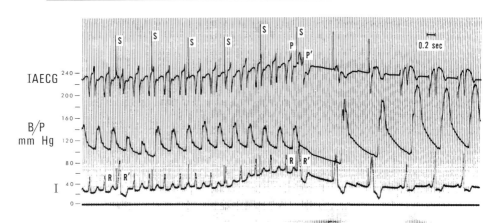

Figure 2A. Simultaneous lead I, intra-atrial electrocardiogram (IAECG), and brachial artery pressure recording illustrate reversion of supraventricular tachycardia induced by the sixth pacemaker stimulus (S). Pacemaker stimulus was introduced from a transvenous demand pacemaker with a fixed rate mode magnetic switch. sR-R' time of this beat is 280 msec with an R'-P' time of 170 msec. The first pacemaker stimulus with an R-R' time of 320 msec does not terminate the tachycardia. (Reproduced with permission from Ryan et al. *Circulation* 1968;38:1039).

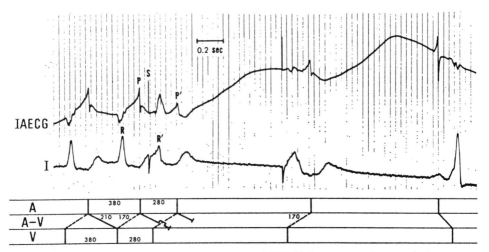

Figure 2B. Intra-atrial electrocardiogram (IAECG) in same patient and standard ECG lead I with pacemaker stimulus (S) inducing a VPB (R') at 280 msec from the previous QRS that caused early retrograde activation of the atria (R'-P' time of 170 msec). In this case the antegrade pathway following P' was refractory and the tachycardia terminated. (Reproduced with permission from Ryan et al. *Circulation* 1968;38:1039).

or the degeneration of tachycardia into faster forms causing hemodynamic complications, or ventricular fibrillation. Although Fisher[8] initially reported an incidence of adverse results to be only 4%, other researchers[9] have observed an incidence of induced accelerated ventricular tachycardia or ventricular fibrillation between 18% and 35%. This high risk of accelerated ventricular tachycardia led to the withdrawal of antitachycardia pacemakers as the only treatment for patients with malignant ventricular arrhythmias. However, this technology has been implemented to the new automatic implantable cardioverter defibrillators (ICD) that are coupled with both defibrillators and pacemakers.

Implantable Cardioverter Defibrillator

The resuscitation of patients experiencing sudden cardiac death depends on the time elapsed between onset of the malignant arrhythmia and the application of defibrillation. Since most of those events occur outside the hospital, the only available method to treat patients with out-of-hospital malignant ventricular arrhythmia prior to the development of the implantable cardioverter defibrillator (ICD) was to maintain the patient with cardiopulmonary resuscitation until an external defibrillator could be applied. This depended on the prompt arrival of mobile coronary units. These units are available in very few cities, and when available, their arrival time can be relatively long. Because of this, investigations were begun in the 1960s into the development of an automatic implantable cardioverter defibrillator for patients with a high risk of sudden death. The first studies demonstrating the efficacy of implanted defibrillators appeared in 1970, with the works by Mirowski et al.[10] (Fig. 3) and Schuder et al.[11] Mirowski et al. later improved the device and developed the first automatic implantable defibrillator for experimental[12] and clinical use.[13] The first human implantation took place in February, 1980, at the Johns Hopkins Hospital in Baltimore.[13,14] The initial implanted human device identified only ventricular fibrillation or sinusoidal ventricular tachycardia above 200 beats per minute. Clinical trials using this device began in 1982, and the United States Food and Drug Administration (FDA) approved the ICD for broad clinical use in patients with refractory malignant ventricular arrhythmias on November 15, 1985. Since then,

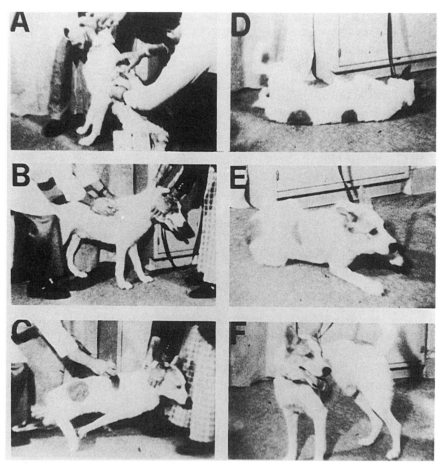

Figure 3. Selected frames from a motion picture of a typical automatic defibrillation episode. (A) Defibrillator testing procedure with the external analyzer. (B) Ventricular fibrillation is induced by magnetic activation of an implanted fibrillator. (C) Loss of consciousness secondary to the arrhythmia. (D) Delivery of the defibrillatory shock, 15 seconds after the onset of fibrillation. E and F show the animal 5 and 15 seconds, respectively, after automatic defibrillation (Reproduced with permission from Mirowski et al. Miniaturized implantable automatic defibrillator for prevention of sudden death from ventricular fibrillation. Amsterdam, Excerpta Medica International Congress Series 1978;458:660.)

there has been a progressive increase in the annual number of implants (> 10,000 units during 1992).

The initial ICD device had three components: a pulse generator, defibrillating leads, and rate-sensing leads. Cardiac electrical activity is continuously monitored by implanted electrodes. Arrhythmia recognition is based on two parameters: signal morphology and rate. Dual recognition parameters allow higher specificity for ventricular tachyarrhythmias. However, "spikey" ventricular tachycardias, which are typically nonsinusoidal, may not satisfy the morphology criteria and may be missed if the morphology criteria alone is used. Devices based on rate parameter alone provide more sensitivity with faster arrhythmia recognition. However, their specificity is low, since any tachycardia above the rate cut-off, such as atrial fibrillation, can satisfy arrhythmia detection criteria of the device. Once arrhythmia recognition criteria are satisfied after a tachycardia detection window of 5 to 20 seconds, the device's arrhythmia termination cycle is initiated (Fig. 4).

In the majority of current units, once tachycardia detection is met, capacitors were charged and shock delivered (committed discharge). In some patients with nonsustained ventricular tachycardia, the device discharged after spontaneous termination of the arrhythmia. Newer ICDs are programmably noncommitted and permit sensing throughout the time it takes for capacitor charging. If the arrhythmia spontaneously terminates during this time, shock is aborted.

Newer ICDs also have the capability of antitachycardia pacing for patients with sustained ventricular tachycardia. If antitachycardia pacing is not successful or accelerates the arrhythmia, a low-amplitude cardioversion is attempted. Most malignant ventricular arrhythmias are aborted with this shock. If arrhythmia persists, a maximal rescue shock of approximately 30 J is administered. If bradycardia is present after reversion of the arrhythmia, back-up pacing is initiated. The actual life span of currently available ICDs is approximately five years.

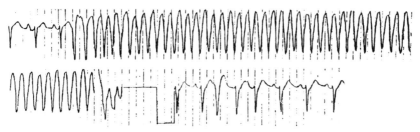

Figure 4. Continuous ECG tracing of spontaneous ventricular flutter terminated by AICD discharge.

Indication for ICD Implantation

The indications for ICD implantation are not totally defined and vary among researchers.[15,16] At present, patients who are considered definite candidates for ICD therapy are those who have survived an episode of cardiac arrest due to malignant ventricular arrhythmias without concomitant acute myocardial infarction, and patients with recurrent ventricular tachyarrhythmias in whom hemodynamically significant sustained ventricular tachycardia or ventricular fibrillation was induced during electrophysiological study.

Guidelines of the ACC/AHA for ICD implantation are summarized in Table 1. With the development of more sophisticated defibrillator devices, which incorporate overdrive pacing and demand pacemaker function, a wider variety of clinical arrhythmias have come under therapy. These developments, together with the percutaneous nonthoracotomy implantation, have increased the scope of patients who can benefit.

Preimplantation Evaluation

Before ICD implantation, patients with malignant ventricular arrhythmias should undergo evaluation to exclude potentially correctable causes of the arrhythmia. Adequate control of the arrhythmia with pharmacological therapy and identification of possible indications for concomitant surgical intervention should be accomplished. This is important since some antiarrhythmic agents, especially amiodarone, may interfere with the ICD functioning and increase the defibrillation threshold.[17,18] Other interactions of antiarrhythmic drugs and ICD include: 1) the appearance of proarrhythmia induced by an antiarrhythmic drug; 2) alteration in the morphology of the tachycardia, with the risk that new morphology is not identified by the ICD device; 3) slowing the tachycardia rate below the cut-off of the device; and 4) transient depression of excitability following ICD discharge, requiring concomitant pacemaker support.

Patients with permanent pacemaker interaction must also be evaluated before ICD implantation.[19] Patients with malignant ventricular arrhythmias frequently have conduction disturbances or significant sinus dysfunction. If the patient has a pacemaker implanted, there may be a transient failure to sense or capture immediately af-

Table 1

ACC/AHA Guidelines for Implantation of Implantable Cardioverter Defibrillator (ICD)

Class I. Conditions for which there is general agreement that ICD should be implanted.

    A)   One or more documented episodes of hemodynamic significant ventricular tachycardia or ventricular fibrillation in patients in whom electrophysiological testing and ambulatory monitoring cannot be used to accurately predict efficacy of therapy.

    B)   One or more documented episodes of hemodynamically significant ventricular tachycardia or ventricular fibrillation in a patient in whom no drug was found to be effective or no appropriate currently available drug was tolerated.

    C)   Continued inducibility at electrophysiological study of hemodynamically significant ventricular tachycardia or ventricular fibrillation despite the best available drug therapy or despite surgery or catheter ablation if drug therapy failed.

Class II. Conditions for which ICD is frequently used but there is divergence of opinion with respect to the necessity of its insertion.

    A)   One or more documented episodes of hemodynamically significant ventricular tachycardia or ventricular fibrillation in a patient in whom drug efficacy testing is possible.

    B)   Recurrent syncope of undetermined origin in a patient with hemodynamically significant ventricular tachycardia or ventricular fibrillation induced at electrophysiological study in whom no effective drug or no tolerated drug is available or appropriate.

Class III. Conditions for which there is general agreement that ICD is unnecessary.

    A)   Recurrent syncope of undetermined cause in a patient without inducible arrhythmias.

    B)   Arrhythmias not due to hemodynamically significant ventricular tachycardia or ventricular fibrillation.

    C)   Incessant ventricular tachycardia or fibrillation found to be effective or no appropriate currently available drug was tolerated.

(From Dreifus LS, et al. *Circulation.* 1991;84:455.)

ter the ICD discharge. Oversensing of the pacemaker stimulus by the ICD may also occur, leading to double-counting, and inappropriate ICD discharge.[19] In addition, the ICD may fail to sense ventricular fibrillation or ventricular tachycardia as a result of pacemaker stimulus oversensing. Of all these interactions, the most severe is the failure of pacemaker inhibition during ventricular fibrillation, leading to ICD inhibition. To prevent this risk, the amplitude of the pacemaker signal should be minimized, the distance between pacemaker and sensing leads maximized, and the setting of the pacemaker should be at the highest sensitivity setting in order to increase the chance of arrhythmia detection by the pacemaker. Fortunately the newer ICD devices incorporate this technology within their intelligence.

Implantation Approaches

There are currently two alternative approaches: thoracotomy or transvenous. Although during the past years, thoracotomy implants account for the majority of procedures,[20] currently the transvenous approach is the treatment of choice due to its lower operative risk and higher efficacy.[21] The transthoracic approach is presently reserved for patients in whom other cardiac surgery is planned (e.g., aneurismectomy or coronary artery bypass graft surgery), or when transvenous implantation has been unsuccessful. Bardy et al.[21] demonstrated that successful implantation of a transvenous cardioverter-defibrillator is possible in most patients (95%); the implant defibrillation threshold is usually low (mean 10.9 ± 4.8 J), surgical morbidity and postoperative complications are modest since most patients can be discharged three days after surgery, and results are excellent with no surgical deaths or sudden deaths occurring in a mean follow-up of 11 months.

Clinical Efficacy

There is presently little doubt about the clinical efficacy of ICDs. The reported incidence of sudden cardiac death at one year is 1% to 4.6%, whereas at five years of follow-up, it is 4% to 20%.[20,22] The seven-year cumulative mortality, excluding operative deaths, was 25%.[22] In the same series, sudden death was 1.5% at one year and 4.1% at two years, and cardiac death was 8.2% and 17.4% at one and two years, respectively. Deaths included documented or presumed ventricular tachycardia or ventricular fibrillation (10%), refractory heart failure (9.6%), myocardial infarction (2.2%), bradyarrhythmia (0.5%), and noncardiac death (2.7%).

The low incidence of sudden cardiac death in patients treated with ICDs contrasts with an incidence of 10% to 30% of patients with malignant ventricular arrhythmias treated with antiarrhythmic drugs only. When efficacy of the ICD is measured by the number of ICD discharges, Mercando et al.[23] reported a potential for freedom from sudden death at one year of 56% and at 4 years of 14% in their ICD recipients. Nevertheless, it should be emphasized that an ICD discharge may be inappropriate in many patients.[24] Newer devices provide monitoring information about the discharge event. Nonetheless, a clear reduction in the incidence of sudden death seems evident in recipients of ICDs.

Tchou et al.[25] observed that the ICD is effective in preventing sudden cardiac death in patients regardless of the severity of left ventricular function (Fig. 5). In 70 consecutive patients with sustained ventricular tachycardia or ventricular fibrillation who did not respond to antiarrhythmic drugs, the two-year survival was 93.4% with only one case of sudden death. Recently, Axtell reported a benefit in a long-term follow-up at five years of 60%; 79% of patients were free of sudden death [26] (Fig. 6).

The clinical efficacy of ICDs in patients with left ventricular dysfunction has been challenged, however. In a study of 197 patients with ICDs, only 53.3% experienced a discharge during 9.1 months of follow-up.[27] The survival for those patients with a discharge was no different from those who did not experience a discharge, 32.8 ± 19.5 months versus 28.0 ± 19.9 months, respectively. Predictors of survival were the concomitant coronary bypass surgery and advanced heart failure. The probability of survival after ICD implantation was better in patients with ejection fraction greater than 25% and higher heart failure class (Fig. 7). The data emphasize that a variety of factors related to left ventricular function affect survival in spite of successful ICD implantation.

There continues to be an expansion of indication for ICD implantation. Recent studies suggest that ICDs may be useful in survivors of out-of-hospital cardiac death without inducible sustained arrhythmias[28] and in patients with ventricular fibrillation but without significant structural heart disease.[29]

In spite of the reduction in the incidence of sudden death attributed to ICDs, it is important to appreciate that patients with an ICD apparatus still present considerable limitations. The inappropriate discharge in conscious patients, although rare in the newest devices, can cause severe psychological disturbances (Fig. 8). It is also important to note that there are presently many patients

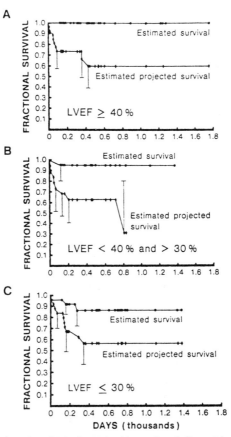

Figure 5. Survival and projected survival based on left ventricular ejection fraction (LVEF) when the automatic cardioverter defibrillator was implanted. The number of subjects at 6 months, 1 year, and 2 years survival and projected survival estimates, respectively, are indicated together with group identification. Patients with left ventricular ejection fraction of 40% or more (Group A; n = 22, 16, 7; 16, 11, 4) (panel A). Patients with left ventricular ejection fraction between 30% and 40% (Group B; n = 16, 13, 5; 13, 9, 3) (panel B). Patients with left ventricular ejection fraction less than 30% (Group C; n = 21, 17, 5; 15, 11, 6) (panel C). Note marked difference between survival (circles) and projected survival (diamonds) in each group of patients. These differences were all statistically significant. Vertical bars indicate one side of the 95% CI related to the survival estimate (from Tchou et al[25]).

(15%–20%) considered as "high risk of sudden death" in whom ICDs are implanted but never used.[30] It is necessary to emphasize that the ICD treats the expression of a primary disease state which is usually progressive, and total cardiac mortality remains high in spite of

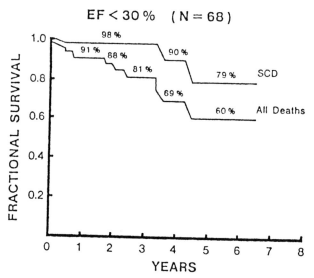

Figure 6. The actual death rates from SCD and all causes are shown (from Antell, et al.[26]).

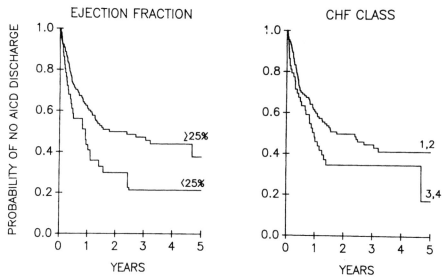

Figure 7. The probability of the AICD discharge related to ejection fraction or NYHA classification of heart failure (from Levine et al[27]).

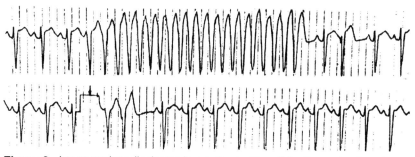

Figure 8. Inappropriate discharge in a patient with self-limiting episodes of ventricular flutter. In this case, discharge appears after the crisis terminates (arrow).

ICDs.[31] Although there is some doubt about the impact of ICDs on total mortality,[31] recent prospective studies suggest that ICDs not only preclude sudden death but also prolong life.[32] Powell et al.[33] demonstrated that in survivors of out-of-hospital cardiac arrest, the implantable defibrillator is associated with a significant reduction in cardiac mortality, particularly in patients with impaired left ventricular function.

There are several ongoing clinical trials that will provide answers to important questions about the real benefit of ICDs. In the Cardiac Arrest Study—Hamburg (CASH),[34] survivors of cardiac arrest are randomized to metoprolol, amiodarone, propafenone, or ICD therapy. After inclusion of 230 patients, the propafenone trial was stopped due to a significantly higher incidence of total mortality and recurrent cardiac arrest.[34]

Studies are now being done to investigate the benefit of prophylactic ICD implantation in patients at high risk of sudden death. These include the Multicenter Automatic Defibrillator Implantation Trial (MADIT),[35] the Multicenter Unsustained Tachycardia Trial (MUSTT),[35] and the Coronary Artery Bypass Graft Patch (CABG-Patch) trial[36] in patients with coronary artery disease, and the Defibrillator Implantation as Bridge to Later Transplantation (DEFIBRILAT), and the Cardiomyopathy Trial (CAT)[37] in patients with advanced heart failure.

Cardiac Surgery

Although ICDs significantly reduce the incidence of sudden cardiac death, neither antiarrhythmic drug therapy nor the ICD cure the malignant arrhythmias. Surgical and catheter ablation therapy, however, provide the opportunity for a radical solution.

The aim of surgery is to remove the arrhythmogenic substrate. In postmyocardial infarction patients, the substrate for arrhythmias is believed to be located in the border zones between viable and necrotic myocardium.

The ideal candidate for direct surgical treatment has the following characteristics:

1. Sustained ventricular tachycardia refractory to medical treatment
2. Ventricular tachycardia with a stable rhythm and without accompanying hemodynamic compromise which allows for preoperative endocardial mapping
3. Left ventricular aneurysm, preferably anteroapical with good contractility in the remaining myocardium
4. Ventricular arrhythmias originating from one, and no more than two, areas of the myocardium.

The only absolute contraindication for surgery of the arrhythmogenic focus is the existence of extremely depressed left ventricular function. In these circumstances, the treatment of choice may be an ICD. Percutaneous catheter ablation or cardiac transplantation may also be indicated in some circumstances.

Surgical Treatment for Ventricular Arrhythmias in Patients with Ischemic Heart Disease

Multiple surgical procedures have been attempted in recent years for patients with ischemic heart disease who have malignant ventricular arrhythmias. Sympathectomy, coronary arterial bypass, aneurysmectomy, or infarctectomy, alone or in combination, are surgical procedures that have been used. The results of these interventions have been unsatisfactory[38] (Table 2).

Sympathectomy

Although sympathectomy is usually used for treatment of patients with long QT syndrome, it has also been tested in patients

Table 2

Results of Indirect Surgical Procedures for the Treatment of Refractory Ischemic Ventricular Tachycardia

Procedure	Patients (n)	Operative Mortality (%)	Intractable Arrhythmia Recurrence (%)	Overall Success (%)
Sympathectomy	12	25	17	58
Coronary arterial bypass	45	22	22	56
Aneurysmectomy or infarctectomy	95	24	17	59
Aortocoronary bypass plus aneurysmectomy	27	41	4	55
Total	179	26	16	58

(From Boineau JP.[38])

with ischemic heart disease. Minardo et al.[39] demonstrated, in an animal model, that myocardial infarction may interrupt epicardial neural pathways, create heterogeneous zones of sympathetic innervation, and predispose to ventricular arrhythmias. The hypothesis on which sympathectomy is proposed is the elimination of these areas of heterogeneous innervation. The Sudden Death Italian Prevention Group[40] randomized 144 patients with anterior myocardial infarction complicated by early ventricular tachycardia or ventricular fibrillation to placebo, oxprenolol, and high thoracic left sympathectomy. Over a mean follow-up of 20 months, the incidence of sudden death was 22% in the placebo group, 3.6% in patients treated with sympathectomy, and 2.7% in patients who received oxprenolol. In spite of these suggestive findings, sympathectomy is not currently being used for the prevention of ventricular arrhythmias. Cardiac denervation has also been advocated for the treatment of ventricular arrhythmias associated with coronary artery vasospasm[41] but in general has been unsuccessful.

Coronary Artery Bypass Grafting

It seems logical to believe that coronary artery bypass could be effective in the prevention of sudden death. Although bypass surgery can affect total mortality, the effect on sudden death is only marginal. There are, however, selected groups of patients in which coronary artery bypass grafting may be useful in the prevention of sudden cardiac death. The Coronary Artery Surgery Study[42] assessed the value of medical and surgical treatment for the prevention of sudden cardiac death in 13,476 patients with significant coronary artery disease and operable vessels. During a mean follow-up of 4.6 years, sudden death occurred in 3.4% and was more frequent in medically treated patients, 4.9%, than in those who received surgical treatment, 1.6%, ($P < 0.0001$). This reduction was most pronounced in patients with three-vessel disease and history of congestive heart failure in whom sudden death occurred in 8%, compared with 31% of medically treated patients. Coronary artery bypass grafting was also beneficial in patients with two-vessel disease without congestive heart failure (Fig. 9). In the European Coronary Surgery Study[43], which included patients with two- or three-vessel disease and preserved ventricular function, surgical therapy was associated with a reduction in sudden cardiac death during five-year follow-up. At 12 years, however, survival rates were similar in the surgical and medical patients.[43] The superiority of surgical revascularization over medical treatment in prolonging survival in patients with left mainstem coronary artery disease in even asymptomatic individuals, has also been demonstrated.[44,45]

Patients resuscitated from out-of-hospital cardiac arrest frequently present with severe coronary artery lesions. The role of coronary artery bypass grafting in these patients is unclear. Kelly et al.[46] studied 50 survivors of cardiac arrest who were surgically revascularized. None of the 10 patients with inducible ventricular fibrillation in preoperative electrophysiological study had inducible ventricular arrhythmias at the time of the postsurgical study. In contrast, 16 of the 20 patients (80%) with inducible sustained ventricular tachycardia before coronary artery bypass grafting had sustained ventricular tachycardia or ventricular fibrillation when studied postoperatively. Kron et al.[47] performed coronary artery bypass grafting in 8 patients with out-of-hospital cardiac arrest secondary to ventricular fibrillation. After surgery, 5 patients had neither spontaneous nor inducible arrhythmias, although 3 patients had spontaneous ventricular fib-

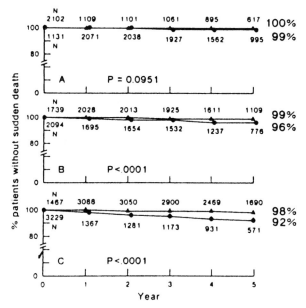

Figure 9. Percent of patients without sudden cardiac death in surgically treated group (▲) compared with that in medically treated group (●). None of the patients had a history of CHF. (A) Patients with one-vessel disease. (B) Patients with two-vessel disease. (C) Patients with three-vessel disease. The actual number of patients are given for each survival curve. (From Holmes et al.[42])

rillation. The Seattle study [48] also suggests surgery in patients resuscitated from out-of-hospital ventricular fibrillation with coronary artery bypass reducing the incidence of sudden death. In a mean follow-up of 4.9 years, 11 (13%) of 85 patients had coronary bypass surgery, and 76 (42%) of 180 medically treated patients had a second cardiac arrest ($P < 0.04$).

Aneurysmectomy

Aneurysmectomy or infarctectomy, alone or in combination with coronary artery bypass grafting, has been used to treat intractable arrhythmias with unsatisfactory results.[49] An in-hospital mortality of 24% and intractable arrhythmia recurrence rate of 17% resulted in an overall success rate of approximately 59%. The failure to achieve better results is probably related to failure to excise the border zone of the aneurysm where ventricular tachycardia begins.

Thus, simple aneurysmectomy without electrophysiological guidance only cures ventricular arrhythmias fortuitously, and arrhythmia recurrence rates are unacceptably high.

The results of electrophysiologically guided aneurysmectomy[49,50] have been shown to be superior to simple aneurysmectomy. In 1978, Guiraudon et al.[51] developed encircling endocardial ventriculotomy for the treatment of malignant ventricular arrhythmias in patients with previous myocardial infarction. This was usually carried out after a standard ventriculotomy through the infarction or aneurysm zone. The ventriculotomy is extended around the border of subendocardial fibrosis, sparing the epicardium and coronary arteries. The area of scar thought to contain the arrhythmogenic focus is isolated with this technique. Of 21 patients surviving the operation, 95% were free of further ventricular tachycardia, although 23% required concomitant antiarrhythmic drugs. Nevertheless, this procedure is followed by a loss of both systolic contraction and diastolic compliance[52], and a surgical mortality rate of 9%.

The extended endocardial resection, a further development of surgical therapy, carries the incision to visible endocardial fibrosis which is resected from the underlying myocardium.[53] This procedure is useful in patients in whom intraoperative mapping is not possible or cannot be completed. The operative mortality and morbidity of this technique is similar to that of map-guided subendocardial resection, and the incidence of arrhythmia recurrence is slightly greater. The operative mortality is reported at 10%; 7.6% of the surviving patients had inducible ventricular tachycardia at the time of postoperative electrophysiological study.[53]

Map-guided electrophysiological procedures are the most sophisticated surgical intervention, designed to precisely locate the region of origin of the ventricular arrhythmias. Epicardial mapping is the initial intraoperative procedure used for the localization of the site of origin of ventricular tachycardia.[54] The earliest site of ventricular activation is considered to represent the region of origin of ventricular tachycardia. Several variations of ventricular mapping techniques have been used, including activation sequence mapping,[55] fragmentation mapping,[56] pace mapping,[57] and cryothermal mapping.[58] The resection of the precise subendocardial zone is the aim of all these techniques and requires the availability and experience of the electrophysiology laboratory. The Collaborative Registry collected information from eight centers[59] and 665 patients. The operative mortality was 12% and survival was 72% at two years and 57% at five years. Over a mean follow-up of 27.4 months, 68 patients (10.5%) experienced recurrent ventricular tachycardia. Sudden cardiac death occurred in 5.7% of patients. The overall out-of-hospital recurrence of arrhythmic events was 16%.

Hargrove and Miller reported the experience of the Hospital of the University of Pennsylvania using map-guided subendocardial resection.[60] In 68% of the patients, tachycardia was totally noninducible without antiarrhythmic drugs. The incidence of noninducibility increased to 93% when antiarrhythmic drugs were administered. Noninducibility was directly proportional to the percentage of tachycardias mapped at operation (Fig. 10). The three factors which significantly increased operative mortality included: severely depressed left ventricular function with ejection fraction less than 20%, emergency operations, and prior heart surgery. Five-year survival was approximately 60%.

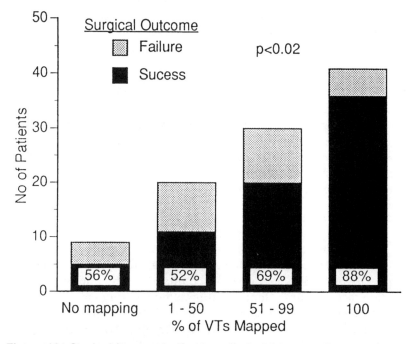

Figure 10. Stacked bar graph showing effect of intraoperative mapping on surgical success of subendocardial resection. VT = ventricular tachycardia. (From Hargrove.[60])

Surgical Treatment for Ventricular Arrhythmias in Patients with Nonischemic Heart Disease

Valvular Heart Disease

Critical valvular aortic stenosis is a well-recognized risk factor for sudden cardiac death (see Chapter XI). In patients with hemodynamically significant valvular stenosis and well-preserved ventricular function, aortic replacement is associated with improved prognosis.[61,62]

Malignant ventricular arrhythmias and sudden cardiac death are occasionally reported in patients with mitral valve prolapse (see Chapter XI). The origin of the tachyarrhythmia has been localized in the mitral valve area. Ventricular tachycardia has been reported to be effectively controlled after mitral valve replacement.[63,64] Candidates for surgery have significant valvular regurgitation and left ventricular dysfunction. In the absence of hemodynamically significant mitral regurgitation or proven ventricular tachycardia originating from the mitral apparatus, replacement of the mitral valve is not indicated.

Hypertrophic Cardiomyopathy

Patients with hypertrophic cardiomyopathy are at high risk of sudden cardiac death (see Chapter X). Although cardiac surgery including myotomy or myomectomy is useful to improve symptoms, its role in the prevention of sudden cardiac death is controversial.[65] Furthermore, map-guided surgery is not useful.

Dilated Cardiomyopathy

Ventricular arrhythmias and sudden cardiac death are frequent in patients with dilated cardiomyopathy (see Chapter X). Since the disease involves diffuse myocardial damage, a single focal arrhythmogenic focus is rarely found and map-guided surgical resection is rarely effective. In patients with severely depressed ventricular function, surgery is associated with a high operative mortality. For this reason, an ICD is a better choice for most patients with dilated cardiomyopathy and malignant ventricular arrhythmias and may be used as a "bridge" to cardiac transplantation[66] (see above).

Orthotopic heart transplantation has become the definitive surgical procedure in patients with severely depressed ventricular function and is occasionally indicated for the treatment of refractory malignant ventricular arrhythmias.[67] Sudden cardiac death, however, has been reported occasionally in some patients as a manifestation of acute transplant rejection (see Chapter X).

Arrhythmogenic Right Ventricular Dysplasia

Patients with arrhythmogenic right ventricular dysplasia occasionally experience sustained ventricular arrhythmias (see Chapter X). Map-guided surgery is frequently difficult and is associated with increased incidence of recurrences due to the diffuse involvement of the right ventricle and the presence of multiple arrhythmogenic foci.[68] Guiraudon[69] advocates the total disconnection of the right ventricle from the left heart. Clinical experience is, however, quite limited and requires demonstrated benefit in larger series and by other surgeons.

Long QT Syndrome

Patients with long QT syndrome who do not respond to β-blocking agents may be candidates for high cervicothoracic sympathectomy (Chapter XII).[70,71] Experience is based on 67 patients with syncopal episodes despite full doses of β-blockers[71] in whom the incidence of sudden cardiac death was 8% at 5 years, an incidence of sudden death which is relatively low considering these patients represent a subgroup at high risk of sudden death. The combination of β-blocker and high thoracic left sympathectomy in symptomatic long QT syndrome results in an incidence of sudden cardiac death of approximately 3%. When a patient with long QT syndrome continues to have syncopal episodes despite β-blockers or high thoracic left sympathectomy, the implantation of the ICD device is the most rational approach. Patients with long QT syndrome can experience frequent episodes of ventricular fibrillation, causing severe psychological problems, particularly in young individuals.

Wolff-Parkinson-White Syndrome

Patients with Wolff-Parkinson-White syndrome are at increased risk of malignant arrhythmias and sudden death (Table

2)(see Chapter XIII). Treatment is presently indicated in symptomatic patients with Wolff-Parkinson-White syndrome and rapid antegrade pathway conduction.[72] Surgery was the treatment of choice for symptomatic patients with reciprocating tachycardias due to its excellent results. Surgery is technically simple and offers better results for free-wall than for septal pathways. Guiraudon et al.[73] reported successful results using an external close-heart approach in conjunction with cryoablation of the left free-wall accessory pathways. Gallagher et al.[74] reported a success rate in their first 267 patients of 98% for right pathways, 94% for left free-wall pathways, 85% for anteroseptal pathways, and 81% for posteroseptal pathways. After several modifications of the technique, these researchers reported 100% efficacy in 118 operative cases.[75] Mortality was approximately 5%, and only 1% in patients without associated cardiac abnormalities.[75] Nevertheless, surgical therapy for Wolff-Parkinson-White syndrome has now been replaced almost completely by radiofrequency catheter ablation.

Catheter Ablation

Catheter ablation using DC intracardiac countershock for patients with ventricular tachycardia remains an investigational procedure. Although some investigators have obtained successful results,[76] this technique should be applied with caution in patients with ventricular tachycardia considering the low efficacy reported in most series, and the serious complications involved.

The procedure involves induction of tachycardia and localization of the arrhythmogenic foci using standard methods in the catheterization laboratory. Once the putative site of ventricular tachycardia origin is located, varying energy sources are then applied to this site to ablate the foci. The greatest experience has been gathered using high-energy DC shocks applied to the endocardial site by a standard defibrillator.[77] The Percutaneous Cardiac Mapping and Ablation Registry[78] included 164 patients with ventricular tachycardia. This registry reported an overall complete cure of tachycardia of 18%. An additional 41% appeared to improve with drug therapy. In contrast to this low efficacy, there was a high incidence of serious procedure-related complications. A total of 11 procedure-related deaths including electromechanical dissociation, induction of nonresuscitable ventricular arrhythmias, and progressive intractable heart failure have been reported. Other serious complications can include major cerebrovascular accidents, myocardial perforation, or arterial thrombosis. During long-term follow-up there is a small but significant risk of sudden death.[79] With radiofrequency techniques, better results have been reported, with fewer complictions in patients with idiopathic, incessant, and sustained ventricular tachycardias, and recently also in patients with coronary artery disease.[80,81] Radiofrequency energy has been successfully applied to control ventricular tachycardia when the right bundle branch is a critical component of the tachycardia circuit.[82]

Other catheter ablation procedures have recently been investigated.[83–86] Lawrie et al.[83] reported a cryoablative technique that avoids ventriculotomy. Brugada et al.[84] reported three patients with incessant ventricular tachycardia successfully treated with transcoronary chemical ablation with 2 mL of 99% ethanol infusion. After coronary arteriography was performed to identify the coronary artery supplying the arrhythmogenic focus, the artery was then selectively cannulated and an ice saline infusion applied through a catheter to temporarily terminate the arrhythmia. Catheter laser ablation is also presently being investigated for the treatment of malignant ventricular arrhythmias, although it is presently only applicable in humans during open heart surgery.[85,86] Radiofrequency ablation procedures for the treatment of patients with ventricular tachycardia are still investigational, but will probably be used more in the future.

Radiofrequency catheter ablation now plays a key role in patients with Wolff- Parkinson-White syndrome. Kuck et al.[87] reported that this technique is successful in almost all patients treated. These results have been confirmed by many other researchers. It is now the technique of choice for the treatment of Wolff-Parkinson-White syndrome with symptomatic arrhythmias. In patients with drug-resistant intranodal tachycardias, radiofrequency ablation is probably the first choice.[88] Thus, with this technique an important problem related to sudden death in young people has been solved.

In conclusion, major strides have been accomplished in the development of implantation devices for the treatment and prevention of cardiac arrest. Our current devices are merely the most primitive expression of more sophisticated and intelligent devices yet to come. These devices will have the potential to change our approach to the treatment of patients at risk of sudden death. New automatic antitachycardia devices are rapidly being developed and tested. The circuitry, sensitivity, and logistic flexbility will expand their clinical application. At the same time, catheter ablation techniques using a variety of energy sources, hold promise for wider use in the interruption of reentrant tracts and arrhythmic foci.

References

1. Zehender M, Buchner C, Meinertz T, et al. Prevalence, circumstances, mechanisms and risk stratification of sudden cardiac death in unipolar single-chamber ventricular pacing. *Circulation* 1992;85:596.
2. Johnson RA, Hutter AM, DeSanctis RW, et al. Chronic overdrive pacing the control of refractory ventricular arrhythmias. *Ann Intern Med* 1974;80:380.
3. Eldar M, Griffin JY, Abbot JA, et al. Permanent cardiac pacing in patients with long QT syndrome. *J Am Coll Cardiol* 1987;10:600.
4. Rosenthal ME, Josephson ME. Current status of antitachycardia devices. *Circulation* 1990;82:1889.
5. Wellens HJJ, Lie HI, Durrer D. Further observations on ventricular tachycardia as studied by electrical stimulation of the heart. *Circulation* 1974;49:647.
6. Almendral JM, Rosenthal ME, Stamato NJ, et al. Analysis of the resetting phenomenon in sustained uniform ventricular tachycardia: Incidence and relation to termination. *J Am Coll Cardiol* 1986;8:294.
7. Wyndham CRC. Antitachycardia pacing: Clinical aspects. In: El-Sherif N, Samet P, eds. *Cardiac Pacing and Electrophysiology.* Philadelphia: WB Saunders;1991;706.
8. Fisher JD, Mehra R, Furman S. Termination of ventricular tachycardia with bursts of rapid ventricular pacing. *Am J Cardiol* 1978;41:94.
9. Roy D, Waxman HL, Buxton AE, et al. Termination of ventricular tachycardia: Role of the tachycardia cycle length. *Am J Cardiol* 1982;50:1346.
10. Mirowski M, Mower MM, Staewen S, et al. Standby automatic defibrillator. *Arch Int Med* 1970;126:158.
11. Schuder JC, Stoeckle H, Gold JH, et al. Experimental ventricular defibrillation with an automatic and completely implanted system. *Trans Am Soc Artif Organs* 1970;16:201.
12. Mirowski M, Mower MM, Langer A, et al. A chronically implanted system for automatic defibrillator in active conscious dogs. *Circulation* 1978;58:90.
13. Mirowski M, Reid PR, Mower MM, et al. Termination of malignant ventricular arrhythmias with an implanted automatic defibrillator in human beings. *New Engl J Med* 1980;303:322.
14. Holmes DR. The implantable cardioverter defibrillator. In: Furman S, Haynes DL, Holmes DR, eds. *A Practice of Cardiac Pacing.* Armonk: Futura Publishing Company; 1993;465.
15. Lehmann MH, Saksena S, for the NASPE Policy Conference Committee. Implantable cardioverter defibrillators in cardiovascular practice: Report of the Policy Conference of the North American Society of Pacing and Electrophysiology. *PACE* 1991;14:969.

16. A Task Force of the Working Groups on Cardiac Arrhythmias and Cardiac Pacing of the European Society of Cardiology. *Eur Heart J* 1992;13:1304.

17. Guarnieri T, Lenine JH, Veltri EP, et al. Success of chronic defibrillation and the role of antiarrhythmic drugs with the automatic implantable cardioverter-defibrillator. *Am J Cardiol* 1987;60:1061.

18. Haberman R, Veltri EP, Mower MM. The effect of amiodarone on defibrillation threshold. *PACE* 1987;10:406.

19. Calkins H, Brinker J, Veltri EP, et al. Clinical interactions between pacemakers and automatic implantable cardioverter-defibrillators. *J Am Coll Cardiol* 1990;16:666.

20. Winkle RA, Mead RH, Ruder MA, et al. Long term outcome with the automatic implantable cardioverter-defibrillator. *J Am Coll Cardiol* 1989;13:1353.

21. Bardy GH, Hofer B, Johnson G, et al. Implantable transvenous cardioverter-defibrillators. *Circulation* 1993;87:1152.

22. Veltri EP, Mower MM, Guarnieri T, et al. Clinical efficacy of the automatic implantable defibrillator: 7 year cumulative experience. *Chest* 1987;92:975.

23. Mercando AD, Furman S, Johnston D, et al. Survival of patients with the automatic implantable cardioverter defibrillator. *PACE* 1988; 11:2059.

24. Hook BG, Callas DJ, Kleiman RB, et al. Implantable cardioverter-defibrillator therapy in the absence of significant symptoms. Rhythm diagnosis and management aided by stored electrogram analysis. *Circulation* 1993;87:1897.

25. Tchou P, Kadri N, Anderson J, et al. Automatic implantable cardioverter defibrillators and survival of patients with left ventricular dysfunction and malignant ventricular arrhythmias. *Ann Intern Med* 1988;109:529.

26. Axtell K, Tchou P, Akhtar M. Survival in patients with detressed left ventricular function treated by implantable cardioverter-defibrillator. *PACE* 1991;14:291.

27. Levine JH, Mellits ED, Baumgardner RA, et al. Predictors of first discharge and subsequent survival in patients with automatic implantable cardioverter-defibrillators. *Circulation* 1991;84:558.

28. Crandall BG, Morris CD, Cutler JR, et al. Implantable cardioverter-defibrillator therapy in survivors of out-of-hospital sudden cardiac death without inducible arrhythmias. *J Am Coll Cardiol* 1993;21:1186.

29. Meissner MC, Lehmann MH, Steinman RT, et al. Ventricular fibrillation in patients without significant structural heart disease: A multicenter experience with implantable cardioverter-defibrillator therapy. *J Am Coll Cardiol* 1993;21:1406.

30. Saksena S, Camm J. Implantable defibrillators for prevention of sudden death. Technology at a medical and economic crossroad. *Circulation* 1992;85:2316.

31. Kim SG. Implantable defibrillators therapy: Does it really prolong life? How can we prove it? *Am J Cardiol* 1993;71:1213.

32. Bocker D, Block M, Isbruch F, et al. Do patients with implantable defibrillator live longer? *J Am Coll Cardiol* 1993;21:1638.

33. Powell AC, Fuchs T, Finkelstein DM, et al. Influence of implantable cardioverter defibrillators on the long-term prognosis of survivors of out-of-hospital cardiac arrest. *Circulation* 1993;88:1083.
34. Siebels J, Cappato R, Ruppel R, et al, and the CASH Investigators. ICD vs. drugs in cardiac arrest survivors: Preliminary results of the Cardiac Arrest Study—Hamburg. *PACE* 1993;16:552.
35. Klein H, Trappe HJ, Fieguth G, et al. Prospective studies evaluating prophylactic ICD therapy for high risk patients with coronary artery disease. *PACE* 1993;16:564.
36. Brachmann J, Freigang K, Saggau W. Coronary Artery Bypass Graft Patch Trial. *PACE* 1993;16:571.
37. The Cardiomyopathy Trial Investigators. Cardiomyopathy Trial. *PACE* 1993;16:576.
38. Boineau JP, Cox JL. Rationale for a direct surgical approach to control ventricular arrhythmias. *Am J Cardiol* 1982;49:381.
39. Minardo JD, Tuli MM, Mock BH, et al. Scintigraphic and electrophysiological evidence of canine myocardial sympathetic denervation and produced by myocardial infarction or phenol application. *Circulation* 1988;78:1008.
40. Schwartz PJ, Motolese M, Pollavinni G, et al. and the Sudden Death Italian Prevention Group. Surgical and pharmacological antiadrenergic interventions in the prevention of sudden death after a first myocardial infarction. *Circulation* 1985;72:III-358.
41. Grondin CM, Limet R. Sympathetic denervation in association with coronary artery bypass grafting in patients with Prinzmetal's angina. *Ann Thorac Surg* 1977;23:111.
42. Holmes DR, Davis KB, Mock MB, et al. The effect of medical and surgical treatment on subsequent sudden death in patients with coronary artery disease: A report from the Coronary Artery Surgery Study. *Circulation* 1986;73:1254.
43. Varnauskas E and the European Coronary Surgery Study Group. Twelve year follow-up of survival in the randomized European Coronary Surgery Study. *New Engl J Med* 1988;319:332.
44. Takaro T, Hultgren H, Lipton M, et al. and participants in the Veterans Administration Cooperative Study Group. VA cooperative randomized study for coronary arterial occlusive disease. II. Left main disease. *Circulation* 1976;54:III-107.
45. Taylor HA, Deumite J, Chaitman BR, et al. Asymptomatic left main coronary artery disease in the Coronary Artery Surgery Study (CASS registry). *Circulation* 1988;79:1171.
46. Kelly P, Ruskin JN, Vlahakes GJ, et al. Surgical coronary revascularization in survivors of prehospital cardiac arrest: Its effects on inducible ventricular arrhythmias and long-term survival. *J Am Coll Cardiol* 1990;15:267.
47. Kron IL, Lerman BB, Haines DE, et al. Coronary artery bypass grafting in patients with ventricular fibrillation. *Ann Thorac Surg* 1989;48:85.
48. Every NR, Fahrenbruch CE, Hallstrom AP, et al. Influence of coronary bypass surgery on subsequent outcome of patients resuscitated from out of hospital cardiac arrest. *J Am Coll Cardiol* 1992;19:1435.

49. Harken AH, Horowitz LN, Josephson ME. Comparison of standard aneurysmectomy and aneurysmectomy with directed endocardial resection for treatment of recurrent sustained ventricular tachycardia. *J Thorac Cardiovasc Surg* 1980;80:527.
50. Mason JW, Stinson EB, Winkle RA, et al. Surgery for ventricular tachycardia: Efficacy of left ventricular aneurysm resection with operation guided by electrical activation mapping. *Circulation* 1982;65:1148.
51. Guiraudon G, Fontaine G, Frank R, et al. Encircling endocardial ventriculotomy: A new surgical treatment for life-threatening ventricular arrhythmias resistant to medical treatment following myocardial infarction. *Ann Thorac Surg* 1978;26:438.
52. Ostermeyer J, Breithardt G, Borggrefe M, et al. Direct operations for management of life-threatening ischemic ventricular tachycardia. *J Thorac Cardiovasc Surg* 1987;94:848.
53. Moran J, Kehoe R, Loeb J. Extended endocardial resection for the treatment of ventricular tachycardia. *Ann Thorac Surg* 1982;34:538.
54. Horowitz LN, Josephson ME, Harken AH. Epicardial and endocardial activation during sustained ventricular tachycardia in man. *Circulation* 1980;61:1227.
55. Josephson ME, Horowitz LN, Farshidi A, et al. Recurrent sustained ventricular tachycardia. 2. Endocardial mapping. *Circulation* 1978;57:440.
56. Wiener I, Mindich B. Fragmented endocardial electrical activity in patients with ventricular tachycardia: A new guide to surgical therapy. *Am Heart J* 1984;107:86.
57. Josephson ME, Waxman HL, Cain ME, et al. Ventricular activation during ventricular endocardial pacing. II. Role of pace-mapping to localize origin of ventricular tachycardia. *Am J Cardiol* 1982;50:11–22.
58. Gallagher JJ, Del Rossi AJ, Fernandez J, et al. Cryothermal mapping of recurrent ventricular tachycardia in man. *Circulation* 1985;71:733.
59. Borggrefe M, Podczeck A, Ostermeyer J, et al. Long-term results of electrophysiologically guided antitachycardia surgery in ventricular tachyarrhythmias: A collaborative report on 665 patients. In: Breithardt G, Borggrefe M, Zipes DP, eds. *Nonpharmacological Therapy of Tachyarrhythmias.* Armonk: Futura Publishing Company; 1987;102.
60. Hargrove WC, Miller JM. Risk stratification and management of patients with recurrent ventricular tachycardia and other malignant ventricular arrhythmias. *Circulation* 1989;79:I-178.
61. Henry WL, Bonow RO, Borer JS, et al. Evaluation of aortic valve replacement in patients with valvular aortic stenosis. *Circulation* 1980;61:814.
62. Rahimtoola SH. Valvular heart disease: A perspective. *J Am Coll Cardiol* 1983;1:199.
63. Ross A, de Weese JA, Yu PN. Refractory ventricular arrhythmias in a patient with mitral valve prolapse: Successful control with mitral valve replacement. *J Electrocardiol* 1978;11:289.
64. Kay HJ, Krohn BG, Hoffman RL. Surgical correction of severe mitral valve prolapse without mitral insufficiency but with pronounced cardiac arrhythmias. *J Thorac Cardiovasc Surg* 1979;78:259.

65. Mohr R, Schaff HV, Danielson GK, et al. The outcome of surgical treatment of hypertrophic cardiomyopathy. *J Thorac Cardiovasc Surg* 1989;97:666.

66. Stevenson LB, Fowler BM, Schroeder JS, et al. Poor survival of patients with idiopathic cardiomyopathy considered too well for transplantation. *Am J Med* 1987;83:871.

67. Stevenson LW, Miller LW. Cardiac transplantation as therapy for heart failure. *Curr Prob Cardiol* 1991;16:219.

68. Fontaine G, Guiraudon G, Frank R, et al. Surgical management of ventricular tachycardia unrelated to myocardial ischemia or infarction. *Am J Cardiol* 1982;49:397.

69. Guiraudon GM, Klein GJ, Gulamhusein S, et al. Total disconnection of the right ventricular free wall: Surgical treatment of right ventricular tachycardia associated with right ventricular dysplasia. *Circulation* 1983;67:463.

70. Moss AJ, McDonald J. Unilateral cervicothoracic sympathetic ganglionectomy for treatment of the long QT interval syndrome. *New Engl J Med* 1971;285:903.

71. Schwartz PJ, Locati E, Priori SG, et al. The Long Q-T Syndrome. In: Zipes DP, Jalife J, eds. *Cardiac Electrophysiology: From Cell to Bedside.* Philadelphia: WB Saunders Co; 1990;589.

72. Sealy WC, Gallagher JJ, Wallace AG. The surgical treatment of the Wolff-Parkinson-White syndrome. Evolution of improved methods for identification and interruption of the Kent bundle. *Ann Thoracic Surg* 1975;22:443.

73. Guiraudon GC, Klein GC, Gulamhusein S, et al. Surgical repair of Wolff-Parkinson-White syndrome: A new closed-heart technique. *Ann Thorac Surg* 1984;37:67.

74. Gallagher JJ, Sealy WC, Cox JL, et al. Results of surgery for preexcitation caused by accessory atrioventricular pathways in 267 consecutive cases. In: Josephson ME, Wellens HJJ, eds. *Tachycardias: Mechanisms, Diagnosis, Management.* Philadelphia: Lea and Febiger; 1984;259.

75. Cox JL, Gallagher JJ, Cain ME. Experience with 118 consecutive patients undergoing operation for the Wolff-Parkinson-White syndrome. *J Thorac Cardiovasc Surg* 1985;90:490.

76. Fontaine G, Cansell A, Frank R, et al. Catheter ablation techniques for ventricular tachycardia. In: El-Sherif N, Samet P. *Cardiac Pacing and Electrophysiology.* Philadelphia: WB Saunders Co; 1991;471.

77. Scheinman MM. Catheter ablation: Present role and projected impact on health care for patients with cardiac arrhythmias. *Circulation* 1991;83:1489.

78. Evans GT, Scheinman MM, Zipes DP, et al. The Percutaneous Cardiac Mapping and Ablation Registry: Final summary of results. *PACE* 1988;11:1621.

79. Hindricks G, Haverkamp W, on behalf of the Multicenter European Radiofrequency Survey (MERFS) Investigators. The Multicenter European Radiofrequency Survey: Summary of heart complications of radiofrequency catheter ablation of cardiac arrhythmias in 4372 patients. *Eur Heart J* 1993;14:A256.

80. Morady F, Harvey M, Kalbfleisch S, et al. Radiofrequency ablation of ventricular tachycardia in patients with coronary heart disease. *Circulation* 1993;87:363.
81. Klein LS, Shih HT, Hackett K, et al. Radiofrequency ablation of ventricular tachycardia in patients without structural heart disease. *Circulation* 1992;85:1666.
82. Langberg JJ, Desai J, Dullet N, et al. Treatment of macroreentrant ventricular tachycardia with radiofrequency ablation of the right bundle branch. *Am J Cardiol* 1989;63:1010.
83. Lawrie GM, Pacifico A, Kaushik RR. Transannular cryoablation of ventricular tachycardia. *J Thorac Cardiovasc Surg* 1989;98:1030.
84. Brugada P, de Swart J, Smeets J, et al. Transcoronary chemical ablation of ventricular tachycardia. *Circulation* 1989;79:475.
85. Saksena S, Hussain SM, Gielchinsky I, et al. Intraoperative mapping-guided argon laser ablation of malignant ventricular tachycardia. *Am J Cardiol* 1987;59:78.
86. Svenson RH, Littmann L, Splinter R, et al. Application of laser for arrhythmia ablation. In: Zipes DP, Jalife J, eds. *Cardiac Electrophysiology: From Cell to Bedside.* Philadelphia; WB Saunders; 1990;986.
87. Kuck KH, Geiger M, Schluter M, et al. Radiofrequency current ablation of left-sided accessory pathways. The single catheter technique. *J Am Coll Cardiol* 1991;17:108A.
88. Yeung-Lai-Wah JA, Alison JF, Lonergan L, et al. High success rate of atrioventricular node ablation with radiofrequency energy. *J Am Coll Cardiol* 1991;18:1753.

Chapter XIX

Mobile Coronary Care Units and Out-Of-Hospital Resuscitation

The knowledge gained from hospital coronary care units and the establishment of effective pharmacological and electrical intervention for cardiac arrhythmias represent important advances in clinical cardiology. The realization, however, that in spite of the success of these units, many patients still die outside the hospital, has led to the extension of coronary care units into the community either as mobile or satellite facilities. These units were developed in an attempt to bring the highly specialized medical facility to patients rather than awaiting their uncertain arrival at the hospital. The initial efforts by Pantridge and Geddes[1] in Belfast were followed quickly by the development of a number of mobile units in the United States.[2-5] These programs were developed initially to respond to patients who were experiencing symptoms of an acute myocardial infarction. Soon it was evident that in spite of the effectiveness of these units in treating the early arrhythmias of acute myocardial infarction, many patients experienced major delay prior to calling for assistance and were dying suddenly. This led to the development of more rapid rescue facilities. The second generation of mobile units began to more directly address the problem of sudden collapse and death rather than specifically to the problems of an acute myocardial infarction. This effort ultimately led to the development of the wide use of cardiopulmonary resuscitation and automatic defibrillators by both the lay public and the semitrained and trained emergency technicians.

From: S. Goldstein, A. Bayés-de-Luna, J. Guindo-Soldevila: *Sudden Cardiac Death.* Armonk, NY: Futura Publishing Co., Inc., © 1994.

Delaying Decision

One of the most significant problems in expediting patient hospitalization is the delay in seeking medical care. Initial studies by Moss and coworkers[6,7] observed that it took almost five hours to reach the hospital after the onset of symptoms; two and one-half hours were made up of the patient's decision-making process to seek help. A number of demographic and clinical factors appeared to influence the patient in delaying the decision to seek medical help, including the nature of the symptomatology.[8–10] Those individuals who experienced syncope or shortness of breath had a much shorter decision-making time than those with chest pain. Chest pain, nevertheless, was the main symptom in 80% of patients with infarcts. Those individuals with a previous history of angina or acute infarction had a longer decision time, since they appeared to have difficulty distinguishing something new in their symptoms from the usual episode of angina. The decision time has been modified to some extent over the last 20 years but still represents a continuing issue. Studies by Kenyon and associates[11] identified certain psychological characteristics of patients which impact on this decision-making process. The sense of body awareness and responsiveness to physiological phenomena are important factors affecting response time to myocardial infarction symptomatology.

It is estimated that between 60% to 70% of sudden death caused by cardiac arrest occurs before hospitalization. Simon[12] noted that because of the problems inherent in instantaneous cardiac arrest and the delay in calling for emergency aid, only 22% of the patients could be helped by mobile coronary care units. Of those dying of acute coronary events, Simon noted that 36% of the deaths were unwitnessed, and in 28% cardiac arrest occurred before an ambulance was called. In an additional 14%, cardiac arrest occurred either after the ambulance was called or during transit, and 8% occurred in the emergency department of the hospital.

Wikland[13] studied the records of 84 cases in which an attempt to call for help, using a highly developed telephone communication center in Stockholm, occurred during an acute coronary attack. Medical assistance was primarily sought by the witness in 81 cases and in 2 cases by relatives of the patient. In only one case was assistance sought by the patient alone. When help was called during the acute attack, 49% of the deaths occurred before the arrival of a physician or an ambulance, 37% during transit to the hospital, and 14% after examination by a physician. In Belfast, 73% of the patients came under intensive medical care within four hours of their hospitalization. The mean arrival time to a hospital emergency department in Rochester, New York, reported by Moss et al.,[6,7] was only slightly longer than the mobile units in Belfast. The experience of the Belfast group demonstrated that cardiac arrest could be treated effectively outside the hospital. In addition, many of these patients could be returned, after recovery and hospitalization, to normal activities. The inordinate decision delay led Greene[14] to suggest that high-risk patients should participate in a buddy system, which could expedite their decision-making process. He proposed that the patient's spouse or coworkers be advised in conjunction with the patient to seek medical care early when unusual symptoms occurred.

Efforts at educating patients to call for emergency facilities earlier and to improve the quality of emergency care are important. These efforts can have an effect on the overall mortality of acute coronary artery disease, but their total effectiveness is questionable. At best, they will be able to expedite arrival time in those people who do not die instantaneously and who may previously have delayed their entry into the medical care system. This will, however, leave a large group who die instantaneously in whom a mobile rescue facility may be effective. Friedman et al.[15] observed that of those individuals dying instantaneously, the focus of the mobile resuscitation units, usually do not have prodromal symptoms and therefore do not experience decision delay. Those dying suddenly, not instantaneously, are more likely to have prodromal symptoms and a moderate delay and can be affected by educational programs. The best teacher, however, a previous myocardial infarction, appears to have a negative effect on delay.[10]

Mobile Units

The early proponents of the mobile coronary care unit demonstrated that not only were they able to resuscitate and prevent cardiac arrest in transit, but that early recognition and treatment of cardiac arrhythmias in the mobile unit decreased the morbidity and long-term mortality of patients experiencing acute myocardial infarction. These advantages of mobile units were to be used later to initiate medical therapy including thrombolytic agents. The importance of the pioneering efforts of Pantridge and his group[1] cannot be underestimated. Not only did they clarify some of the early phenomena of acute myocardial ischemia, but demonstrated that the logistics of providing out-of-hospital medical care can be met in urban societies.

The second generation of mobile units directed its efforts to the problem of cardiac arrest rather than to early treatment of acute myocardial infarction. Well-trained mobile coronary care units can arrive at the patient's side within minutes. Dr. Leonard Cobb, the director of the Seattle unit, reported that approximately 30% of patients found in ventricular fibrillation by the mobile coronary facility could be successfully resuscitated.[16] Lewis et al.[3] reported that 20% of the out-of-hospital patients who were resuscitated from ventricular fibrillation were long-term survivors. In addition, 43% of patients with other forms of cardiac arrest were long-term survivors. These researchers stated, "While early coronary care by mobile ambulance undoubtedly is beneficial to patients . . . the vehicle must be able to reach the patient in four minutes to save lives." From these reports it is clear that the development of expeditious arrival of trained personnel is crucial for the effective treatment of cardiac arrest. The effect of arrival time on long-term survival is shown in Figure 1 from our study of out-of-hospital resuscitation.[17] Eisenberg et al.[18] reported that long-term survival is directly related to the time of early arrival of the mobile coronary care unit. Several studies indicate that

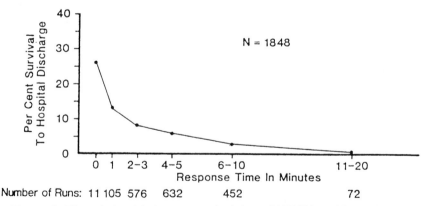

Figure 1. The relationship between arrival time of MCCU to ultimate hospital discharge. The number of individual emergency medical service runs for each response time is listed below each time frame (from Goldstein.[17]). MCCU = mobile coronary care unit.

patients with cardiac arrest due to ventricular fibrillation can be re-suscitated in the field if the unit arrives within four minutes of the event. Approximately 25% of those resuscitated will be discharged from the hospital alive. Fewer will be resuscitated if the event is characterized with ventricular asystole. The arrival time of mobile units is related to the geography of the community and the density of the population. Therefore, rural and suburban communities are clearly at a disadvantage.

The operation of mobile units in various communities differs. Some are primary response systems and others are secondary responders. Primary systems respond to a broad variety of medical and surgical conditions in addition to cardiac arrest. Cardiac runs represent approximately 10% of all emergency runs provided by primary response systems. It is therefore difficult to measure their specific effect on the successful resuscitation of cardiac arrest alone since they also respond to noncardiac events. Secondary responders are called after the primary response team ascertains that a cardiac arrest or a significant cardiac event has occurred. They apply their expertise more specifically to the cardiac patient and their effect can measure the success of resuscitation after cardiac arrest more directly. Cardiac runs for mobile secondary responders may represent as many as 50% of calls. In Columbus, Ohio[19] the secondary response units saw approximately 57% of patients with acute myocardial infarction who did not experience sudden death, and 59% of all cardiac arrest patients. In addition, units differ in their ability to initiate therapy. Some are trained for major resuscitation including endotracheal intubation, while others may be limited by their training and their ability to initiate therapy.

Pozen et al.,[20] in an attempt to evaluate adequacy of training, studied the accuracy of the paramedic arrhythmia diagnoses and the medical control at the receiving hospital. Incorrect diagnosis and treatment of cardiac arrhythmias was common when they were later reviewed and evaluated by a cardiologist. Only 39% of the life-threatening arrhythmias were correctly diagnosed, whereas 64% of those without life-threatening arrhythmias were correctly diagnosed. Incorrect responses may have an adverse effect on outcome since the mortality rate was 43% in the incorrectly treated group and 20% in the correctly diagnosed and treated patients. It is clear that medical surveillance and quality control of mobile coronary care units is critical for the achievement of maximum efficacy.

Success of Mobile Units

The incidence of cardiac arrest in the mobile coronary care unit itself varies between 5% and 10%. Defibrillation was carried out in 7% to 11% of runs by vehicles dedicated to cardiac problems.[21] The hospital discharge rates of those successfully defibrillated range between 7% to 30%, whereas the rates for those with asystole on arrival approached zero.

The success of out-of-hospital cardiac arrest depends on the definition of the event and the outcome measured (Fig. 2). In a study carried out by Valenzuela et al.,[21] survival measured in a series of

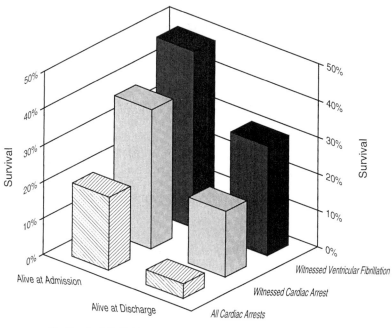

Figure 2. Survival after out-of-hospital cardiac arrest as a function of case definition and survival definition. The case definitions are as follows: all arrests, all cases meeting study entry criteria, witnessed arrest, witnessed cardiac arrest in adults, and witnessed ventricular fibrillation, witnessed cardiac arrest in adults, with initial monitored cardiac rhythm of ventricular fibrillation. The survival definitions are as follows: alive at admission, vital signs present, patient admitted to cardiac care unit; and alive at discharge, patient discharged alive from initial hospitalization for cardiac arrest (from Valenzuela et al.[21]).

372 patients varied from 6% to 15%. Twenty percent of all arrests survived to hospital admission and 6% were discharged from the hospital. Of adults who had a witnessed arrest, 26% survived to hospital admission and 10% were discharged. Patients whose collapse was witnessed and in whom initial rhythm was ventricular fibrillation survived to hospital admission in 38% and to discharge in 11%. It is therefore important to clarify the definition used in these studies.[22]

The extent of residual neurological damage of discharged patients has been assessed by Nagle et al.[23] They reported that 12% of patients discharged alive had significant central nervous system defects. Abramson[24] observed that in patients without purposeful response to pain 10 to 15 minutes after resuscitation, only 9% survive three months and of these, 43% were arousable, 36% had good cerebral function, and 25% regained previous cerebral status. Of 40 patients who were resuscitated after five minutes of arrest, 15% recovered good cerebral function. A study of the neuropsychological sequelae and cardiac arrest examined the effect of the intravenous administration of nimodipine immediately after restoration of spontaneous circulation.[25] At 12 months after resuscitation, 48% of the survivors had persistent moderate to severe cognitive defects. Nimodipine, a calcium entry blocking agent, had no effect on the neuropsychological sequelae.

The health status of long-term survivors of out-of-hospitalization was studied six months after the event, using a sickness impact profile.[26] Fifty percent of those who had been working prior to their cardiac arrest were working six months later. Most survivors were living at home and operating independently. The survival of resuscitated patients was related not only to age and the use of cardiopulmonary resuscitation, but also to the etiology of cardiac arrest. Those with acute myocardial ischemia or infarction as their entry had a one-year mortality rate of 15%. Patients with coronary heart disease but without any evidence of associated acute ischemia or infarction are at a very high risk of recurrent arrest, approaching 25% within one year.

The importance of bystander cardiopulmonary resuscitation was investigated by Ritter and associates[27] (Fig. 3). In a study of over 2000 emergency medical runs, cardiopulmonary resuscitation was administered in 23% of the individuals who survived and were admitted to the hospital, of whom 12% were discharged alive. In comparison, 14.6% of the cardiac arrest victims did not receive cardiopulmonary resuscitation and 4.7% were discharged alive. An important factor in patient survival was the amount of time that elapsed before the emer-

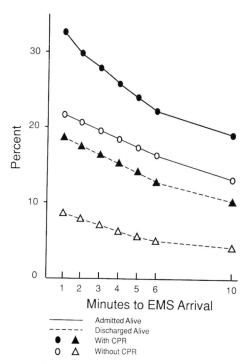

Figure 3. Minutes to emergency medical system (EMS) arrival. Least squares regression model relating the dichotomous survival outcome to quadratic functions of EMS response time separately for those with and without CPR. There was no evidence of a significant lack of fit for any of the four models ($P > 0.05$) (from Ritter et al.[27]).

gency medical system (EMS) personnel arrived and whether or not cardiopulmonary resuscitation was initiated. Patients who received bystander cardiopulmonary resuscitation were more likely to have ventricular fibrillation when the EMS arrived. Another factor related to patient survival was the location of the victim at the time of cardiac arrest. Arrest victims who were at work or in a public place had a better chance of survival in cardiopulmonary resuscitation than those at home. Although bystander cardiopulmonary resuscitation provides a window of effectiveness, it is a narrow window of less than five minutes' duration. Efficacy is determined by the rapid arrival of the emergency medical care definitive therapy.

Survival from out-of-hospital cardiac arrest results from a complex interplay between the patient's age, sex, response times, and the early administration of cardiopulmonary resuscitation. The survival of women after cardiac arrest associated with acute myocardial infarction is somewhat less than men.[28] The racial incidence of cardiac arrest and subsequent survival indicates a significantly worse outcome in African-Americans than in whites.[29] African-Americans were less likely to have witnessed cardiac arrest, bystander-initiated cardiopulmonary resuscitation, or a favorable initial rhythm. In addition, once admitted to the hospital, survival was also worse in African-Americans than whites. Cummins[30] observed that when cardiopulmonary resuscitation was initiated by a bystander, it had a significant effect on survival rate, 32% when compared to 22% who did not have bystander efforts (Fig. 4). The neurological dysfunction which occurs in patients receiving cardiopulmonary resuscitation was examined in Seattle. Anoxic coma occurred in 11% of bystander cardiopulmonary resuscitation and in 22% in those who received delayed resuscitation. The percent of patients who were conscious on admission was 50% after bystander cardiopulmonary resuscitation and only 6% in those who had a delayed response. Although bystander cardiopulmonary resuscitation resulted in more patients being discharged alive, these investigators found no effect on long-term survival associated with bystander resuscitation.[27]

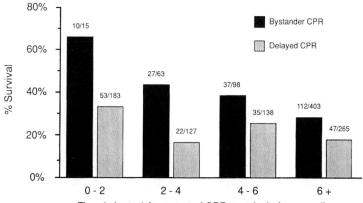

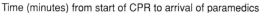

Figure 4. Time (minutes) from start of cardiopulmonary resuscitation (CPR) to arrival of paramedics (duration of CPR). Comparison of survival in the by-stander-CPR group and the delayed-CPR group stratified by the duration of CPR performed before the arrival of the paramedics. (Witnessed arrests only, all rhythms, cardiac etiology.) (From Cummins et al.[30])

Satellite Coronary Care Units

Other approaches to cardiac resuscitation have led to fixed life support systems located in airports, athletic stadiums, and large industrial plants. There is little question that the ability to provide cardiopulmonary resuscitation and speedy defibrillation for patients who have experienced cardiac arrest can be effective. There will be, in these settings, even more patients who can be resuscitated effectively if trained medical personnel are present. The logistic problems of providing trained personnel and maintaining their skills is of considerable importance. Goldstein et al.[31] compared the effectiveness of a satellite industrial coronary care unit in a large industrial population to the general medical care experienced in the same population when off work. They observed that in spite of the availability of highly trained staff present in an industrial coronary care unit, the mortality of the workers in the plant who had a satellite unit available to them was no different than the mortality of the patient who was at home and dependent upon the usual community facilities. Most of the deaths observed were instantaneous and the patients were dead on arrival to the satellite unit. Unless trained personnel were available to move throughout the plant and resuscitate patients, fixed coronary care units, either within a plant or in a hospital, were of limited value and did not significantly change the mortality rate. This does not deny the fact that this type of unit can be effective in some patients who might respond to symptoms and seek early medical observation. It does emphasize the fact that fixed units will have a minimal effect on sudden cardiac arrest. The problem of instantaneous death requires the mobilization of a resuscitation team to the side of the victim.

Efforts in education, training, and improvement of emergency medical care logistics are imperative and should be a high priority in approaching the problems of sudden death. The efforts of voluntary health organizations such as the American Heart Association and the Red Cross in teaching cardiopulmonary resuscitation are important steps in public awareness of cardiac arrest problems. They also help the public handle the problems more effectively. These efforts can do nothing but improve the overall mortality rates. In the meantime, the development of highly mobile and rapid emergency units must be continued. Their effectiveness has been proven in field trials and must be translated into a nationwide community effort.

Defibrillation in the Field

The success of early defibrillation not only led to the dissemination of defibrillators into mobile coronary care units, but also to the extensive use of emergency medical technicians in the field, trained in early cardiac care. The success of emergency medical technicians to defibrillate patients in the field with remote medical supervision achieved significant success, particularly in rural communities. In communities where early defibrillation by medical technicians was available, 19% of patients found in ventricular fibrillation were resuscitated and discharged alive from the hospital[32]. In communities where emergency medical technicians trained in defibrillation were not available, only 3% survived. Eighty-three percent of the long-term survivors received electric shocks administered solely by technicians. These observations enforced the fact that early defibrillation by minimally trained technicians can be effective for emergency cardiac care. Similar attempts using transcutaneous pacing by emergency medical technicians were not as effective. A study of this strategy failed to demonstrate any beneficial results in patients with asystolic arrest.[33]

Automatic external defibrillators which have the ability to diagnose and terminate arrhythmias were subsequently developed. These devices are sufficiently simple and allow for a training time of less than 16 hours. It was also possible to relax the stringent requirements for maintenance of defibrillation skills. Studies carried out in Iowa[32,34] and later in Seattle[35] confirmed the benefit of these devices (Figs. 5 and 6). The automatic defibrillators were able to convert ventricular fibrillation in 97% of the patients treated, compared to 70% of the patients in the control population not treated with automatic defibrillators. Hospital admissions and discharge rates were similar in the two groups. However, of the 29% of patients managed with the external defibrillator who were admitted alive, 17% were ultimately discharged. This compared to 33% and 13%, respectively, who did not use the automatic defibrillator.[32] In 276 patients treated by firefighters using automatic defibrillators in Seattle, 30% survived to hospital discharge, compared to an expected rate of 17% in the control study.[35] A statewide program using automatic defibrillators was initiated in California, using basic emergency medical technicians and public safety personnel.[36] In the first 46 months of this study, 1487 patients received defibrillator shocks; 68% of these had witnessed ventricular fibrillation. Of that group, 191 patients were

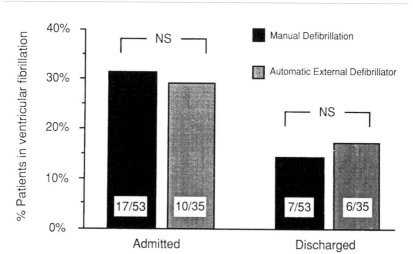

Figure 5. Patients in ventricular fibrillation. Hospital admission and discharge comparisons for patients with an initial rhythm of VF treated with either the automatic external defibrillator (AED) or standard manual defibrillation (from Stults et al.[32]).

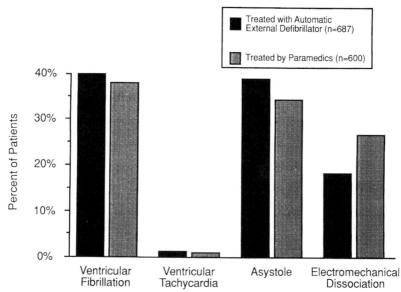

Figure 6. Condition of patients on the arrival of the first responding unit. Of 1287 patients with cardiac arrest, 687 received treatment first from firefighters who were equipped with automatic defibrillators, whereas the other 600 were first treated with cardiopulmonary resuscitation only by firefighters before the arrival of paramedics. About 40% of each treatment group were discovered to be in ventricular fibrillation. Only 16 patients were discovered in cardiac arrest with ventricular tachycardia (from Weaver et al.[35]).

discharged from the hospital, representing 19% of those who had witnessed ventricular fibrillation and 13% of all patients who had shocks. Using this program, the number of rescuers trained in defibrillation tripled in the four-year period.

The major success of out-of-hospital resuscitation must, however, be tempered by the realization that many individuals cannot be successfully restored to life. Prediction of the failure of out-of-hospital resuscitation attempts indicate that inability to restore circulation before transport was almost always associated with hospital failure.[37,38] There is little to be gained from rapid transport of nonresuscitated adults to the hospital. Excluding adult patients with persistent ventricular fibrillation, resuscitation can be terminated out-of-hospital if circulation does not return within 25 minutes. Resuscitation was most successful with cardiopulmonary resuscitation of ventricular fibrillation.

The continued success of these programs led to even further extension of these devices, namely, to transtelephonic defibrillation. The cellular transtelephonic defibrillator makes it possible to achieve rhythm diagnosis and defibrillation in remote areas. With this device, cardiac rhythm is telephonically transmitted to a receiving station which can then activate a self-contained defibrillator. In a study of 211 calls responded to by a physician over a distance of up to 15 miles, satisfactory electrocardiographic transmission and voice communication was established in 81.5%.[37] One hundred direct-current shocks of 50 to 360 joules were effectively administered to 22 patients with 48 episodes of ventricular fibrillation and ventricular tachycardia.

The technological and logistical developments in the last 20 years have enabled physicians and technicians to provide defibrillation at the bedside in urban, rural, and remote locations all over the world. Their success has been proven, yet it remains for government to distribute these devices throughout the community to achieve universal success.

References

1. Pantridge JF, Geddes JS. A mobile intensive-care unit in the management of myocardial infarction. *Lancet* 1967;2:271.
2. Nagle EL, Hirschman JC, Nussenfeld JD, et al. Telemetry-medical command in coronary and other mobile emergency care systems. *JAMA* 1970;214;332.
3. Lewis RP, Schaal SF, Frazier JT, et al. Mobile cardiac care: A community approach. *Ann Intern Med* 1972;76:865.

4. Graf WS, Polin SS, Paegel BL. A community program for emergency cardiac care: A three-year coronary ambulance/paramedic evaluation. *JAMA* 1973;226:156.

5. Crampton RS, Stillerman R, Gascho JA, et al. Prehospital coronary care in Charlottesville and Albemarle County. *Virginia Med Monthly* 1972; 99:1191.

6. Moss AJ, Goldstein S. The pre-hospital phase of acute myocardial infarction. *Circulation* 1970;41:737.

7. Moss AJ, Wynar B, Goldstein S. Delay in hospitalization during the acute coronary period. *Am J Cardiol* 1969;24:659.

8. Simon AB, Feinleib M, Thompson HK Jr. Components of delay in the prehospital phase of acute myocardial infarction. *Am J Cardiol* 1972;30:476.

9. Duggan JJ, Schiess WA, Hilfinger MF Jr. Unheeded signals of fatal coronary artery disease. *NY J Med* 1971;71:2639.

10. Goldstein S, Moss AJ, Greene W. Sudden death in acute myocardial infarction: Relationship to factors affecting delay in hospitalization. *Arch Intern Med* 1972;129:720.

11. Kenyon LW, Ketterer MW, Gheorghiade M, et al. Psychological factors related to prehospital delay during acute myocardial infarction. *Circulation* 1991;84:1969.

12. Simon AB, Alonzo AA. Sudden death in nonhospitalized cardiac patients. *Arch Intern Med* 1973;132:163.

13. Wikland B. Medically unattended fatal cases of ischaemic heart disease in a defined population. *Acta Med Scand*(suppl)1971;524:9.

14. Greene WA, Goldstein S, Moss AJ. Psychosocial aspects of sudden death. *Arch Intern Med* 1972;129:725.

15. Friedman M, Manwaring JH, Rosenman RH, et al. Instantaneous and sudden deaths: Clinical and pathological differentiation in coronary artery disease. *JAMA* 1973;225:1319.

16. Cobb LA, Alvarez H, Copass MK. A rapid response system for out-of-hospital cardiac emergencies. *Med Clin N Am* 1976;60:283.

17. Goldstein S. Cost effectiveness of mobile intensive care unit for an entire community. In: Califf RM, Wagner GS, eds. *Acute Coronary Care: Principles aand Practice.* Boston, Dordrect, Lancaster: Martinus Nijhoff Pub; 1985;281.

18. Eisenberg M, Hallstrom A, Bergner L. Long-term survival after out-of-hospital cardiac arrest. *N Engl J Med* 1982;306:1340.

19. Lewis R, Lanese R, Stang J, et al. Reduction of mortality from prehospital myocardial infarction by prudent patient activation of mobile coronary care system. *Am Heart J* 1982;103:123.

20. Pozen M, D'Agostino R, Sytkowski P, et al. Effectiveness of a prehospital medical control system: An analysis of the interaction between emergency room physician and paramedic. *Circulation* 1981;63:442.

21. Valenzuela TD, Spaite DW, Meislin HW, et al. Case and survival definitions in out-of-hospital cardiac arrest: Effect on survival rate calculation *JAMA* 1992;267;272.

22. Cummins RO, Chamberlain DA, Abramson NS, et al. Recommended guidelines for uniform reporting of data from out-of-hospital cardiac arrest: the Utstein style. *Ann Emer Med* 1991;20:861.

23. Nagle R, Gangola R, Picton-Robinson I. Factors influencing return to work after myocardial infarction. *Lancet* 1971;2:454.

24. Abramson N, Safar P, Detre K, et al. Neurological function in CPR survivors. *Circulation* 1982;66:II-350.

25. Roine RO, Kajaste S, Kaste M. Neuropsychological sequelae of cardiac arrest.

26. Bergner L, Bergner M, Hallstrom AP, et al. Health status of survivors of out-of-hospital cardiac arrest six months later. *Am J Public Health* 1984;74:508.

27. Ritter G, Wolfe RA, Goldstein S, et al. The effect of bystander CPR on survival of out-of-hospital cardiac arrest victims. *Am Heart J* 1985;110:932.

28. Orencia A, Bailey K, Yawn BP, et al. Effect of gender on long-term outcome of angina pectoris and myocardial infarction/sudden unexpected death. *JAMA* 1993;269:2392.

29. Becker LB, Han BH, Meyer PM, et al, and the CPR Chicago Project. Racial differences in the incidence of cardiac arrest and subsequent survival. *N Engl J Med* 1993;329:600.

30. Cummins RO, Eisenberg MS, Hallstron AP, et al. Survival of out-of-hospital cardiac arrest with early initiation of cardiopulmonary resuscitation. *Am J Emerg Med* 1985;3:114.

31. Goldstein S, Greene W, Moss AJ. Lack of effectiveness of a satellite industrial CCU in reducing mortality from acute myocardial infarction. *Circulation* 1971;44 (suppl II):II-171.

32. Stults KR, Brown DD, Kerber RE. Efficacy of an automated external defibrillator in the management of out-of-hospital cardiac arrest: Validation of the diagnostic algorithm and initial clinical experience in a rural environment. *Circulation* 1986;73:701.

33. Cummins RO, Graves JR, Larsen MP, et al. Out-of-hospital transcutaneous pacing by emergency medical technicians in patients with asystolic cardiac arrest. *N Engl J Med* 1993;328:1377.

34. Stults KR, Brown DD, Schug VL, et al. Prehospital defibrillation performed by emergency medical technicians in rural communities. *N Engl J Med* 1984;310:219.

35. Weaver WQD, Hill D, Fahrenbrugh CE, et al. Use of the automatic external defibrillator in the management of out-of-hospital cardiac arrest. *N Engl J Med* 1988;319:661.

36. Haynes BE, Mendoza A, McNeil M, et al. A statewide early defibrillation initiative including laypersons and outcome reporting. *JAMA* 1991;266:545.

37. Dalzell GW, McKeown PP, Roberts JD, et al. A cellular transtelephonic defibrillator for management of cardiac arrest outside the hospital. *Am J Cardiol* 1991;68:909.

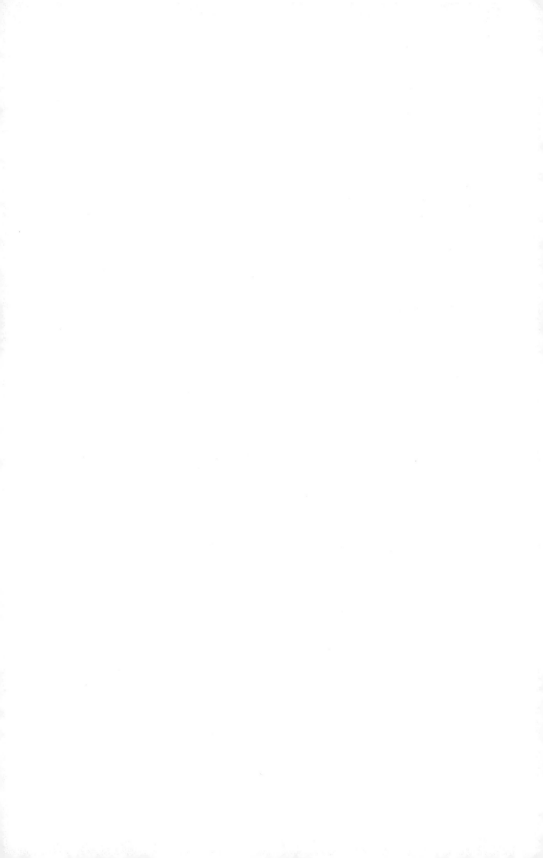

Chapter XX

Future Directions in the Treatment and Prevention of Sudden Death

Sudden death may not be the knotted skein so often discussed today if we but unravel and study those threads comprising electrical stability of the heart.

Thomas James, MD[1]

This monograph represents our current understanding of the etiology, mechanism, and prevention of sudden death due to cardiovascular disease. Past clinicians have provided a rich history of investigations for the last 2000 years. It is evident that significant information has been collected in the last 30 years since Lewis Kuller[2] called our attention to this issue as it particularly relates to coronary heart disease. We can see more clearly some of the specific issues relative to its solution. Nevertheless, that this is a problem of worldwide importance dominated by, but not exclusive to, ischemic heart disease forces us to appreciate its universality.

The prevention of ischemic heart disease will clearly address, in a large part, the problems of sudden death. The progressive decrease in ischemic heart disease mortality in the United States (Fig. 1) and a number of other countries provides optimism that both sudden and nonsudden death mortality is achievable in the future. At the same time, there has been a measurable decrease in out-of-hospital deaths[3] (Fig. 2). This progress has occurred due to progress in primary prevention including smoking cessation and improved dietary

From: S. Goldstein, A. Bayés-de-Luna, J. Guindo-Soldevila: *Sudden Cardiac Death.* Armonk, NY: Futura Publishing Co., Inc., © 1994.

Per cent Change

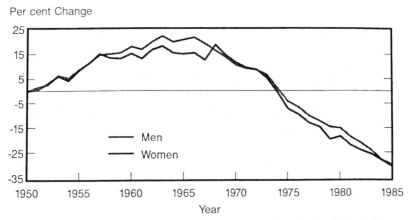

Figure 1. Change in coronary heart disease mortality, in the United States, from 1950 to 1985.

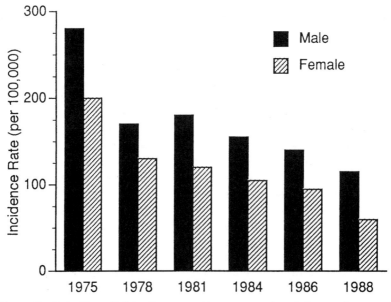

Figure 2. Out-of-hospital deaths caused by coronary heart disease by sex and by time period (Worcester Heart Attack Study). (From Goldberg et al.[3])

habits, all of which have had an important effect on the mortality rate. The success of these antismoking campaigns in the United States can be seen in Figure 3. Since 1955 there has been a 50% decrease in the prevalence of cigarette smoking in males, from 56.9% to 28.1%. There are still 46 million Americans who smoke cigarettes, and a total of 52.5 million who use some form of tobacco. The progress in the battle against cigarette smoking is unique to the United States. With the exception of a few European countries, there has been little progress in the rest of the world. In the third world, particularly in Asia and Africa, cigarette smoking continues at a catastrophic rate.

Major risk screening and primary prevention therapy for hypertension were also important factors in this downward trend in the incidence of stroke, coronary heart disease mortality, and sudden death. At the same time, major interventions in out-of-hospital cardiac care, with improved care both in the ambulance and the emergency room, have accelerated the application of new treatment for serious arrhythmias, acute myocardial infarction, and cardiac collapse. It is also clear that there is no single factor that has resulted in this improvement. This decrease in mortality in the United States is a result of a wave of interventions resulting from the explosion of research in the last part of the 20th century.

Other forms of heart disease, of course, continue to be problematic. Although valvular heart disease has diminished largely as a

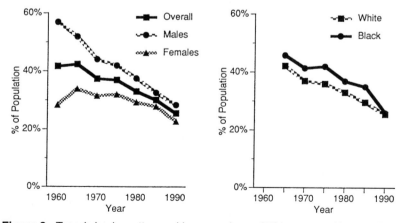

Figure 3. Trends in cigarette smoking prevalence (%) by sex and by race in the United States. (Current Population Survey, 1955; National Health Interview Surveys, 1965–1991; Data compiled by the Office on Smoking and Health, CDC.)

result of the prevention of rheumatic heart disease in the developing countries, the poorly defined pathogenesis of cardiomyopathies remains a continuing dilemma. It is more than likely that within this heterogeneous group, a number of specific etiologic phenomena will be identified as being related to genetic, environmental, or acquired factors. The dysfunctional ventricle is fertile ground for the development of life-threatening arrhythmias and sudden cardiac arrest. In order to understand this dysfunctional process we must learn more about the contractile phenomenon of the ventricle and its interrelationship to the electrical integrity of the heart. The understanding of the relationship between impulse propagation and contraction lies at the cellular and subcellular level. The degeneration of pump function and the dysfunction of the myocyte appear to be closely related to the loss of the heart's electrical integration and the precipitation of cardiac arrest. In the understanding of these interrelated processes lies the answer to the prevention of cardiac arrest in this disease state.

As basic research explores the mechanism by which ventricular dysfunction occurs and ischemic heart disease progresses, new methods of providing care of patients who experience cardiac arrest must be developed. The number and distribution of trained personnel to provide rapid support for the cardiac arrest victim must be made more widely available. The remarkable developments in defibrillation technology have restored life to thousands of cardiac arrest victims. The success of these units proves that effective resuscitation can be achieved outside the hospital environment. The extension of defibrillation technology to implantable devices initiated by Mirowski[4] added further dimension to the potential treatment of cardiac arrest. The current technology has the ability to recognize, record, and respond to a variety of electrical phenomena including bradycardia, asystole, ventricular tachycardia, and fibrillation in one implantable device. It also provided a conceptual basis for the treatment of a variety of potentially lethal arrhythmic phenomena and has led to expanded research in the electrophysiology of the heart. At the same time, the use of ablation techniques for the treatment of Wolff-Parkinson-White preexcitation syndrome provided a bridge into our understanding of atrial and ventricular depolarization. Corrective ablation can now be accomplished to interrupt the pathological pathways that heretofore have led to cardiac collapse. This technology has found ready application to the treatment of supraventricular arrhythmias and is now being applied to ventricular arrhythmias.

The final approach to the prevention of sudden death rests upon the appropriate therapy for individuals identified at increased risk for cardiac arrest. It is clear from the epidemiologic studies that, in a large part, the cardiac arrest victim is identified long before sudden death. Expanded identification of patients at risk of cardiac arrest can be achieved with the widespread development of primary health facilities and early identification of cardiac dysfunction by primary practitioners. The identification of gene localization of familial-transmitted cardiac diseases may provide an opportunity to prevent its expression and calls for more aggressive approaches to families with both acquired and congenital defects.

Major strides have, however, occurred in a number of cardiac disease states. β-adrenergic blocking agents and antiplatelet agents have been shown to significantly modify the risk of sudden death in coronary heart disease. Angiotensin-converting enzyme inhibitors also have the potential to prevent sudden death in patients with heart failure. The early enthusiasm for antiarrhythmic agents for the suppression of ventricular ectopy unfortunately met with near disaster. Yet, the potential for modifying the metabolic environment in which cardiac dysfunction occurs has the potential to decrease arrhythmic sudden death mortality. Observations that β-adrenergic blocking agents, for instance, appear to increase the threshold for the development of ventricular fibrillation provide support for this hypothesis. It is therefore possible that other drugs can be identified to achieve similar effects. The ability to modify the electrophysiology of the dysfunctional cardiac remains an important area of productive investigation.

The further development of bioengineering and genetic modeling of the cells also provides an opportunity to prevent cardiac arrest in both ischemic heart disease and other forms of ventricular dysfunction. It is clear, however, that the answer to the prevention of sudden death lies not so much in the event itself, but in the understanding and prevention of the underlying dysfunctional heart. Once our understanding of these phenomena is achieved, cardiac death, either sudden or nonsudden, can be prevented.

References

1. James TN. Mysterious sudden death. *Chest* 1972;62:454.
2. Kuller L. Sudden and unexpected non-traumatic deaths in adults: A review of epidemiological and clinical studies. *J Chronic Dis* 1966;19:1165.

3. Goldberg RJ, Gorak EJ, Yarzebski J, et al. A community-wide perspective of sex differences and temporal trends in the incidence and survival rates after acute myocardial infarction and out-of-hospital deaths caused by coronary heart disease. *Circulation* 1993;87:1947.
4. Mirowski M, Reid PR, Mower MM, et al. Termination of malignant ventricular arrhythmias with an implanted automatic defibrillator in human beings. *N Engl J Med* 1980;303:322.

Index